Forgotten Traditions of Ancient Chinese Medicine

A CHINESE VIEW FROM THE
EIGHTEENTH CENTURY

The *I-hsüeh Yüan Liu Lun* of 1757
by Hsü Ta-Ch'un

Translated and Annotated by

PAUL U. UNSCHULD

PARADIGM PUBLICATIONS
Brookline, Massachusetts
1998

Forgotten Traditions of Ancient Chinese Medicine

The I-hsüeh Yüan Liu Lun of 1757 by Hsü Ta-Ch'un

translated by

Paul U. Unschuld

©1998 Paul U. Unschuld

ISBN 0-912111-56-9

Library of Congress Cataloging-in-Publication Data:

Hsü, Ta-ch'un, 1693–1771

          p. cm.

Chinese and English

Translation of: I-hsüeh Yüan Liu Lun.

Includes Index.

ISBN 0-912111-24-0 (hardcover)

ISBN 0-912111-56-9 (paperback)

1. Medicine, Chinese – Early works to 1800. I. Unschuld, Paul U.
(Paul Ulrich), 1943– . II. Title

R127.1.H7513   1989   89-3001

710 – dc19   CIP

Printed in the United States of America

PARADIGM PUBLICATIONS

http://www.paradigm-pubs.com

44 Linden Street, Brookline, Massachusetts 02445 USA

Publisher: Robert L. Felt

Cover Design by Laura Shaw Design

To the memory of Anna Helene Szymanski, 1894-1990.

Acknowledgments

Parts of the manuscript have been discussed with Hermann Kogelschatz, Ma Kanwen, and Zheng Jinsheng. The entire translation was compared to the original Chinese text by Rupprecht Mayer. I am most grateful for all the suggestions and constructive criticisms I have received from these colleagues.

The portrait of Hsü Ta-ch'un was kindly supplied for publication by the Medical History Teaching and Research Section of the Guangzhou College of Chinese Medicine; I am obliged to Prof. Zhou Jingping for her assistance.

Also, I should like to thank Dr. Wu Mengchao, Chief of the Department of Hepatobiliary Surgery of Changhai Hospital, 2nd Military Medical College, Shanghai, for providing photographs taken of Hsü Ta-ch'un's grave in Wu-chiang county, Kiangsu province.

Paul U. Unschuld
Munich, March 1990

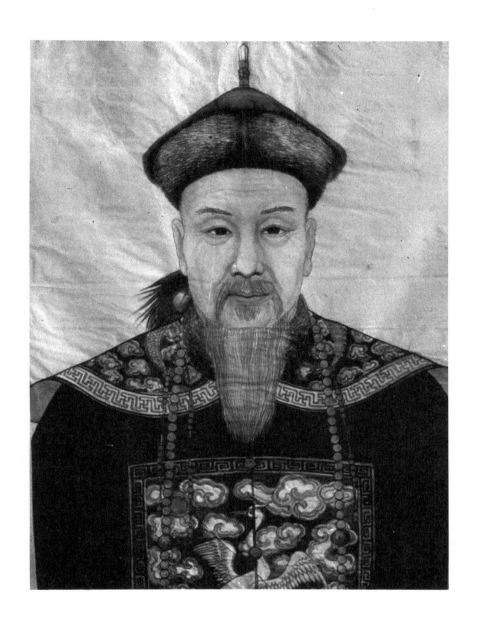

Hsü Ta-ch'un (1693-1771). Portrait by Sung Ta-jen
after an original kept by the Hsü family.

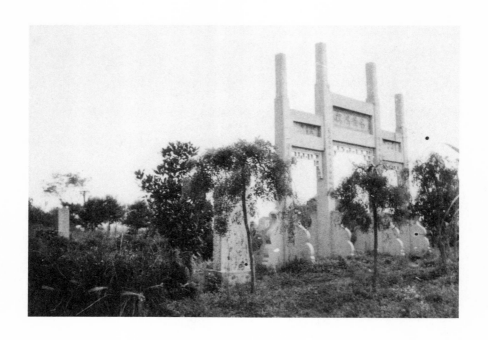

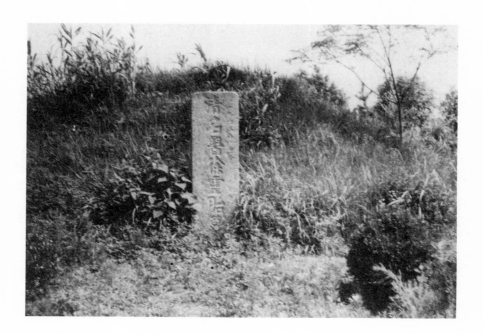

The tomb of Hsü Ta-ch'un in Wu-chiang county, Kiangsu.

Table of Contents

Prolegomena

Chinese Text and Translation

IV. Prescriptions and Drugs

V. Therapeutic Patterns

Prolegomena

1. Introductory Remarks

Hsü Ta-ch'un (1693-1771) was an outstanding Chinese intellectual, physician-scholar and medical writer of the second millennium A.D. As the author of the *I-hsüeh Yüan Liu Lun* and other works he is still present to us, not in person but in his ideas. In Hsü Ta-ch'un we encounter a highly educated representative — one to date virtually unknown in the West — not only of traditional Chinese medicine but also of the upper echelons of Chinese culture prior to the impact of Western civilization. Hsü Ta-ch'un speaks to his readers, now as in the eighteenth century, in easily understandable language. His book, *I-hsüeh Yüan Liu Lun,* translated and edited herewith into a Western language for the first time, and published with its Chinese original text, is a remarkable document without known parallel in the history of Chinese medical literature. Its author reflected, in one hundred short essays, on a wide range of essential aspects of medicine, and left us a unique source not only for an appreciation of the ideas of an individual Chinese physician living more than two centuries ago, but also for better penetration of the contents and history of traditional Chinese medicine preceding its contact with European medicine. Hsü Ta-ch'un's thoughts and arguments should serve as a stimulus to reassess at least some of the assumptions characterizing the reception of Chinese medicine in current Western culture.

Traditional Chinese medicine has a documented history comparable in length to the documented history of European medicine, and the former has developed, at least until the end of the imperial age, as rich a body of knowledge as the latter. In previous monographs and essays, I have analyzed and described various more or less isolated aspects of traditional Chinese medicine and pharmaceutics, marking my own way through a vast source of untapped data. With the present book I continue this work, and here, as earlier, I should like to emphasize that no single monograph will adequately convey the entirety of the Chinese traditions of health care, first because, of the more than twelve thousand works extant from earlier centuries, not even a handful have been translated in a philologically serious manner, and second because the wealth of the history of traditional Chinese medicine requires a library of Western secondary literature, and not just footnotes. This translation of the *I-hsüeh Yüan Liu Lun* is annotated to a degree that is necessary to clarify some of its more special statements and to enable Western readers to study it as an independent work. In writing secondary literature on Chinese medicine we should have progressed beyond the stage where it is necessary to elucidate the theories of yin-yang and five-phases theories and the fundamental tenets of Chinese philosophy in each book anew. For a more comprehensive analysis of the history and conceptual background of fundamental thoughts referred to by Hsü Ta-ch'un, readers might benefit from consulting introductory studies of traditional Chinese medicine.

2. Biographical Data on Hsü Ta-ch'un

The history of Hsü Ta-ch'un's family has been traced back to the Sung dynasty, at which time Hsü's ancestors appear to have left Kiangsi for Chekiang. During the Ming dynasty, the family moved to Kiangsu and settled in the city of Wu-chiang 吳江. A paternal great-grandfather of Hsü Ta-ch'un, Hsü Yün-ch'i 徐韞奇, was a man of letters and author of several works, including at least one medical title. His grandfather, Hsü Chiu 徐釚 (1636-1708), a poet, landscape painter, and also a man of letters, was chosen to participate in the compilation of the official history of the Ming dynasty. Hsü Ta-ch'un's father, Hsü Yang-hao 徐養浩 (d. ca. 1721), was an expert in the water systems of Kiangsu. He was recommended for the position of Department Vice Magistrate at one time, but was not chosen.[1]

Hsü Ta-ch'un was born in 1693 in the city of Wu-chiang. In a gazetteer of his native district, printed in 1747, which he helped a friend to compile, Hsü's personal name is listed as Ta-yeh 大葉.[2] Later, in a preface to a reprint of the *Pen-shih shih* written by his grandfather Hsü Ch'iu, Hsü signed his name Ta-ch'un 大椿.[3] His style-name, Ling-t'ai 靈胎, by which he is best known, appeared first in an imperial decree summoning him to Peking.[4] Later in his life Hsü Ta-ch'un 徐大椿 adopted the sobriquet Hui-hsi lao-jen 洄溪老人 (The old man from Hui-hsi), referring to a village where he had taken up residence.

Never having competed in the official examinations, Hsü Ta-ch'un, whose family appears to have been rather poor when he was young, became a famous scholar and physician nevertheless.[5] He continued his father's expertise on his native province's water system, and was asked at least twice to offer his opinion on major water control projects undertaken by the administration. Also, he was twice called to the capital, once in 1761 for consultations with regard to the illness of the Grand Secretary Chiang P'u 蔣溥, and again in 1771 to help in the treatment of another official. Hsü Ta-ch'un died three days after his second arrival in the capital; his remains were brought back to his native place by his son Hsü Hsi 徐爔, who was also a physician. After Hsü Ta-ch'un's death, the poet, literary critic and essayist Yüan Mei 袁枚 (1716-1798), a patient and acquaintance, wrote a biography characterizing the departed as an outstanding medical scholar and practitioner. The entire text of this biography is quoted in Appendix A to this Introduction.

2

Hsü Ta-ch'un wrote books, essays, and poems on subjects including medicine, philosophy, river control, music, and other topics, reflecting some areas of his broad interest. His fame as a physician was sufficiently acknowledged to have several authors publish their medical works later under his name. Hsü Ta-ch'un mentions in his own writings only four medical titles written by himself, i.e., commentaries on the *Nan-ching* 難經, the [*Shen-nung*] *Pen-ts'ao Ching* 神農本草經, and the *Shang-han Lun* 傷寒論, as well as the *I-hsüeh Yüan Liu Lun* 醫學源流論, a discussion of one hundred issues from virtually all realms of medicine, including also ethical and sociological essays. Further works attributed to his authorship with some certainty are the *I-kuan Pien* 醫貫砭, a critique of the *I-kuan* by Chao Hsien-ko 趙獻可, a physician and medical author of the second half of the 16th century, the *Lan-t'ai Kuei-fan* 蘭臺軌范, a comprehensive collection of prescriptions, and the *Shen-chi Ch'u-yen* 愼疾芻言, a short text with essays on various subjects, similar to the *I-hsüeh Yüan Liu Lun*. A complete list of all works associated with his name is given in Appendix B at the conclusion of this introduction.

Hsü Ta-ch'un must be grouped among the conservatives of his time in that he identified many current weaknesses and problems as unavoidable consequences of deviation from what he considered the correct paths pointed out by the Sages of antiquity. He voiced harsh criticism against most of the theoretical innovations introduced into medicine since the Sung era, and he despised the standards of medicine practiced by many of his contemporaries. He idealized the "ancients" as almost perfect examples for all future generations, and he recommended the *Huang-ti Nei-ching* as the most authoritative source of wisdom for health care. And yet, from the thoughts he published, especially in the *I-hsüeh Yüan Liu Lun*, it is obvious that Hsü Ta-ch'un, despite his emphasis on "Han-learning," was far from being an inflexible admirer of things past and gone forever. It appears as if his argumentation is often much more modern than one might be tempted to expect in view of his polemics against additions to medicine in "later times," and on the basis of his mourning after "forgotten traditions" of some ancient classic age.

3. Characteristic Thoughts in the
I-hsüeh Yüan Liu Lun

Hsü Ta-ch'un finished the *I-hsüeh Yüan Liu Lun* in 1757 when he was 65 years old. Thirty years earlier he had published his first known medical work, a commentary on the *Nan-ching* of about the first century A.D.[6] This commentary shows Hsü already an advocate of a return to the sources; he did not acknowledge any of the innovative ideas proposed in that classic on pulse diagnosis and acupuncture treatment as progress beyond the teachings of the *Nei-ching*, the "real classic" of Chinese

3

medicine. Rather, he praised the *Nan-ching* only for those of its contents that agreed with the *Nei-ching*, while he criticized it for anything he interpreted as a deviation. Already, by the age of thirty-five, Hsü Ta-ch'un had in the realm of medical opinions obviously found a political stance that he was to adhere to until the end of his life. Also, from the sophistication of his arguments and from the depth of his knowledge, apparent from his *Nan-ching* commentary, we may assume that by the time he wrote the *I-hsüeh Yüan Liu Lun,* Hsü Ta-ch'un must have been able to reflect on at least forty years of medical erudition and, possibly, clinical experience. Even though he was to live for another fourteen years, we may regard the *I-hsüeh Yüan Liu Lun* as a summary of his experiences and insights as a physician and medical scholar.

Hsü Ta-ch'un may be counted among the foremost advocates of the political movement known as han-hsüeh p'ai 漢學派, the "school of Han learning." Earlier than political philosophy itself, medicine became an arena for the propagation of arguments against the massive changes introduced into Chinese philosophical and political life as a result of so-called "Sung learning," or, in Western terms, Neo-Confucianism.[7] In a noteworthy similarity to trends in Europe, where during the first millennium Christian fundamentalism proved antagonistic to ancient European science, and played a role in pushing Galenic-Hippocratic medicine into temporary oblivion, Chinese naturalism may have been stymied during the same period by a contradiction between Confucianist emphasis on man as a social being, and Taoist understanding of man as an integrated aspect of nature. It was only during the Sung, with theoretical foundations laid by such T'ang intellectuals as Han Yü 韓愈 (768-824) and Li Ao 李翱 (d. 844), that the rift between Taoist ideals and Confucian ethics was bridged to such an extent that creative thoughts were allowed to roam freely through all aspects of human existence, and to devote themselves to all kinds of scientific as well as technological issues without risking a confrontation with ideological barriers. Not surprisingly, the Sung era was to become a most innovative period with respect to many levels and facets of Chinese culture.

This development may, with all due caution, also be seen as paralleling certain aspects of European history. Beginning with the twelfth century, the influence of the Christian dogma on intellectual affairs began to slowly wane again under the impact of various political and economic tendencies competing, with an ever greater success, with the power of the Church. Emperors like Frederic II (1194-1250), whose youth in Sicily was apparently influenced by the fruitful shadow of nearby Arabic culture, as well as the growth of cities and wealthy independent traders, were some of the forces increasingly denying supreme authority to biblical doctrine. It may have been a major historical precondition for the kind of European culture developing following the Renaissance, that a compromise was reached early — even though not without great pains — between the interests of the Church, and those of its secular adversaries. Truth was separated into two distinct realms, including the primary truth of divine revelation and the secondary truths found by man himself, through research and investigation. This development foreshadowed the separation of human existence into mind and body by Descartes, and opened a path for a coexistence of science with religion, which appears to have exerted a similar effect on European culture as the Sung teaching in China: it enabled creative minds to address any issue lending itself to research. Ideological confrontations between the Church as a guardian of truth gained from revelation, and scientists as propagators of a truth gained from their own investigations, decreased in number and severity from century to century.

A difference from China, though, is obvious too. The European compromise held through the phases of inquisition and counter-reformation, and European science and technology have benefited from a split culture ever since. With the demise of Sung culture, though, and despite such fascinating periods as those guided by the initial Ch'ing rulers, Chinese science and technology lost much of their creative spirit, and numerous Ch'ing era Chinese nationalists, who remembered the intrusion of the Mongols and a similarly autocratic Ming government, and who had to live now under Manchurian rule themselves, saw no other way into the future than to return to the ancient past; the very coexistence of Confucianist and Taoist ideas, and the freedom of the mind permitted by this coexistence, were for them not the reason for a blossoming of Chinese civilization, but the starting point of decline. Hsü Ta-ch'un was one of these conservative intellectuals, and the focus of his criticism was the realm of medicine.

3.1. The General Medical World View of Hsü Ta-ch'un

Hsü Ta-ch'un's notions of health and illness encompass many levels of understanding, and yet, an unprepared Western reader of his *I-Hsüeh Yüan Liu Lun* may be surprised by his familiarity with Hsü's thoughts. In fact, virtually none of the concepts outlined in his *I-hsüeh Yüan Liu Lun* could support the widespread argument that fundamental differences exist between traditional Chinese medical thinking on the one side and traditional or modern Western medicine on the other side. Hsü Ta-ch'un, it appears from his essays in the present text, would have had no real difficulty discussing basic issues concerning prevention and therapy with contemporary or twentieth century Western colleagues. While Western secondary literature on traditional Chinese medicine has emphasized, over the past two decades, an incompatibility between

Eastern and Western thought, Hsü Ta-ch'un has left us, with his *I-hsüeh Yüan Liu Lun,* reconciliatory statements documenting common ground across cultural boundaries.

In the preface to the *I-hsüeh Yüan Liu Lun,* Hsü attributed to man a place in the hierarchy of beings that was as prominent as that assigned to man in the Judaeo-Christian tradition of Europe:

> Mankind occupies the most important position in the world.
> (Preface, p. 52)

With such a statement, Hsü Ta-ch'un contradicted a more ecological world view held by early Taoists who had compared the importance of man to that of any ant. In China, as in Europe, medicine was not a tool of ecological thinking; rather, medicine employed its knowledge of the workings of nature to separate man from the laws of ecology. Medicine, in China as in Europe, developed as an ally in man's attempt to leave nature, and to secure for himself what no other species can claim, i.e., a right to health, and the right to die old. The *Huang-ti Nei-ching, Su-wen,* defined a normal, healthy life as spanning a period of 100 years, and it is man's own fault, the author of the respective passage wrote, if he succumbs to death earlier.[8] Health, then, was regarded, in China as in Europe, as a possession, as a resource, that was given to man for a fixed period. Hsü Ta-ch'un likened health to a fixed share of influences already given to man at the moment of his birth, and he compared this "fixed share" to a certain amount of firewood that is cast on a fire — if there is more, the fire will burn longer; if there is less, the fire will die out earlier. That is, in contrast to the *Huang-ti Nei-ching,* Hsü Ta-ch'un did not assume identical periods of longevity as granted to everyone. He pointed out, instead, that a person's lifespan is individually determined, and he thereby implicitly excused medicine for not being able to rescue old age for every patient.

> At the moment we get our lives, we have already received a
> fixed share. (I.1, p. 56)

In other words, man, in a certain way, is comparable to summer insects existing for a predetermined lifespan through a very short period of the year. The difference from these insects, or any other species of animal life, is to be seen in the ability of man to defend his fixed share (and I shall return to the militaristic metaphors of health care implied here) against the enemies of a fulfilled life. These enemies, however, are, basically, man himself, if he behaves destructively, as well as nature, when it causes conditions that are detrimental to health. Medicine has to assist the owners of health, first, to avoid harm caused by themselves and, second, to cure themselves of the effects of their own or nature's "misbehavior." It should not be surprising that traditional Chinese medicine, similar to European medicine prior to bacteriology and the discovery of antibiotics, placed strong emphasis on the prevention of illness. And yet, medicine's primary task, in China as in Europe, has been to cope with illnesses in their earlier or later stages, and to give advice on how to escape from self-inflicted problems or problems caused by some external factor.

Hsü Ta-ch'un realized the existence of a phenomenon that was called *vis medicatrix naturae* in Europe since antiquity; that is, a tendency of nature to cure certain problems by itself.[9] It was the belief in a self-interest of nature to return from crisis to harmony that guided Hippocratic medicine in ancient Greece and has influenced so-called natural health care in central Europe especially since the nineteenth century. In the words of Hsü Ta-ch'un:

> Also, if an illness is not accompanied by fatal pathoconditions, any external affection will slowly retreat, and any internal damage will gradually recover. [That is, the illness] will heal by itself. (V.22, p. 301)

> When pathoconditions emerge as a result of affections from outside, or of harm from inside, they heal by themselves, even though one devotes [only] little attention to their treatment. This is even more true for minor illnesses; they may heal gradually even without any intake of drugs. Even in cases [where] the strength of the illness is quite dangerous, the evil influences will recede gradually, and a state of normalcy will return by itself, if the physician in charge does not commit too great a mistake. (III.10, p. 124)

Similar to the ancient Hippocratic authors who realized that certain illnesses take characteristic courses, Hsü stated:

> But, there are cases where [an illness] heals after a fixed period of time no matter whether the treatment is started early or late. (V.17, p. 285)

The success of treatment may, therefore, be an illusion. It is not to the physician's but to nature's credit when the patient improves again:

> But the reason [for such successes] must be sought in facts such as that the illness was basically minor anyway, and had a tendency towards healing by itself, . . . (IV.7, p. 166)

Medicine, therefore, in the opinion of Hsü Ta-ch'un and paralleling the tradition of Europe, is not to intervene in each and every case. It is the physician's task to closely monitor the course of an illness, and to support a natural tendency towards self-healing with milder or stronger stimuli. Much further research is needed, though, to allow for an assessment of whether these thoughts were introduced into Chinese medicine by Hsü, or were adopted by him from insights gained in former times.

3.2. The Foundations of Life

Most important for a healthy life is an availability of correct ch'i 氣, that is, of those influences that all the functional segments of the organism need in order to fulfill their proper tasks. The "fixed share" referred to above is an initial allotment of "original influences," forming, essentially, the basis of human existence.

> This so-called fixed share is the original influences. If one were to look for them, one would not see them. If one were to search for them, one would not find them. They are attached to the interior of the influences and the blood, but they already govern [life] prior to [the existence of] influences and blood. (I.1, p. 56)

> In general, whether a person will die [or not] is determined by the presence or loss of his original influences. If, therefore, someone's original influences have received harm in the course of an illness, [his situation] may become quite dangerous. The reason is [that] as soon as one's original influences are lost, none of the five viscera and six bowels is supplied with influences any longer. (I.8, p. 78)

The influences and the blood circulate through the body, reaching everywhere:

> Man's influences and his blood penetrate every [region of his body]. (I.6, p. 72)

Under normal, i.e., healthy, conditions, this circulation occurs in a specific direction. In case of illness, though, there are changes:

> At first, [the situation may] appear peaceful, but after a while the influences [in the body] will move contrary to their proper direction, and phlegm will rise. (III.5, p. 111)

Also, in case of illness, entire functional regions may be cut off from the circulatory flow of influences.

> If, for instance, the heart has been cut off [from the circulation of influences], that person is benighted and will not recognize anything. . . . only when the lung has been cut off [from the circulation of influences] will the moment of death very soon follow. (I.8, p. 78)

Not only an interruption of the lung from its supply of influences is to be considered very dangerous; the patient's chances for survival are not much better if the stomach has been cut off.

> One considers the influences of the stomach as the basis [of life]. . . . As long as they are present, [the patient] will survive. If they are lost, [the patient] will die. (II.1, p. 86)

An indicator of an impending life crisis is the appearance of the so-called "true influences" of any of the viscera; they are deployed by the viscera when their supply with stomach influences stops.

> [Movements in the] vessels [indicating the presence of] the true influences of a viscus occur when the [flow of the] influences of the stomach has already been cut off, and hence fails to circulate through all the five viscera. (II.1, p. 86)

It may well be that concepts of suffocation and starvation have contributed to the prominent roles assigned to the influences received by the lung, and emitted by the stomach.

In addition to blood and the influences, a third vital substance found in the organism is *ching* 精, i.e., essence.

> Each of the five viscera[1] has its genuine essence; these [essences] are separate materializations of the original influences. (I.1, p. 57)

In the same way as the air needed for breathing may have been decisive in the development of the concept of *ch'i*, the male semen may have been instrumental in the development of this concept of *ching*.

> Everyone knows that the essence is stored in the kidneys, . . . [This] essence is a fatty paste [stored] inside the kidneys. Some of it stays there for a long [time], some of it is generated daily anew. Inside the kidneys is a location where the essence is stored; it is [always] filled and never empty in the same way as a well is filled with water day and night. . . . Essence leaving [the kidneys] as a result of sexual agitation or intercourse, as well as essence that is lost [at night] as a result of illness, are both created daily anew. (I.7, p. 57)

Man's interior economy, and the world surrounding him, are filled with *ch'i* 氣, i.e., with influences emitted and absorbed by virtually every phenomenon. There is no clear difference between "good" and "bad," between "proper" and "evil" influences. Influences that may be proper turn evil when they overstep certain boundaries, and these may be boundaries of quantity or boundaries of location. For instance, wind, a perfectly normal ch'i in man's environment, may enter the human body

9

where it becomes defined as evil, and where it is seen to obstruct the circulation of proper influences.

> . . . and suddenly he is affected by some external evil, as for instance, malign wind, foul influences, demonic evil, or [some other] terrible poison that closes the passageways of his influences. At this moment [the influences] cannot move [through the body], and the vital influences are blocked [in their flow]. (III.11, p. 127)

> Or, it may be that, at one time, [the passage of one's normal influences] is blocked by evil influences, . . . (II.3, p. 94)

As long as these evil influences occupy only specific parts of the organism, a therapy should be successful. Prognosis is rather bleak, though, as soon as they have penetrated to man's original influences.

> The reason is that [if the patient's body] has many areas that have not been affected by illness, while those areas that have been affected are few, it will be quite possible to maintain [the patient's] essence and strength, and to cause his regular influences to gradually reach their fullest extent again. (I.3, p. 63)

> [At that time,] the evil influences have merged with the [patient's] original influences. No drug could be of help here, and death [is inevitable]. (III.5, p. 111)

It may have become obvious already that to Hsü Ta-ch'un, the human organism was certainly no terra incognita, surrounded by skin with abstract processes happening inside. Rather, Hsü Ta-ch'un had a very clear idea, even in the absence of systematic anatomical data, of the body as a territory with distinct sections, interrelated by conduits and network vessels.

> The human body constitutes one single unit, but it has, nevertheless, different [sections that may be categorized as] exterior and interior, or upper and lower. What is meant by "exterior"? ["Exterior" refers to] the skin, the flesh, the sinews, and the bones. What is meant by "interior"? ["Interior" refers to] the viscera, the bowels, essence, and the spirit. The conduits and network [vessels] serve to connect [all these regions of the body]. (I.3, p. 63)

3.3 On the Concept of Illness

Health was, for Hsü Ta-ch'un, a state of normalcy (p. 53), and

> As long as a person's essence and spirits are complete and strong, no external evil will dare to offend [that person].
> (III.12, p. 130)

The concept of illness is referred to by Hsü Ta-ch'un with the term *chi* 疾. This term includes a rather holistic concept focusing on the sufferer and his individual condition, and it covers, in addition, notions of "disease" as an artifact with an inter-individual validity. In the *I-hsüeh Yüan Liu Lun* there is no distinction between an individual's personal experience of well-being or suffering on the one hand, and the medical label offered to a person's condition regardless of his or her personal feelings on the other hand. The term *chi* refers in all cases to a cultural construct, that is, to an external definition of a person's condition.

The holistic dimension of illness in the *I-hsüeh Yüan Liu Lun* is restricted to intra-individual perspectives. Even though external pathogenic factors, as for instance climatic factors, are recognized, both diagnosis and therapy are focused on individual patients and do not take a person's social environment into account.

Man is seen in the *I-hsüeh Yüan Liu Lun,* and in traditional Chinese medicine in general, as a microcosm reflecting a macrocosm of nature and society. Traditional Chinese medicine realizes that the same laws that govern the workings of nature and society are also at work in the human microcosm. In this, there is little difference with traditional European medicine. However, in Europe, ever since Johann Peter Franck (1745-1821), it has become a standard approach in medicine and public health to attempt changes not only in individual but also in social and environmental terms, if social and environmental factors are seen as responsible for the health problems encountered by individuals or entire groups. This kind of socio-environmental holism is nearly entirely absent from traditional Chinese medicine even though the necessary theoretical foundations could be demonstrated.

On the other hand, Western medicine is aware, through its knowledge of cybernetics and biochemical regulatory systems, of the interrelatedness of all the functional subsystems constituting the biological and mental organism as a whole. In daily clinical diagnosis and therapy, however, this knowledge is rarely considered or taken into practical account. In contrast, the theoretical tenets of traditional Chinese medicine demand the interrelatedness of an individual organism's various functional subsystems to form the basis of diagnosis and therapy.

11

The *I-hsüeh Yüan Liu Lun* offers ample evidence for the fact that an intra-individual holistic perspective does not necessarily exclude ontological and localistic perspectives. On the contrary, Hsü Ta-ch'un's holistic notion of illness is essentially ontological and localistic, and it emphasizes cause-effect relationships.

> Whenever an illness emerges, it must have a cause, . . .
> (I.2, p. 60)

> When a person suffers from [an ailment] this is called "illness." The reasons why this illness has emerged is called "cause." Now, identical body heat may be associated with wind or cold, with phlegm or food, with rising fire due to yin depletion, with depression and grief, with fatigue and fear, and with worms occupying [one's body]. All these are to be called causes. (III.8, p. 118)

> If two [persons suffer from] such illnesses, it may be that the physical manifestations of their illnesses are identical, while the causes of their [respective] illnesses are different.
> (III.4, p. 107)

Illnesses are states of being, but they are also entities. That is to say, wind or dampness are external influences that may cause an illness in that, after they have entered, they are the illness. In the same way, weariness or grief may cause an illness, but the resulting illness, such as body heat, is an entity that may become manifest at a very specific location, or affect the entire body.

> All the illnesses man may suffer from [are related either to the] seven emotions or to the six excesses. (II.2, p. 90)

> Illnesses related to the seven emotions are called "harm from inside." [Illnesses caused by] an intrusion of any of the six excesses are called "affection from outside." (III.4, p. 107)

> When an illness emerges from inside [of the body] it must start [its course] from the viscera and bowels. When an illness enters [the body] from the outside, it must start its course from the conduits and network [vessels]. (I.5, p. 69)

> Whenever an illness emerges, it must have a cause, and the locations affected by an illness can always be specified in terms of body sections. (I.2, p. 60)

The paragraph in the *I-hsüeh Yüan Liu Lun* which conveys the most obvious localistic notion of illness is entitled "On Intra-Abdominal Abscesses." We should recall here the new perspective that started with Andreas Vesalius (1514-1564), after extensive anatomical studies, and that gained an enormous momentum in Europe after an initial resistance by authors devoted to humoral pathology and Galenic view was quickly swept away.

Vesalius was the first to demonstrate systematically, and on the basis of genuine research, the relationship between illness and morphological lesions, and it is a noteworthy trans-cultural coincidence that a European contemporary of Hsü Ta-ch'un, Giovanni Battista Morgagni (1682-1771), who died in the same year as Hsü, published in 1761, within four years of the appearance of the *I-hsüeh Yüan Liu Lun*, his *De sedibus et causis morborum*, thereby decisively strengthening the basis of modern anatomical pathology. Morgagni went beyond Vesalius in that he cited specific organs as seats of illnesses; if Morgagni and Hsü Ta-ch'un had had a chance to meet, they would not have regarded each other as strangers, as the following excerpt from the latter's paragraph "On Intra-abdominal Abscesses" may show:

> In the case of liver abscesses, there is a very subtle pain in the flanks. After some time, [the patient] will vomit pus and blood. Abscesses in the small intestine resemble abscesses affecting the large intestine, except that they are located a little higher. Bladder abscesses are accompanied by pain below the lower abdomen, near the [pubic] hair line. They hurt as soon as one touches the skin and urination is difficult and causes pain. (IV.23, p. 304)

Closely related to his localistic perspective, and an indication of Hsü Ta-ch'un's perspective of intra-individual holism, is his emphasis on the concept of illness transmission in the organism.

> Sometimes illnesses are transmitted [from one location in the body to another], and undergo transformations, following definite rules. In other cases, [illnesses] are transmitted and transformed [without] following any fixed rule.
> (III.5, p. 110)

> As soon as a transmission has occurred [one should examine the illness's] secondary and primary locations, . . .
> (III.5, p. 110)

> Only such illnesses that have settled in the skin, the flesh, the sinews, and the bones, and that do not find their way into the [main] conduits and network [vessels], will not be transmitted

further. These are the so-called illnesses of the physical shell.
(I.2, p. 60)

A term often used by Hsü Ta-ch'un is *cheng* 症. The dictionary meaning of *cheng* is "symptom" or "ailment," but both these English concepts fail to cover the entire notion represented by the Chinese term. I have, therefore, suggested a new English term, "pathocondition," as a possible equivalent. A symptom represents, in Western thinking, a sign accompanying an illness; it is generally inconceivable that a patient suffering from diphtheria develops the symptoms of measles, and must be diagnosed as suffering from diphtheria nevertheless. Even though many illnesses with indistinct symptoms are known in Western medicine, and although specific individual symptoms may be indicators of more than one illness, the relationships between illness and symptom in Western medicine, and between illness and *cheng*, or pathocondition, in Chinese medicine are not identical, and overlap only partially.

> Any illness in its entirety is called "illness," but one single illness is inevitably accompanied by several pathoconditions. For instance, when the great-yang [conduit and viscus] have been harmed by wind, that is the illness. An aversion against wind, a hot body, sweating without external reason, and headache are pathoconditions [accompanying this illness]. Together, these [pathoconditions] constitute a great-yang illness; they are the basic pathoconditions of a great-yang illness. (III.7, p. 115)

> Each single illness has a name characterizing this specific illness. For instance, "struck-by-wind" is an encompassing designation. It includes [pathoconditions] such as "partial paralysis," "[limb] paralysis," "wind[-induced] heat," and "[pain] pervading all joints." All these pathoconditions are, in turn, accompanied by numerous [individual] pathoconditions, each of which bears a specific name, and each of which has a master prescription. (IV.7, p. 166)

> Pathoconditions are manifestations of an illness. If the illness is heat, the pathocondition is heat; if the illness is cold, the pathocondition is cold. That is a definite principle. But one should also know that pathoconditions and illnesses may contradict each other — a fact that may very easily lead to a mistaken treatment, and that should be known to everyone. (II.3, p. 93)

> Today, the name of an illness may still be quite similar to that [of an illness in ancient times], but the pathoconditions that

appear in the course of this [illness today] may be very different [from those in ancient times]. (IV.13, p. 187)

An illness, in the medical world view of Hsü Ta-ch'un, is a state defined by a conceptual system. An illness is not realized or experienced as such by a patient; it is identified by the physician in terms of the theories forming the basis of traditional Chinese medicine. All the patient may notice or suffer from in the course of his illness are specific conditions — i.e., the pathoconditions — but these pathoconditions do not necessarily represent clues rigidly corresponding to the illness affecting the patient, and hence indicating the character of the illness. Pathoconditions may be straightforward symptoms allowing for an easy diagnosis; they may, however, contradict the nature of the illness and mislead one to identify a state of health opposite to the real nature of the problem.

Hsü Ta-Ch'un went to great lengths in his *I-hsüeh Yüan Liu Lun* to draw the attention of his contemporaries to the complexity of the relationships between underlying illness and observable conditions, and he repeatedly emphasized the necessity to take all possible parameters into account to arrive at a correct diagnosis, the basis, that is, of an appropriate therapy.

> How, then, does a physician know how to distinguish whether [an illness] is minor or serious, and whether [the patient will] die or survive? He must ask for pathoconditions, and he must press the vessels, and then he will know all this. (II.2, p. 90)

> It is, therefore, essential to employ [also the other three diagnostic methods of] looking [for changes in the patient's complexion, of] listening [to his voice and of smelling his odors, and of] asking [him for his preferences for specific flavors of his food]. If these three [methods] are taken into account together [with an investigation of the movement in the vessels, contemporary healers, too,] will not lose one patient in a hundred. (II.1, p. 88)

In particular, Hsü Ta-Ch'un pointed out that the system of correspondences in traditional Chinese medicine has its limits, and that rather than forming one neatly woven web of linear connections, three sets of phenomena may confuse the physician in his attempts to arrive at a diagnosis, i.e., the illness itself, the movement in the vessels (i.e., the pulse), and the pathoconditions.

> There are even [such illnesses] that are contradicted by the [movement in the patient's] vessels. One and the same

movement in the vessels may appear together with one specific pathocondition that seems fitting, but it may also appear together with another pathocondition, and seem out of place. Or, one and the same pathocondition may be accompanied by one specific [movement in the] vessels that is fitting, but it may also be accompanied by another [movement in the] vessels that seems out of place. One and the same illness may be accompanied by tens of [different movements in the] vessels, and one and the same [movement in the] vessels may be associated with hundreds of pathoconditions. [These relationships] change and are not fixed. If one clings to merely one doctrine, though, one may take a patient's [movement in the] vessels as one's guideline and find that his pathoconditions do not agree. (VI.4, p. 321)

The body may be affected by not just one illness, with its concomitant pathoconditions; different illnesses may exist separately at the same time.

Illnesses and pathoconditions may appear separate or combined in innumerable variations. Hence, it is essential to search for the beginning and to sort out the different ends. (III.7, p. 115)

And it is even possible that

someone suffers at the same time from two illnesses with mutually contradictory causes; . . . (VI.15, p. 279)

3.4 Therapeutic Principles

One of the complaints pervading the entire *I-hsüeh Yüan Liu Lun* (and we shall return to this complaint later when we outline in more detail Hsü's notion of a loss of tradition) focuses on a paucity of therapeutic approaches applied by his contemporaries in the treatment of illnesses. Hsü Ta-ch'un stated his view quite clearly:

The treatment of an illness may follow many principles. (I.6, p. 72)

Here we encounter a second indication of Hsü's intra-individual holism, since illnesses, in contrast to diseases, must be treated with a view toward the condition of the individual sufferer. The entire body of the patient must be taken into regard, because as a result of different preconditions, one and the same illness may take a different course in different individuals, and requires different treatments accordingly:

16

[After such preparations,] I may be confronted with thousands of ends and tens of thousands of beginnings of the illnesses under heaven, and yet I will be able to design [therapeutic] patterns in thousands of adaptations. (VI.7, p. 254)

When [two patients suffer from] an identical illness, it may happen that [the same] treatment is effective in one of these patients, but remains without effect in the other. . . . Well, illnesses may be identical, but the persons [suffering from them] are different. (III.6, p. 113)

If one treats [all those patients who appear to suffer from one identical illness] with one and the same therapy, one may hit the nature of the illness, but [one's approach] may still be exactly contraindicated by the [condition of a] patient's influences and body. (III.6, p. 113)

Equally important as the focus on the specific course an illness may have taken in an individual, is the search for the cause and for the location of a single illness, or various illnesses, affecting the patient.

Causes and illnesses condition each other; they are intertwined in many ways, and the therapeutic patterns [to be employed must] vary [from case to case]. (III.4, p. 107)

If someone fails to inquire about the cause of the original illness, and about the cause of a concomitant illness, and if he simply states, "Such and such an illness is to be treated with such and such drugs," his [therapy] may hit [the illness] by chance, and the drugs tossed [into the patient] may indeed sometimes effect a cure. But, if he uses them again . . .
(III.8, p. 118)

If one disregards the location of an illness entirely and employs drugs to attack, contrary [to what would be correct], a place that is absolutely free of illness, this is what the *Neiching* calls "punishing the innocent." (I.5, p. 69)

Once this moment has arrived, the physician must] examine where an illness is located, and apply the treatment with all due consideration. Then the illness will not be able to hide away. (IV.14, p. 190)

To discover the whereabouts of an illness is not always easy because:

Furthermore, it may well be that the viscera and bowels have an illness — while, contrary [to what one might expect], the illness appears in the [patient's] limbs and joints. (I.5, p. 69)

In the biography of Pien Ch'io 扁鵲 in the *Shih-chi* 史記, Pien Ch'io is reported to have left the court of the Marquis of Ch'in after the latter's illness had moved into the bones and their marrow.[10] He explained to a messenger, who had been sent to follow him and obtain his reason for leaving, that an illness enters the body through the skin. As long as it remains located in the skin, it may be eliminated by different means than those used when the flesh and muscles, the conduits, the "depots" and "palaces" have been invaded. Death is inevitable when the illness has reached the bones and their marrow. Similarly, treatment is different in Hsü's view depending on where the evil influences settle after invading the organism.

> If evil [influences] have entered the sinews, the bones, the muscles or the flesh, then the illness [resulting from this intrusion] is a morphological one, and the [thermo-]influences and flavor [influences] of drugs will show no effect.
> (IV.14, p. 190)

> . . . man's illnesses proceed from the outside [of the body] to its internal regions. As long as they flow through the [main] conduits and the network [vessels], as well as through the viscera and bowels, there is no other way to eliminate them except through an intake of drugs. However, once an illness has settled down at a specific location, and when it can be felt in the region between skin, sinews, and bones, one applies a paste there to seal up the [illness's] influences, and to let the qualities of the drugs proceed through the pores of the hair into the *ts'ou-li* [area between skin and flesh], penetrate the conduits and their network [vessels], pick up [the illness] there and move it out [of the body], or attack and disperse it.
> (IV.23, p. 219)

> If the poisons have already gathered together and cannot leave [the body] through the skin, they will spread in all directions and cause harm everywhere. Only encircling drugs are able to tie them together and prevent them from spreading. They cause the influences to gather together and leak to the outside. This way, the [resulting abscesses] are small in size but [they accumulate and] rise as a bump. They easily develop pus, and [this pus] easily leaks out. (V.24, p. 307)

> Sometimes it is advisable to treat [different pathoconditions] separately; sometimes it is advisable to treat them jointly.
> (III.3, p. 104)

3.5 On Drugs

Hsü attributed to the ancients a very careful application of drugs:

> Not a single substance was arranged [in a prescription]
> without specific purpose, and the application of such a
> prescription left absolutely no room for compromise.
> (IV.13, p. 187)

Virtually all facets of Hsü Ta-ch'un's medical views so far discussed
are reflected in the ideas underlying his statements on the use of drugs.
One of the reasons for the broad spectrum of curative approaches recommended by Hsü may be seen in his approach to both illnesses and
diseases.

Illnesses, as I have outlined above, may take a different course in different individuals, and have to be treated with regard to the respective
condition of a given patient. For their treatment (in contrast to the treatment of diseases), Hsü Ta-ch'un recommended more or less complicated
prescriptions made up from several drugs. In general, a prescription is an
entity designed to cope with a specific illness. Since identical illnesses
may manifest themselves differently, individual ingredients may have to
be increased or decreased, others may have to be added or even left out,
in the treatment of specific cases. Illnesses manifest themselves as pathoconditions. One drug may be suited to eliminate one or several pathoconditions. The drugs in a prescription therefore mirror the pathoconditions to be treated. Hsü Ta-ch'un assumed that there was little need for
the physicians of his time to establish new prescriptions themselves
because the ancients had already designed appropriate prescriptions for all
illnesses. It is the task, in Hsü Ta-ch'un's eyes, of a physician of later
times, first, to search for a well-established prescription covering an illness he is confronted with, and, second, to modify this prescription
according to the individual requirements of his patient. He should be
aware of how far the adaptive modification of a prescription may be
stretched, and where he has to switch to an entirely different prescription.

> If [a physician] is brilliant in his considerations and perfect in
> his skills, he will adapt his [treatment] to the [individual] cir-
> cumstances [of each illness]. And, since the circumstances of
> an illness may vary one thousandfold, he will establish ten
> thousand different [therapeutic] patterns. (III.3, p. 105)

Illnesses may be basically identical, but the pathoconditions
accompanying them may vary. In such cases, it is not necessary to compose separate prescriptions. Rather, one increases
or reduces [the number of drugs] in a particular prescription

in accordance with the different pathoconditions that have become apparent. (IV.2, p. 150)

If the pathoconditions of a specific [patient] differed slightly [from those covered by a particular well-established prescription], patterns were available to add or leave out [certain drugs from this prescription], and [these patterns] were added to the prescriptions [as an appendix]. (IV.13, p. 187)

Single[-substance] prescriptions are composed of no more than one or two substances. They cure no more than one or two pathoconditions, and their effects are very swift. If their application fails to hit [the illness, single-substance prescriptions] may cause harm to the person [treated]. . . . When a person suffered from no more than one or two pathoconditions, the [ancient Sages] treated [that person] with but one drug. Since such drugs had special [therapeutic abilities], their power was rather strong, and they produced, therefore, extraordinary effects. However, when an illness resulted in several simultaneous pathoconditions, [the ancients] always combined several drugs and created a [complex] prescription. (IV.4, p. 157)

This latter quotation may lead to Hsü's notions on a medicinal treatment of diseases. Traditional Chinese medicine was well aware, from the beginning of its documented history, that there are certain ailments that take virtually identical courses in each patient afflicted. The treatment of these ailments, which we may call diseases, focuses on the disease as an identifiable entity, not on the patient as a sufferer. An example is leprosy. Reliable reports on the presence of leprosy in China date back as far as the Han dynasty. Of course, given all the difficulties of retrospective diagnosis, not all persons described as having been afflicted with *lai* 癩, *li yang* 癘瘍 or *ta ma feng* 大麻風 may indeed have suffered from Hansen's disease. Still, the terms mentioned, and others as well, have undoubtedly included leprosy, and the Chinese have recognized that this is a disease standing apart from other ailments as a separate nosological entity requiring a specific treatment regardless of the constitution of the patient.[11]

Reading through Hsü Ta-ch'un's *I-hsüeh Yüan Liu Lun* and other medical texts, one realizes that the distinction between illnesses and diseases is not as clear-cut as our use of two different terms might suggest. In fact, "illness" and "disease" should be seen as merely marking the ends of a continuum termed *chi* 疾. The existence of prescriptions allows both for an adaptation of flexible formulas to cases of individual "illness," and for an application of standardized medication against "disease:"

> It is for this reason that the people of ancient times had ready-made cure-all prescriptions, such as the "dark-red golden ingot" or the "extremely valuable pills," [prescriptions] that cured very many illnesses and that achieved miraculous successes in all cases. (I.6, p. 72)

Hsü, as an opponent of Sung learning, rejected the notion, introduced by Chang Yüan-su 張元素 (with the sobriquet Chieh-ku 潔古) (ca. 1180), that drugs enter specific conduits and exert their effects only at specific locations.[12] In a sophisticated discourse, Hsü Ta-ch'un notes that certain illnesses appear at very specific locations or in very specific conduits; he warned, however, against the assumption that those drugs that cure illnesses emerging at such locations cure illnesses only at these specific locations:

> Man's influences and his blood penetrate every [region of his body]. . . . similarly, when [a drug] enters the human body, its effects will reach every [region]. How could it be that a particular drug enters only a particular conduit? (I.6, p. 72)

Hsü Ta-ch'un conveyed, in his *I-hsüeh Yüan Liu Lun,* very clear notions on the inherent qualities of drugs. He was aware of a close relationship between geography and active ingredients, and it might have been only a minor step for him to accept the view that there are methods to search for these active ingredients and define their nature.

> When, in [ancient] times, [the drugs] came into use, there were specific areas where [specific drugs] grew. These, then, were their native places. Hence, [each drug] was rich in influences and full of strength. (IV.16, p. 197)

> Even [in case a drug remained without effect] if the substance itself was not a false substitute, the variety may have been different. (IV.16, p. 197)

> When drugs cure an illness, in some cases this can be explained, in others not. . . . or when [drugs are] identical in their [abilities to] dissolve poison [but differ in their actual effects] — such as *hsiung-huang,* which dissolves the poisons of snakes and insects, and *kan-ts'ao,* which dissolves the poisons of foods and beverages — [then these are] already [some examples of therapeutic drug effects] that cannot be explained entirely. . . . But when it comes to . . . [the ability of] *shih-chün-tzu* to kill *hui* worms, or to [the ability of] *ch'ih-hsiao-tou*

to eliminate skin swellings, [these are examples of drug effects] that are even harder to explain. (IV.17, p. 200)

Aside from the addition or deletion of ingredients to or from a prescription, Hsü Ta-ch'un was well aware of possibilities of modifying natural effects of individual drugs by two methods. In his essays "On the Patterns of Drug Boiling" and "On Patterns of Drug Intake," Hsü Ta-ch'un cited many examples where differences in the processing of specific substances, and also in their intake before or after meals, resulted in different therapeutic abilities:

> The patterns of drug boiling need a very thorough discussion, because whether a drug has an effect or not is entirely dependent upon these patterns. Poultry, fish, sheep, and pork, if cooked improperly, may harm man, and it should go without saying that this applies all the more to drugs whose special [virtue] lies in the curing of illness. (IV.18, p. 203)

> Whether [the treatment of] an illness results in a cure or not, requires more than [a composition of drugs in a] prescription that hits the illness. Although a prescription may [be well suited to] hit an illness, it will not only fail to exert any effect, but will — on the contrary — even cause harm, if its intake did not correspond to an appropriate pattern. It is absolutely essential to be aware of this. (IV.19, p. 206)

A second mode of modifying the effects of individual substances was already described in the Han dynasty *Shen-nung Pen-ts'ao Ching* 神農本草經. In the introductory section of the *Hsin-hsiu Pen-ts'ao* 新修本草 of 659, quoting the *Shen-nung Pen-ts'ao Ching*, T'ao Hung-ching 陶弘景 detailed the "seven emotions" that drugs could harbor toward each other, if combined in one prescription.[13] Hsü Ta-ch'un repeated some of these compatibility rules as examples (see p. 175), and the important aspect of this to be noted here is that he essentially reversed the Sung-Chin-Yüan integration of drug application into the theoretical realms of the medicine of systematic correspondence.

Prior to the Sung, pharmaceutics had remained virtually untouched — with the exception of the *Shang-han Lun* — by the yinyang and five-phases theories.[14] The application of drugs, the definition of their effects, and compatibilities as well as incompatibilities, had not been explained on the basis of thoughts of systematic correspondence but on the basis of experience, and of metaphors taken from the social environment. Hsü Ta-ch'un, as a representative of Han learning, despised the efforts of the Sung-Chin-Yüan era to develop a pharmacology of systematic correspondence, and argued, once again, in favor of an empirically and metaphorically legitimated application of materia medica. His open criticism of

Sung influences in medical theory appears in many statements; one example may suffice here:

> By the time of the Yüan, when Liu Ho-chien,[5] Chang Chieh-ku[6] and others appeared, the study of the *Nei-ching* was emphasized by everyone. Each time these [authors] discussed an illness [in their books], they first quoted from the text of the Classic; then they took into account what all the experts [of later centuries] had said; and, finally, they added a therapeutic pattern which seemed to be the very best. But these people were not accomplished scholars; they were unable to penetrate deeply the meaning of the classics and they failed to investigate thoroughly the conceptual origins underlying the design of prescriptions by [Chang] Chung-ching. Hence their doctrines showed no effects [in actual therapy]; they were irrelevant. Each of these [author-physicians] was preoccupied with merely his own biases, and none of them found his way back to the central stream [of ancient medicine].
> (VII.3, p. 364)

3.6 Metaphors in the *I-hsüeh Yüan Liu Lun*

The use of metaphors in the realm of medicine is part of cognitive dialectics. On the one hand, theoretical knowledge cannot develop out of nothing, and in medicine the human quest for a better understanding of the functions of the organism is guided by stimuli received from one's social and/or physical environment. The ideas of the nature of a healthy organism, of illness, and of appropriate therapeutic interventions that develop in medical systems have been, in China as in Europe, highly reflective of the social and physical environment of the thinkers who developed these systems. Systems of medical ideas are, therefore, metaphors in themselves, revealing at least as much of the world where their authors lived, or would have preferred to live, as of what they tried to explain.

On the other hand, it is a general characteristic in the advancement of any knowledge that explanations of the new and unfamiliar employ a language referring to the familiar. Hence, plausible metaphors are borrowed from man's environment to explain new notions developed in medicine and science. Galen adopted images taken from the kitchen and from winepresses. Paracelsus compared human physiology with the processes he had witnessed in the Carynthian foundries, Descartes likened the organism to the mechanism of a clock-work, Virchow explained the coexistence of cells on the basis of the coexistence of people with equal rights in the democratic society that he envisaged, and so on.

Similar examples could be quoted from Chinese medical literature, and may also be found in Hsü Ta-ch'un's work. When such metaphors are unavailable, or transcend readily available experiences, (as for instance when scientists speak of a "curved space"), then it is most difficult for the layperson to follow the progress of knowledge, and a gulf develops between those who understand and others who do not.

Metaphors, then, are both complimentary and antagonistic to scientific theory; the more strongly developed, and the more accepted by the general public, the abstract theoretical foundations of a given knowledge are, the less resort should be necessary to environmental metaphors. The rejection of Sung-Chin-Yüan theoretical pharmacology by Hsü Ta-ch'un required, therefore, a return to ancient metaphors in order to make the function of the drugs in the organism plausible to the readers of the I-hsüeh Yüan Liu Lun.

Even the most advanced realms of Western medicine are occasionally explained to outsiders by means of environmental metaphors. For example, when in November 1987, a Nobel Prize was awarded for the first time to a Japanese researcher, his findings in immunology were described, in the international press, in terms that could have been written by Hsü Ta-ch'un. "The man who explained the war in our body" and "The struggle fought in our body" were the most succinct headlines formulated by newspapers to emphasize the proximity between immunological and military responses to unwanted intruders into one's territory.[15] Another newspaper reported, "The defensive system of the living organism has to cope with millions of different intruders all the time. The cells and molecules of this immune system patrol through the body unceasingly, always in search of pathogenic agents. It is most fascinating that a specifically trained trackhound, an antibody, is aimed at each intruder."[16]

Hsü Ta-ch'un appropriately wrote:

> If, however, those agents that are responsible for warding off [evil intruders] fail to do so, those [intruders] attacking them will gather in their place. (III.12, p. 130)

Hsü Ta-ch'un devoted an entire essay to "parallels in the use of drugs and the use of soldiers," and he outlined a perspective on drug use that is, first, disease-oriented and, second, localistic. Some of his arguments could well have survived into the era of bacteriology.

> Now, the rationale of having soldiers is to eliminate violence, and if there is no other way, military operations must be started. Similarly, the rationale of having drugs is to attack

illnesses, and if there is no other way, they must be employed. (III.12, p. 183)

To suffer from an illness . . . is as if one were confronted with a hostile country. . . . One must know the foreign [territory], and one must know one's own [territory]. And, if one checks the [enemy] at many places, there will be no grief over a destroyed body or over losses of life afterwards. (III.12, p. 183)

If a physician discovers what has caused the attack, and if he treats the [patient] according to a [proper] method, letting [the patient's] influences pass through [the body again], and expelling the evil, then [the patient] will be cured immediately. (III.11, p. 127)

Militaristic metaphors do appear in the *I-hsüeh Yüan Liu Lun* not only in the immediate context of drug use, but are an essential facet of the ontological perspective complementing Hsü's functional view of illness:

[Superior practitioners] see to it that the original influences are complete and remain in control, so that [the original influences] themselves may keep the evil [influences] outside. If, however, evil influences gain the upper hand and cause harm, the [superior practitioners] activate original influences that remained untouched so far; they have them fight with their back toward the city wall and enter a decisive struggle, and thus they avoid the shame that follows the death [of a patient]. (I.1, p. 58)

Quite elucidating, in this context, is Hsü's discussion of how to proceed when evil influences have invaded the body. Evil influences, he pointed out, are like thieves entering a house. Hsü Ta-ch'un criticized as entirely inappropriate the popular therapeutic approach of his time, supplementing a patient's proper influences, to strengthen them to an extent where they could expel the evil influences themselves. Rather, Hsü emphasized, "It is essential in such a situation to apply drugs that attack the evil influences directly." To strengthen the patient's proper influences during an illness is, he notes, as if one were to strengthen the walls of a house after thieves had already broken in. Hsü refuted the argument that supplementation was the same as sending enforcements to the inhabitants of the house, pointing out that such enforcements would know no difference between thieves and inhabitants and support both. (III.1, p. 98)

Further metaphors employed by Hsü Ta-ch'un include those taken
from the physical environment, from household experiences, from the
arts, and various other areas that Hsü Ta-ch'un deemed obvious enough
to elucidate physiological and pathological processes:

> Inside the kidneys is a location where the essence is stored; it
> is [always] filled and never empty in the same way as a well is
> filled with water day and night. (I.7, p. 75)

> The pattern employed here is identical with that of Yü the
> Great when he regulated the flood. When a great flooding
> occurs, [large streams such as the Ch'ang]-chiang, the Wei, the
> [Huang-]ho, and the Han will drain [the water from the
> smaller] rivers nearby into the ocean. It would be absolutely
> impossible to cause all the water covering the land to find a
> course to the ocean through only one river. (V.6, p. 251)

> When evil influences are present in abundance, and when the
> original influences are strong, the evil influences and the origi-
> nal influences will merge with each other. It is like oil poured
> into flour; once [the oil and flour] have merged, they cannot
> be separated again, . . . (III.10, p. 125)

> Furthermore, there are illnesses that have been cured already
> and, nevertheless, before long will end in death, because the
> evil influences have left together with the illness. For a time
> everything appears normal, but the true influences cannot
> recover — just as in a fight between two tigers, one wins but
> has exhausted all his strength. (III.10, p. 125)

> One may compare this to calligraphy. Someone may already
> be quite an expert in using the brush, but his composition [of
> characters] is unbalanced; or the form of the characters is
> complete, but the individual strokes are not accomplished. In
> all these cases one could not state that [this person] was an
> able calligrapher. (IV.1, p. 147)

3.7 "Psychological" and "Sociological" Views in the *I-hsüeh Yüan Liu Lun*

Hsü Ta-ch'un must have been a keen observer of his fellow men.
The *I-hsüeh Yüan Liu Lun* contains, in its final chapter, a number of
essays that can only be termed sociological today. Hsü knew the
psychology of physicians and patients, and even though we may read

between the lines of various ethical exhortations published in centuries prior to Hsü's work of problems of physician behavior, and in the patient-physician relationship, I know of no other pre-twentieth-century Chinese text with a similar depth and broadness of reflection on these issues.

Before we take a closer look at some of his statements in this regard, Hsü's definition of an ideal physician should be quoted:

> Therefore, only such people who are critical and go for genuine knowledge should study [medicine]. Hence anyone taking up the profession [of medicine] must surpass others in his natural gifts, and he must leave others behind in his knowledge. He should be able to leave all common affairs aside, and concentrate his mind [on his study] for many years. And if he is, in addition, taught by an [expert] teacher, he will be able to reach a secret penetration and tacit understanding of the intentions of the ancient Sages. (VII.5, p. 371)

Hsü Ta-ch'un was well aware that few of his contemporaries could come up to the ideals listed here, and even though, as we shall see later, he accused many of his colleagues of simply being of bad character, he also realized the constraints affecting both physicians and patients in their encounter. An example is his warning against speeding up a treatment unnecessarily where it should be clear, at least to the physician, that the ailment will heal only after a set period of time. Here, as in other essays, Hsü Ta-ch'un noted the intense stress under which physicians and the patients or their relatives are placed in their relationships.

> Given that physicians know of all this and that the patients, as is unavoidable, demand that we speed up the effects [of a treatment], then we should clearly tell them the reason [for their slow recovery], and identify in advance the time [when] they will be healed. If they do not believe, and if they demand that the physician design another good prescription, then one employs drugs that are balanced and light in their qualities, and neutral in flavor — simply to respond to the demands of the patient — and waits until [the illness] heals by itself. If the [patient] still does not believe [that enough has been done], one must firmly decline [to meet the patient's demands]. It is definitely impossible to give in to do him a favor and thus cause harm to that person through an inappropriate treatment. If one acts like this, the patient may well develop hatred [for a physician] and malign him for a while. But later, when the [physician's] words have come true, the [patient] will realize that our knowledge is great and our rank high. (V.17, p. 286)

27

Hsü Ta-ch'un voiced several arguments that may be interpreted as supporting professionalization. He criticized his "colleagues" for not being independent enough from their patients, and he defended expert physicians against accusations when a patient died. His point (raised in the final essay of *I-hsüeh Yüan Liu Lun*) that physicians who kill patients through their treatment should be seen as agents of fate is quite innovative and was, to my knowledge, never previously raised. On the other hand, though, Hsü despised all physicians who studied and practiced medicine to earn a living, and he provided his readers with many details of how practitioners attempted to betray their clients.

> Ever since, though, most of the physicians have been unsuccessful students [for an official career], and they lacked the capital to become traders. Hence they had no other way but to [take up medicine for] earning their livelihood.
> (VII.4, p. 368)

> First, they cause the ulcers [of their patients] to develop as large as possible, so that these people are frightened to hell, and only then do they treat them. . . . Such people have nothing in mind but to cheat the people and to acquire riches.
> (VII.2, p. 360)

> Three out of ten patients die as a result of mistakes committed by physicians; three out of ten patients die as a result of mistakes committed by themselves; and another three out of ten patients die as a result of mistakes committed by outsiders who happen to have browsed through medical literature.
> (VII.8, p. 381)

> Well, this has its origin in the physicians of today who prefer to make lofty speeches, to betray the people. (IV.24, p. 180)

> Ginseng, then, is a sacred drug employed by physicians who practice with an eye to reward, and who wish to avoid accusations. (IV.11, p. 180)

> Physicians who kill someone through a mistaken therapy may still be excused; but those who harm people at liberty and destroy families day after day, they are worse than thieves and robbers! One must be cautious [about such practitioners]! (IV.11, p. 180)

Interestingly enough, when the Ssu K'u Ch'üan-shu 四庫全書 edition of 1778 was prepared, from which the calligraphy of the present text was selected, lengthy passages were omitted (but are again appended in the present edition) from the final two paragraphs "On Patients" and "On the Fact that It Is Not a Crime When Physicians [Harm Patients through] Mistaken Treatments." The passages omitted are those most critical of contemporary physicians and one might surmise that they were censored as having gone too far. Still, sufficient open criticism was left in the preceding essays to convey Hsü's basic message.

If we cannot be sure whether Hsü's critical remarks concerning his colleagues were censored, or were shortened for some other editorial reason, the omission of two complete essays from the edition of 1778 is difficult to explain except by the political annoyance caused by their contents. The two essays "On Similarities between the Ways of Medicine and the Ways of Government" and "On Parallels between [the Emergence of] Illnesses and the Changing [Condition] of States" are based on thoughts and analogies that demonstrate close relationships between therapeutic activities in medicine and governmental activities in the state:

> To order the body is like ordering the empire. . . . When rebellions occur at any of the four frontiers, an appropriate [defense] is to choose a general and to dispatch troops to quickly drive away [all rebels]. If, however, one were to go into the Hall of Learning, to discuss ceremonies and music, then the enemy would [advance quickly] to the gates [of the city]. If therefore [for an illness caused by evil influences that have entered the body from outside] one carelessly employs supplementing [drugs] before the evil influences have been eliminated completely, this will cause these evil influences to proceed deeper into [the patient's body, causing him to] die. (V.2, p. 233)

It may well have been that a medical intellectual was granted by the editors of the 1778 version of the *I-hsüeh Yüan Liu Lun* a right to resort to household and military metaphors to elucidate basic physiological, pathological, and therapeutic processes. Here, though, Hsü made use of outright political metaphors, and it is by no means clear whether he wrote a medical message illustrated by parallels from the area of government, or whether he intended a political message hidden in a medical document. The latter possibility would not have been a novelty in China. Li Ao's "Report on [the Drug] *Ho-shou-wu*"[17] most likely a parable referring to the situation of Confucianism at this time, and suggesting solutions for the future, and Chang Yüan-su's statement "Old prescriptions cannot be used to treat the illnesses of today" are merely two examples from a long tradition of concealing risky political ideas under a disguise of medical argumentation.[18] Even though Hsü Ta-ch'un attested his own dynastic period "a time of great prosperity. Sage after Sage follow each other. A strong central authority exists. The morality

of the court is upright and deserves respect, and favors flow everywhere"
(V.2, p. 240), his general conclusions may have irritated those responsible
for editing his texts.

These conclusions show Hsü Ta-ch'un to be an intellectual who
demanded flexibly adapted solutions for medical as well as political issues.
Just as it would be inappropriate to employ identical therapeutic patterns
against all illnesses alike, political response to social or national crises also
must vary according to the nature of the problem. Hsü recommended,
both in medicine and in politics, the strengthening of a hard-line
approach. In his eyes, his contemporaries were too weak to attack and
fight whatever enemy jeopardized their bodily health or their national
peace. They preferred, he complained, what we might call a policy of
appeasement, based on a belief in a moral basis common to attackers and
defenders alike. Even though Hsü Ta-ch'un must be seen as a representative of the Han-learning movement — a movement carried mainly by
persons to be considered as Confucians — his contempt for a belief in the
strength of morals and of an adherence to the Confucian rites under all
circumstances may hint at the independence of this thought.

4. The Loss of Tradition

On the preceding pages, I have summarized what I consider to be
basic thoughts pervading Hsü Ta-ch'un's book *I-hsüeh Yüan Liu Lun.* A
literal rendering of this title would read "On the Origin and Further
Course of Medicine." This is, indeed, the framework in which Hsü
presented his thoughts. However, he conveys a characteristic message in
almost all of the one hundred short essays that constitute the book. It is
for this message that I have given the book the English title of "Forgotten Traditions of Ancient Chinese Medicine."

Hsü's argumentation maintains a persistent structure. Again and
again he compares the dismal state of the art of his time with what he
assumes to have been the standard of the past, and reaches the conclusion
that little, if anything, is left of that standard. He observes decline in virtually every respect. Some of his summarizing statements are rather
direct:

> Today's physicians . . . have given up the good [old] methods
> of the Sages entirely. (IV.14, p. 190)

> The tradition of the [true] teachings of medicine has been lost.
> (V.10, p. 264)

> The physicians of later times do not even know the general
> names of the illnesses. (V.20, p. 295)

In recent times, however, those who select a physician, and those who practice medicine, they are all equally ignorant and have no way to distinguish [good and bad]. (V.18, p. 289)

The unfounded statements now in fashion are not worth listening to. (II.1, p. 88)

I myself consider it most regrettable that since the T'ang and Sung, scholars have no longer contributed to a [continued] prospering [of medicine]. Rather, they regarded [the practice of medicine] as a lower occupation. Hence step by step the [ancient] traditions were lost. (Preface, p. 52)

Hsü devoted his attention both to acupuncture and to materia medica. The longest essay included in the *I-hsüeh Yüan Liu Lun* is entitled "On the Loss of Tradition in Needling and Cauterization," and offers ten detailed reasons for his conclusion that the practice of needling in his own days was a far cry from its beginnings during the Han. Hsü Ta-ch'un realized that needling had flourished in earlier times, but in Chinese medicine it had become secondary to the application of drugs because both doctors and patients were more comfortable with prescriptions and drugs. Here, too, he notes decline rather than progress:

When the people in ancient times composed a prescription, the underlying rationale was both sophisticated and subtle to a degree that is inconceiveable [today]. (IV.2, p. 150)

As a result, [physicians of recent times] warn each other and believe that the application of ancient prescriptions is difficult, while, in fact, they simply do not know that they no longer have access to the subtle rationale underlying these ancient prescriptions. (IV.2, p. 151)

All the masters of the T'ang era used drugs extensively, but they lacked adaptive ingenuity. The people of the Sung, then, did not know anything about drugs. Their prescriptions were stiff like boards and superficial like skin. The Yüan era is said to have been extremely flourishing. Everyone established his personal school, vainly hastening to put forward his private views. And the Ming, finally, did nothing but plagiarize the leftovers of the Yüan people. (IV.3, p. 154)

Hsü's critique centers around two major shifts he noticed in the application of drugs. First, he regretted that the physicians of "later times" were no longer courageous enough to focus their drugs on illnesses or their various pathoconditions directly. They relied, Hsü complained, on "warming" and "supplementing" approaches, rather than on "attack," and he compared the inappropriateness of such an approach, as I have already shown, with attempts to strengthen the wall of a house when thieves have already got in, and who, as Hsü emphasized, should first be immediately confronted and thrown out. Hsü Ta-ch'un noticed, in this regard, a continuously decreasing variation in the range of therapeutic methods employed:

> Today, the illnesses appear in ever more variations, and the physicians have ever fewer approaches at their disposal.
> (IV.14, p. 191)

Second, Hsü Ta-ch'un fought strongly against what he saw as an undue dominance of theoretical concerns in the application of drugs. The ancients, he pointed out, knew drugs that fought illnesses, and they employed substances that were capable of curing the various pathoconditions accompanying illness. This rather direct approach had become obsolete, in Hsü's view, mainly as a result of Sung-Chin-Yüan theory.

Despite such harsh criticisms, though, Hsü, was quite aware of the fact that the knowledge of the ancients on drugs had been improved in the meantime. Most interesting in this regard is the value he assigned to "trials" and "tests":

> In later times, though, each single drug was employed in the treatment of ever more illnesses, and this with positive results, because what the ancient [physicians] had not yet entirely known became known through many trials to those who lived afterwards. (IV.8, p. 169)

> Still, even among [the prescriptions composed in later times] are some [that display] extraordinary patterns, and a subtle use of drugs, and that may well be suitable to supplement what the ancients had not yet achieved, and that may serve as additional data. (IV.3, p. 155)

Nothing of the more recently acquired knowledge, though, reached the standards of the ancient Sages:

> [Li Shih-chen] studied differences and similarities [among drugs]. He distinguished between false and correct [identification]. He traced the [geographic] origins [of the drugs]; and he collected the sayings of all [the previous] experts. As a result, he brought the materia medica to an even greater degree of completeness [than had existed before]. . . . Here, too, the number of illnesses they could treat successfully increased [with the number of newly introduced drugs]. And yet, none

of these [later additions] reached the purity and authenticity of the [knowledge outlined in] the *Shen-nung Pen-ts'ao*. (IV.15, p. 193)

It would certainly be going too far to conclude that Hsü Ta-ch'un called on a fictitious golden past to criticize his contemporaries and move things ahead — even though this approach is well-documented in earlier Chinese history. And yet, despite his admiration for what he called the Sages of antiquity, Hsü saw a necessity for change not only backwards but forwards. Maybe the fact that he never went through a formal training, and never was compelled to fix his mind on the requirements of a traditional learning, helped him develop the multi-faceted personality that shines through his writings.

5. Epilogue

To present the ideas of Hsü Ta-ch'un to a Western readership more than two hundred years after his death, and almost two and a half centuries after he published his *I-hsüeh Yüan Liu Lun*, may need, at first glance, some justification. The excerpts from the *I-hsüeh Yüan Liu Lun* quoted on the preceding pages, and even more so the entire text itself, should be telling enough that Hsü's words can be regarded not as an outdated, historical document, but as a welcome message for our own time.

Having followed the emerging and broadening interest in traditional Asian health care practices and thoughts in Europe and America over the past few decades, one can hardly escape the impression that much of what has been written, by Western and Asian authors, may have served certain desired ends but failed to provide Western readers with the background information necessary to fully appreciate parallels, overlappings, and outright antagonisms between the history and contents of European and Western medicine in comparison with Chinese and Asian medicine.

Problems have been created, in this regard, by those who abstract some very specific ideas and practices from a rich tradition of Chinese health care, and present them to occidental readers as "Chinese medicine" simply for the fact that they seem to represent what Western medicine appears to lack. It is perfectly legitimate for anyone questioning the basic assumptions of current Western medicine as ultimate wisdom to search the history of European, Asian, or any other culture's health care heritage for traditions that might promise alternative ways of therapy and prevention; that is, towards a definition and handling of illness. Progress, or change, in medicine has, as far as we can see today, never been a happy and harmonious adding of new stones to an edifice of truth and successful healing. Progress and fundamental changes in medicine have been stimulated by the most diverse, and often unexpected and unpredictable, sources — and, the historian may add, have occurred usually against vehement opposition by representatives of established ways. Hence, given a widespread feeling of discontent with high technology and chemistry, and given also an increasing feeling of uneasiness vis-a-vis some of the possibilities opened by the most advanced methods of modern medicine, one may witness today a process that has occurred again and again in the history of medicine, that is, the breaking away of minorities from mainstream practices and thoughts. Whether this movement will lead to any viable alternative is, of course, impossible to predict.

One of the more outstanding parallels history offers in comparison with current developments is the beginning of the reacquisition of ancient European medicine at the peak of the middle ages. A difference, though, may be seen in centuries of philological work opening access to the writings of the ancients and preceding or accompanying an application of knowledge exiled for almost half a millennium in the civilization of Arabia. The encounter with Oriental medicine today has an advantage over learning from ancient Greece and Rome eight or nine hundred years ago in that the interest is focused on a tradition that is still alive. It needs to be emphasized here, though, that "Chinese Medicine" has many facets and levels of theory and practice, and that it is simply inaccurate to assume that so-called "traditional Chinese medicine" today is a mirror image of traditional Chinese medicine as it was propagated or practiced in China centuries or millennia ago.

It is, as our search for an appropriate terminology to render Chinese concepts into modern Western languages demonstrates, quite difficult to open access to ancient primary Chinese sources for an interested European or American readership. The *I-hsüeh Yüan Liu Lun* of Hsü Ta-ch'un, though, should serve as evidence of the necessity, despite our continuing inability to find adequate terminological solutions in all instances, not only to read through and listen to twentieth century interpretations of traditional Chinese medicine but to approach the sources themselves. Without Hsü Ta-ch'un quite a few erroneous distinctions between Western medicine on the one side and Chinese medicine on the other, might be hard to contradict. Hsü Ta-ch'un, in fact, is a fascinating witness of a broadness of learned traditional Chinese medicine that is rarely acknowledged today. He would have been, in many fundamental respects, not only an equivalent interlocutor of Morgagni and other European contemporaries, but from the arguments he advanced in his *I-hsüeh Yüan Liu Lun* we may even go so far as to assume that he would find it difficult to acknowledge a clearcut dichotomy between basic tenets of Western and Asian medical traditions and current realities. This is not to deny that serious differences exist, and one should be aware of the fact that various approaches are emphasized more in one tradition and less in the other. The point is that one should be well aware of the fact that so-called Western medicine did not enter Chinese culture as an entirely alien system of ideas. It was appreciated in China not only because of its promises in terms of disease control, but also because it continued traditions already inherent in Chinese Medicine for a long time. Hsü Ta-ch'un's writing, even though in itself unable to represent traditional Chinese medicine in its entirety, should contribute to a decrease of unjustified antagonism between Eastern and Western medicine, and should support a better understanding of real, not reified, differences.

Notes

1. Sung Ta-jen, 1963, 30 (See Appendix C for full bibliographical data).

2. Arther W. Hummel, *Eminent Chinese of the Ch'ing Period (1644-1912)*, Washington 1943, 323.

3. Ibid.

4. Ibid., 324.

5. Hsieh Sung-mu, 1934, 12 (See Appendix C for full bibliographical data).

6. See Paul U. Unschuld, *Nan-ching: The Classic of Difficult Issues*, Berkeley, Los Angeles, London 1986.

7. Cf. Paul U. Unschuld, *Medicine in China: A History of Ideas*, Berkeley, Los Angeles, London 1985a, 208-210.

8. See *Huang-ti Nei-ching, Su-wen*, first treatise "Shang-ku T'ien-chen Lun" 上古天眞論 translation in Unschuld, 1985a, 277.

9. Henry Sigerist, *A History of Medicine*, New York 1961, 327.

10. See *Shih-chi*, ch. 105.

11. Paul U. Unschuld, "Traditional Chinese Medical Theory and Real Nosological Units. The case of Hansen's Disease," *Medical Anthropological Quarterly* 17 (1985b) 1, 5-8; idem, "Lepra in China," in: J.H. Wolf (ed.) *Aussatz Lepra Hansen-Krankheit. Ein Menschheitsproblem im Wandel. Teil II: Aufsätze.* Würzburg 1986b, 163-183.

12. See also below "On the Origin and History of Medicine," pp. 364.

13. Paul U. Unschuld, *Medicine in China: A History of Pharmaceutics*, Berkeley, Los Angeles, London 1986c, 19, 33, 36.

14. Ibid., 25-27, 85 ff.

15. *Münchener Abendzeitung*, October 13, 1987, 4.; *Time Magazine*, October 13, 1987.

16. *Süddeutsche Zeitung*, October 13, 1987, 13.

17. This is the *Ho-shou-wu Chuan* 何首烏傳. See Unschuld, 1986c, 230-232.

18. Ibid., 102-103.

Appendix A

The Biography of Hsü Ling-t'ai
by Yüan Mei

In the twenty-fifth year of the Ch'ien-Lung reign (1760), the Grand Secretary of the Hall of Literature and Brilliance, Chiang Wen-ch'üeh,[1] suffered from an illness, and the Son of Heaven inquired about famous physicians from all over the country [to attend the patient]. The Minister of Justice, Sir Ch'in,[2] recommended first of all Hsü Ling-t'ai from Wu-chiang, and the Son of Heaven called on him to come to the capital, and ordered him to examine the illness of Sir Chiang. Mr. [Hsü Ling-t'ai] reported that the illness was incurable. The Emperor appreciated his frankness and wanted him to stay in the capital for further services. However, Mr. [Hsü] asked to be allowed to return to his home, and the Emperor gave his permission. Twenty years later,[3] a trusted enuch[4] had an illness, and [Mr. Hsü] was again summoned to proceed to the capital. [By that time,] Mr. [Hsü] was already 79 years old, and because he was quite aware of his frailty and of the possibility that he might not return alive, he took his son Hsi with him and had him carry the piece of wood [that, in the event of his death, was to be placed beneath his body in the coffin.] Three days after they had reached the capital, [Mr. Hsü] died. The Emperor regretted [his death] and granted a gift of gold [to his family]; he ordered [Hsü] Hsi to escort the coffin back home.

Alas! Even though Mr. [Hsü] had only the status of a student in Wu, he received two appointments[5] by the Sage Emperor, with the governor and four high provincial officers coming to the door of his house [to ensure] a speedy journey. All those who heard of this were startled with awe, and praised it as a rare honor.

I am a former historian. I was well acquainted with [Mr. Hsü. For a long time] I had intended to collect his extraordinary prescriptions and unique techniques, and to document them with an enthusiastic pen, so as to hand them on [to posterity] as a medical mirror that would keep the people alive. But I never found the time to obtain [them]. This fall, I went to see [his son] Hsi in Wu-chiang and got his own notes, and I also went to see all those people in Wu who could tell me about Mr. [Hsü's life], so that I might write his biography. This biography reads as follows.

Mr. [Hsü's] personal name was Ta-ch'un; his style name was Ling-t'ai. In later years he adopted the sobriquet "The old man of the Hui creek" (Hui-hsi lao-jen). His family had been respected in the neighborhood for some time already; his grandfather Ch'iu participated, for his great proficiency in literary styles, in the eighteenth year of the K'ang-hsi [reign (1679)] in the compilation of the Ming dynastic history by the Han-lin Academy.

Mr. [Hsü] was of uncommon talents; his intelligence and his physical strength went beyond those of other people. He was well versed in the classics of astronomy, in the annals of geography, in vocal and instrumental music, as well as sword-play, lance throwing, and the [martial] techniques employed by [King] Kou [when his state of] Ying [overcame the state of] Yüeh. His special expertise, though, was in the field of medicine. Whenever he looked at a patient, [his view] penetrated the *kao-huang* region.[6] He was able to call the lungs and enter into dialogue with them. When he employed drugs, it was as if spirits or demons had given them. He sealed passes and occupied strategic straits in the same way as the troops of [the Han general] Chou Ya-fu. All the other followers of Ch'i [Po] and Huang[-ti who watched his therapies] stood there in awe and admiration. Until the end [of a treatment], no one was able to determine how [Hsü Ta-ch'un] had done it.

Tse Keng-shih from Lu-hsü lay down with an illness for six days. He did not speak; he did not eat; and his eyes were clear with their gaze fixed straight ahead. Mr. [Hsü] said, "This is a sign of yin and yang striking at each other." A short while after [Hsü] had given him a first dose [of medicine, the patient's] vision became obscured and he was able to speak. Then he took [another medicine] with some hot liquid, jumped up and said with a sigh, "At the moment when I was critically ill, there were two men, one red and one black, whirling around me to play their game with me. Suddenly the black man was struck dead by a thunderbolt, and immediately afterward the red man was led away by a white tiger. What was it?" Mr. [Hsü] responded with a smile, "the lightening was the *fu tzu* thunder-crash powder given [to you]. The white tiger was the white-tiger-from-heaven decoction I gave you." Tse was startled and thought [Mr. Hsü] to be a spirit!

The child of Chang Yü-ts'un was born without skin. Anyone who saw [the child] felt an urge to vomit, and [the father] intended to do away with it. Mr. [Hsü] ordered a paste to be made from glutinous rice. [The paste was to be smeared on] the [child's] body, which was then wrapped with thin gauze, and buried in the earth with only the head sticking out. [The child] was given milk to drink and after two days and nights had grown skin.

Mrs. Jen suffered from wind-obturation. Both her thighs felt like [they were] pinched with needles. Mr. [Hsü] ordered [her] to prepare a thick bedding and then asked a strong old woman to wrap her and hold her tight, and he warned [the old woman], "No matter how wildly she moves and how loudly she cries, you must not let her go. [Hold her] until she starts sweating!" It was done as he had said, and she was cured without drugs.

A merchant named Wang Ling-men had not had sexual intercourse for ten years. [He suffered from] sudden panting, sweat on his head, and inability to sleep from sunset to dawn. Mr. [Hsü] said, "This is [a case] of violent yang. You have consumed too much ginseng." Then he ordered [the merchant] to have intercourse and he was cured.

There was a certain boxing teacher who received a chest injury during a match. His [flow of] breath was interrupted, and his mouth remained closed. Mr. [Hsü] ordered him to lie upside down, and hit him firmly with his fist on his lower back three times with the result that [the teacher] spat several pints of black blood and was cured.

Other cases include, for instance, Sir Wen-ch'üeh,[7] whose pulse he examined before the time [that Shen had risen to fame], and to whom he predicted noble rank; or Hsiung Chi-hui, whose arm he felt when he was very strong, yet recognizing that he was destined to perish. All these are examples of what is called "to see what has no form, and to hear what leaves no sound." His abilities and the quick effects of his ingenuity were always of this kind.

Mr. [Hsü] was tall in stature, with a broad forehead. His voice sounded like a bell, and his white beard was admirable. The moment one saw him one was aware of his commanding maleness. Ever since his boyhood he had developed a special interest in the study of political economics. He was particularly knowledgeable of the problems of irrigation in the South-East. In the second year of [the reign of] Yung-cheng, the [provincial] administration intended to perform a significant opening of the T'ang river.[8] [The river] was to be dredged to an estimated depth of six feet, with the soil [procured from the river bed] to be piled as an embankment on both sides. Mr. [Hsü] objected saying, "This would be wrong. If one opens [the river bed] too deeply, this will be very costly. Also, the mud [flowing with the river] will stagnate, and easily accumulate. The mud from the river banks comes down, and the dykes may all collapse." The prefect approved of this [objection], and [the plan was] changed. [The depth of the river bed] was not so deeply dredged and the soil was piled at a distance of eighteen feet from the river bank. This way, costs were saved and the dykes were protected.

In the twenty-seventh year of [the reign of] Ch'ien-lung, great floods occurred in [the two provinces of] Chiang[-su] and Che[-chiang]. Sir Chuang, the governor of [Chiang-]su, intended to open [connections between] the seventy-two branch courses of the Chen-tse [river][9] and Lake T'ai so that water from the latter might be drained through the former. Mr. [Hsü] objected again, stating, "This could be wrong. The water of Lake T'ai does not flow through the seventy-two branch courses of the Chen-tse. Only those ten or so branch courses near the city enter the river. Hence, [I] suggest that only those water courses be dredged where [the water of the lake] indeed flows out. The remaining fifty or more branch courses are more than two hundred miles long. Their embankments are covered with tens of thousands of houses and graves. If one wished to open [these water courses], the costs would be excessive, and the affairs of the people would be much harmed. Also, mud from the lake might pour [into the newly deepened drainage channels, with the effect] that they were opened one moment and blocked the next moment again. This is a river that was dredged by the people themselves. The government has no responsibility in its maintenance." Sir Chuang reported [Mr. Hsü's] words to the throne, and the Son of Heaven approved of them. Hence the work was assigned to the responsible officials, and the people were not disturbed.

Mr. [Hsü] lived secluded in the [village of] Hui-hsi. There were numerous low houses and a spring called Hua-mei, a small bridge, running water, and many pines and bamboo trees. From a tower one could behold Lake T'ai and strange mountain peaks arranged like children and grandchildren standing in a circle ready for service, with Mr. Hsü whistling and swaggering between. Those who saw him suspected he might be an Accomplished Man at the borders of heaven. [Mr. Hsü] wrote six books, including for instance the *Nan-ching Ching-shih*, and the *I-hsüeh Yüan Liu* [*Lun*]. In these [books] he boldly cut out the harmful, and laid open [the secrets of] the conduits and network [vessels]. He took from the medical literature of old and new what was correct, and he eliminated what was wrong. [The results of his work] have already been famous throughout the world for a long time.

His son [Hsü] Hsi had the style name Yü-ts'un. He inherited his father's nonchalance and unconstraint; he gave life to the people and rescued every creature. In [the year] yi-mao [1795] his grandson Yüan earned the degree of *chü-ren*; he had received instruction in poetry by myself.

Eulogy: The [*Li-*]*chi* states, "One's virtue is to be perfected first; one's technical skills are to be perfected next." [This quotation] might leave one with the impression that [the *Li-chi*] highly valued virtue while it regarded lightly technical skills. [Those who get this impression] do not know that technical skills are the perfection of virtue. How could technical skills exist in the absence of virtue? The people see only the perfect technical skills of Mr. [Hsü], but they are not aware of how he served his parents and how he practiced filial piety, as well as how loyal he was to others in his everyday life. He buried the dead and fed the needy. He built and repaired carriages and bridges. Whenever he saw an opportunity to fulfill a public duty, he acted. This shows that he had first internalized virtue and ventured into an application of technical skills afterward. The movement of his hand followed his heart, and he was able to banish demons and spirits. Alas! How could this have been just by accident!

I still remember how in the year ping-hsü [1766] my left arm suddenly drew in, and I was unable to stretch it again. None of the physicians [I consulted] was of any help. Finally I took a boat and went directly to the Hui creek. There was no one who could have introduced me, and I was afraid Mr. [Hsü] might not want to see me. Hence I was surprised when the door was opened and I was asked to come in as soon as I had presented my name card. Mr. [Hsü] took my hand like that of an old acquaintance, and offered me food. Then he asked me to talk and when the day came to its end, he gave me a medicinal pill and let me depart. My old friend Li Ch'un greeted me by the creek and laughed, saying, "You were lucky this time! When other people come here, they spend ten tabloids of gold for one consultation!" This shows how much [Hsü Ta-ch'un] was revered by his contemporaries. Mr. [Hsü] preferred what was old, and did not like the texts of his own time. In this regard he shared my own general sentiments. Hence I have collected a song of his ridicule for [contemporary] learning, and have recorded it in [my] "Talks on Poetry" as a warning for our time.[10]

Notes

1.   Wen-k'o 文恪 is the posthumous name of Chiang P'u 蔣溥 (1708-1761). See Arthur W. Hummel, *Eminent Chinese of the Ch'ing Period (1644-1912),* Washington 1943, p. 143.

2.   This is Ch'in Hui-t'ien 秦蕙田 (1702-1764).

3.   This must be an error. A correct dating should be ''ten years later'' because Hsü Ta-ch'un died in 1771.

4.   *Chung-kuei* 中貴 may stand here for *chung-kuan* 中宮. This latter term was used, throughout history, as a generic term for enuchs. In addition, the term indicated one of the five seasonal offices of calendrical specialists in the Ch'ing Directorate of Astronomy. See Charles O. Hucker, *A Dictionary of Official Titles in Imperial China,* Stanford 1989, p. 191.

5.   Lit.: ''he was twice given [a carriage] with wheels wrapped in rushes [for greater comfort].''

6.   A region above the diaphragm and below the heart which is hidden from the [ordinary] human eye. Illnesses retreating there are considered incurable. See *Tso-chuan* 左傳, Book VIII, 10th year.

7.   Shen Te-ch'ien 沈得潛 (1673-1769), a famous official and literatus, was canonized as Wen-ch'üeh 文愨 after his death.

8.   This is the Ti-t'ang 荻塘 river flowing from Che-chiang into Chiang-su.

9.   Chen-tse 震澤 is an old designation of Ti-t'ang 荻塘 river. See previous note.

10. Yüan Mei 袁枚, *Hsiao-ts'ang shan fang shih-wen chi, Ssu pu pei-yao, Chi pu* 小倉山房詩文集．四部備要集部 Ch. 34, 12b-14b.

Appendix B

The Medical Literary Work of Hsü Ta-ch'un

This list was compiled on the basis of research by Sung Ta-jen 宋大仁 (see Appendix C, Sung Ta-jen 1958, 1963) and Hu Su-hua 呼素華 (1988), and the data provided by the *Chung-i t'u-shu lien-ho mu-lu* 中醫圖書聯合目錄 of 1961, as well as individual editions of Hsü's works.

A. Seven medical titles written by Hsü Ta-ch'un himself and published during his lifetime.

1. *Nan-ching ching-shih* 難經經釋; also named: *Nan-ching ching-chieh* 難經經解, 2 ch., 1727.

2. *Shen-nung pen-ts'ao ching pai chung lu* 神農本草經百種錄, 1 ch., 1736.

3. *I-kuan pien* 醫貫砭, 2 ch., 1741.

4. *I-hsüeh yüan liu lun* 醫學源流論, 2 ch., 1757.

5. *Shang-han lun lei-fang* 傷寒論類方; also named: *Shang-han lei-fang* 傷寒類方, 1 ch., 1759.

6. *Lan-t'ai kuei-fan* 蘭臺軌范; also named: *Chi-ch'eng ts'u-pien* 集成卒編, 8 ch., 1764.

7. *Shen-chi ch'u-yen* 愼疾芻言; amended and edited in the 19th c. by Chang Hung 張鴻 under the title *I pien* 醫砭, 1 ch., 1769.

B. One collection of case histories.

Hui-hsi i-an 洄溪醫案, 1 ch.; published in 1855 with commentaries by Wang Meng-ying 王孟英 on the basis of a manuscript left behind by Hsü Ta-ch'un.

C. Two critical editions of works by other authors.

1. *P'ing-ting wai-k'o cheng-tsung* 評定外科正宗, a critical edition of the *Wai-k'o cheng-tsung* of 1617 by Ch'en Shih-kung 陳實功 (1555 - 1636).

2. *P'ing Yeh-shih lin-cheng chih-nan* 評葉氏臨症指南, a critical edition of the *Lin-cheng chih-nan i-an* 臨症指南醫案 by Yeh Kuei 葉桂 (1667-1746).

D. Twenty three titles compiled or published by later authors under the name of Hsü Ta-ch'un.

1. *Nei-ching ch'üan shih* 內經詮釋, also named: *Nei-ching yao-lüeh* 內經要略.

2. *Shang-han lun lei-fang tseng chu* 傷寒論類方增注.

3. *Shang-han yüeh pien* 傷寒約編.

4. *Liu ching ping chieh* 六經病解.

5. *Tsa ping yüan* 雜病源.

6. *Tsa ping cheng chih* 雜病証治, also named *Cheng chih chih-nan* 証治指南.

7. *Mai chüeh ch'i wu chu shih*, 脈訣啓悟注釋, also named: *Mai chüeh ch'i wu* 脈訣啓悟.

8. *Hui-hsi mai-hsüeh* 洄溪脈學.

9. *She-chien tsung lun* 舌鑒總論 with *She-chien t'u* 舌鑒圖, also named: *She-t'ai t'u-shuo* 舌胎圖説.

10. *Nü-k'o chih-yao* 女科指要 with *Nü-k'o chih yen* 女科指驗.

11. *Nü-k'o i-an* 女科醫案.

12. *Yao-hsing ch'ieh yong* 藥性切用.

13. *Hui-hsi lao-jen erh-shih-liu mi-fang* 洄溪老人二十六秘方 (recorded by Yü Hsiao-sung 余嘯松), also named: *Hui-hsi mi-fang* 洄溪秘方, *Hui-hsi lao-jen erh-shih-liu chung fang* 洄溪老人二十六種方.

14. *Hui-hsi i-an t'ang-jen fa* 洄溪醫案唐人法 (compiled by Huang En-jung 黃恩榮).

15. *(Tseng chu) ku-fang hsin-chieh* (曾注) 古方新解 (compiled by Lu Shih-o 陸士諤).

16. *Ching-yen fang* 經驗方 (compiled by Yeh T'ien-shih 葉天士).

17. *Yao-hsing shih-chieh* 藥性詩解 (compiled by Hsü's second son Hsü Hsi 徐爔).

18. *Ku-fang chi chieh* 古方集解 (compiled by P'an Wei 潘霨).

19. *T'ang yin tsung-i* 湯引總義.

20. *Yeh-an p'i miu* 葉案批謬.

21. *Ching-lo chen-shih t'u* 經絡診視圖.

22. *Chung-feng ta-fa* 中風大法 (this is the chapter "Chung-feng" 中風 of the *Tsa ping cheng chih* 雜病証治; see above 6.).

23. *Chung-tzu yao-fang* 種子要方 (this is the chapter "Chung-tzu men" 種子門 of the *Nü-k'o chih-yao* 女科指要; see above 10.)

E. Ten collections of works written by Hsü Ta-ch'un (most of which also contain work not written by Hsü himself).

1. *Hsü-shih i-shu san chung* 徐氏醫書三種, 1860, three titles: *Shen-chi ch'u-yen* 愼疾芻言, *Hui-hsi i-an* 洄溪醫案, *Ching-yen fang* 經驗方.

2. *I-hsüeh san shu ho-k'o* 醫學三書合刻, 1875, three titles as listed under E.1.

3. *Hsü-shih i-shu liu chung* 徐氏醫書六種, Ch'ien-lung edition (1736-1795), six titles: *Nan-ching ching-shih* 難經經釋, *Shen-nung pen-ts'ao ching pai chung lu* 神農本草經百種錄, *I-kuan pien* 醫貫砭, *I hsüeh yüan liu lun* 醫學源流論, *Shang-han lei-fang* 傷寒類方, *Lan-t'ai kuei-fan* 蘭臺軌范.

4. *Hsü Ling-t'ai i-lüeh liu shu* 徐靈胎醫略六書, 1903, six titles: *Nei-ching yao-lüeh* 內經要略, *Mai chüeh ch'i-wu* 脈訣啓悟 (with *Ching-lo chen-shih t'u* 經絡診視圖), *Yao-hsing ch'ieh yung* 藥性切用, *Shang-han yüeh pien* 傷寒約編 (with *She-chien t'u* 舌鑒圖), *Tsa ping cheng-chih* 雜病証治, *Nü-k'o chih-yao* 女科指要 (with *Nü-k'o chih-yen* 女科治驗).

5. *Hsü-shih i-shu pa chung* 徐氏醫書八種, 1864, eight titles: six titles as listed under E.3, plus *Shen-chi ch'u-yen* 愼疾芻言, *Hui-hsi i-an* 洄溪醫案.

6. *Hsü-shih i-shu shih chung* 徐氏醫書十種, 1864, ten titles: eight titles as listed under E.5, plus: *P'ing-ting wai-k'o cheng-tsung* 評定外科正宗, *Hui-hsi tao-ch'ing* 洄溪道情 (with *Hsü Ling-t'ai hsien-sheng shou-p'ing Yeh-shih lin-cheng chih-nan* 徐靈胎先生手評葉氏臨症指南).

7. *Hsü Ling-t'ai ch'üan-shu shih-erh chung* 徐靈胎全書十二種, 1864, twelve titles: eight titles as listed under E.5, plus: *Tao te ching* 道德經, *Hui-hsi tao-ch'ing* 洄溪道情, *Yin-fu ching* 陰符經, *Tung-fu ch'uan-sheng* 東府傳聲.

8. *Hsü-shih shih-san chung i-shu* 徐氏十三種醫書, 1896, thirteen titles: twelve titles as listed under E.7, plus *Tseng Hsü Ta-ch'un p'ing wai-k'o cheng-tsung* 增徐大椿評外科正宗.

9. *Hsü Ling-t'ai i-hsüeh ch'üan-shu shih-liu chung* 徐靈胎醫學全書十六種, 1893, sixteen titles: eight titles as listed under E.5, plus *Nei-ching ch'üan-shih* 內經詮釋, *Mai-chüeh ch'i-wu chu shih* 脈訣啓悟注釋, *Shang-han yüeh pien* 傷寒約編, *Tsa ping yüan* 雜病源,

Hui-hsi mai-hsüeh 洄溪脈學, *Liu ching ping-chieh* 六經病解, *She-chien tsung-lun* 舌鑒總論, *Nü-k'o i-an* 女科醫案.

10. *Hsü Ling-t'ai i-shu san-shih-erh chung* 徐靈胎醫書三十二種, n.d., Republican edition, thirty-two titles: sixteen titles as listed under E.9, plus: *Yao-hsing ch'ieh-yong* 藥性切用, *Tsa ping cheng-chih* 雜病証治, *Nü-k'o chih-yao* 女科指要, *Liu ching mai-cheng* 六經脈証 (this is the chapter by the same title of the *Shang-han lei fang* 傷寒類方, see above A.5), *Chung-feng ta-fa* 中風大法, *Chung-tzu yao-fang* 種子要方, *Ku-fang chi-chieh* 古方集解, *She-t'ai t'u shuo* 舌胎圖説, *Ching-lo chen-shih t'u* 經絡診視圖, *Yao-hsing shih-chieh* 藥性詩解, *T'ang yin tsung-i* 湯引總義, *Yeh-an p'i-miu* 葉案批謬, *Ching-yen fang* 經驗方, *Hui-hsi i-an t'ang-jen fa* 洄溪醫案唐人法, *Hui-hsi mi-fang* 洄溪秘方, *Kuan-chien chi* 管見集.

Appendix C

Chinese Secondary Literature on Hsü Ta-ch'un and His Contributions to Medicine

Ku Tuan-fu, "Hsü Ling-t'ai I-shih," *Chung-hsi I-hsüeh Pao,* 1911, 11, (not seen) 賈瑞甫 徐靈胎軼事 中西醫學報.

Hsieh Sung-mu, "Hsü Ling-t'ai P'ing-chuan," *Hsien-tai Chung-i,* 1, 1934, 1, 12-15 謝誦穆 徐靈胎評傳 現代中醫.

Wang Chi-min, "Hsü Ta-ch'un Hua-mei-ch'üan Chi Chen-chi Hsü Ping Hsiao-chuan," *Chung-hua I-hsüeh Tsa-chih,* 25, 1939, 11, 864-870 王吉民 徐大椿畫眉泉記眞蹟序並小傳 中華醫學雜誌.

Liu Yüan, "Ch'ing-tai Ming-i — Hsü Ta-ch'un," *Chung-i Tsa-chih,* 1956, 1, 53-55, 39 劉元 清代名醫 徐大椿 中醫雜誌.

Ts'ao Nan-hua, "Ts'ung Hsü Hui-hsi Hsien-sheng I-an Liang Tse T'an Ch'i," *Kuang-tung Chung-i,* 1957, 8, 34 3 曹南華 從徐洄溪先生醫案 兩則談起 廣東中醫.

Sung Ta-jen, "Ch'ing-tai Chiang-su Ming-i Hsü Ling-t'ai Hsien-sheng Hsiang-chuan," *Chiang-su Chung-i,* 1958, 1, 27-28 宋大仁 清代江蘇名醫徐靈胎先生象傳 江蘇中醫.

Sung Ta-jen, "Hsü Ling-t'ai shou-lu wei-k'an kao-pen 'Kuan chien chi' shu-ching," *Chiang-su chung-i,* 1958, 1, (not seen) 宋大仁 徐靈胎手錄未刊稿本《管見集》書影 江蘇中醫.

Liu Po-ling, "Tsu-kuo te I-hsüeh-chia Hsü Ta-ch'un," *Chi-lin Jih-pao,* 1961, 12, (not seen) 劉伯齡 祖國的醫學家徐大椿 吉林日報.

Liu Po-ling, "Ch'ing-tai I-hsüeh-chia — Hsü Ta-ch'un," *Chung-kuo Ch'ing-nien Pao,* 1961, 30 (not seen) 劉伯齡 清代醫學家徐大椿 中國青年報.

Chu K'ung-yang, "Hsü Ling-t'ai chu-shu i-chi - Hua-mei-ch'üan fa-hsien chi," *Chung-i tsa-chih,* 1962, 2, 37-38 朱孔陽 徐靈胎著書遺蹟畫眉泉 發現記中醫雜誌.

Wu Chia-i, "Hsü Ta-ch'un," *Chien-k'ang Pao,* 1962, 7, (pages unclear on electrographic copy) 吳家怡 徐大椿 健康報.

Sung Ta-jen, "Ch'ing-tai Wei-ta I-hsüeh-chia Hsü Ling-t'ai te I-sheng," *Chiang-su Chung-i,* 1963, 11, 30-34 宋大仁 清代偉大醫學家徐靈胎的 一生 江蘇中醫.

Chiang Ch'un-hua, "Tui Hsü Ling-t'ai Hsüeh-shu Ssu-hsiang te P'ing-chia," *Shang-hai Chung-i-yao tsa-chih*, 1964, 3, 36-41 姜春華 對徐靈胎學術思想的評價 上海中醫藥雜志.

Yang Ch'un-po, "Shih-lun Hsü Ta-ch'un te I-hsüeh Ch'eng-chiu," *Ha-erh-pin Chung-i*, 1964, 6, 38-44 楊春波 試論徐大椿的醫學成就 哈爾濱中醫.

Ch'u Chin-hsiang, "Shih-lun 'Hui-hsi I-an'," *Che-ching Chung-i-hsüeh yüan Hsüeh-pao*, 1980 1, 46-47 褚謹翔 試論《洄溪醫案》浙 江中醫學院學報.

Hsü Jung-chai, "Hsü Hui-hsi 'I-lüeh Liu shu' Pien-hsi," *Liao-ning Chung-i Tsa-chih*, 1980, 9, 21-22 徐榮齋 徐洄溪《醫略六書》辨析 遼 寧中醫雜誌.

Kung Shih-ch'eng and Wu Yin-lung, "Hsü Ta-ch'un Hsüeh-shu Ch'u-t'an," *Liao-ning Chung-i Tsa-chih*, 1980, 9, 22-25 龔士澄 吳銀龍 徐 大椿學術初探 遼寧中醫雜誌.

Wang Yü-t'ing, "Hsü Ta-ch'un yü 'Lan-t'ai Kuei-fan'," *Chi-lin Chung-i-yao*, 1982, 1, 17-20 王雨亭 徐大椿與《蘭臺軌范》吉林中醫藥.

Hsü Yung-hao, "Lüeh-lun Hui-hsi te I-hsüeh Ch'eng-chiu," *Che-chiang Chung-i Hsüeh-yüan Hsüeh-pao*, 1982, 1, 17-20 徐湧浩 略論洄溪的醫學 成就 浙江中醫學院學報.

Fei Yüan-tzu, "Hsü Ling-t'ai yü 'Shen-chi Ch'u-yen'," *Chiang-su Chung-i Tsa-chih*, 1980, 6, 7-8. 弗原子 徐靈胎《慎疾芻言》江蘇中醫雜誌.

Hu Su-hua, "Hsü Ling-t'ai I-chu Ch'u-k'ao," *Chung-hua I-shih Tsa-chih*, 18, 1988, 2, 119-121 呼素華 徐靈胎醫著初考 中華醫史雜志.

Hsü Ta-ch'un's Original Preface to the I-hsüeh Yüan Liu Lun

醫學源流論原序

醫小道也精義也重任也賤工也古者大人之學將以
治天下國家使無一夫不被其澤甚者天地位而萬物
育斯學者之極功也若夫日救一人月治數病顧此則
失彼雖數十里之近不能兼及況乎不可治者又非能
起死者而使之生其道不已小乎雖然古聖人之治病
也通于天地之故究乎性命之原經絡臟腑氣血骨脈
洞然如見然後察其受病之由用藥以驅除而調劑之
其中自有玄機妙悟不可得而言喻者蓋與造化相維
其義不亦精乎道小則有志之士有所不屑為義精則
無識之徒有所不能窺也人之所係莫大乎生死王公
大人聖賢豪傑可以旋轉乾坤而不能保無疾病之患
一有疾病不得不聽之醫者而生殺唯命矣夫一人係
天下之重而天下所係之人其命又懸于醫者下而一

國一家所係之人更無論矣其任不亦重乎而獨是其
人者又非有爵祿道德之尊父兄師保之重既非世之
所隆而其人之自視亦不過為衣食口腹之計雖以一
介之微呼之而立至其業不甚賤乎任重則托之者必
得偉人工賤則業之者必無奇士所以勢出于相違而道
連年死亡略盡于是博覽方書寢食俱廢如是數年雖
因之易墜也余少時頗有志于窮經而骨月數人疾病
無生死肉骨之方實有尋本溯源之學九折臂而成醫
至今尤信而竊慨唐宋以來無儒者為之振興視為下
業遂逡巡失傳至理已失良法併亡惻焉傷懷恐自今以
往不復有生人之術不揣庸妄用數厥言倘有所補所
全者或不僅一人一世已乎乾隆丁丑秋七月洄溪徐
大椿書於吳山之半松書屋

Hsü Ta-ch'un's Original Preface to the I-hsüeh Yüan Liu Lun

"Medicine is a petty profession."

"The concepts [of medicine] are subtle."

"[Physicians carry a] heavy responsibility."

"[Physicians practice] an inferior occupation."

The learning of great men in antiquity was aimed at maintaining order in the world and in the state, and [these great men] insured that none were missed by their benevolence. [When they pushed their efforts to the] extreme, [the result was that everything between] heaven and earth was in its place, and that all beings received their proper care. These were the lofty merits achieved by those possessing such learning. Those who save but one person per day, who cure a number of illnesses per month, who — while caring for this [person] — must neglect someone else, who are not even able to cover [with their activities] all those within a distance of some tens of miles, especially so because there are cases that cannot be treated at all, and since they are unable to raise the dead, and bring them to life again, is not theirs [in comparison] a very petty profession?

And yet, when the ancient Sages cured illnesses, they penetrated the facts between heaven and earth, and they sought the origins of life. Once they had understood [the condition of a patient's] conduits and network [vessels], viscera and bowels, influences and blood, bones and [movement in the] vessels, they [proceeded to] investigate the origins of his illness. And then, they applied drugs to eliminate it and to restore harmony [in the patient's organism]. And because in this [therapeutic process] hidden workings were involved, as well as insights into mysteries beyond description, [the wisdom of these Sages] was closely linked with [the forces of] Creation. Are not, [therefore,] the concepts [applied in medicine] also subtle?

A petty profession will never be considered worth practicing by any scholar. Subtle concepts, however, can never be recognized by those who have no knowledge.

Nothing associated with [the existence of] man exceeds life and death in importance. Kings, dukes, and great men, sages, exemplary persons, and heroes may be able to make the universe turn, but they are unable to protect themselves against suffering from illness. As soon as they fall ill,

51

they hand themselves over to a physician, and whether he keeps them alive or kills them is accepted as fate! Mankind has the most important position in the world, and if the fate of all the people in the world rests in the hands of physicians — how much more is this true for all the people in merely one country or one family! Do not [physicians, therefore, carry a] heavy responsibility?

But those [who are physicians today] are not people of rank and emolument, or of morality, and they are not as important as the elderly or the teachers. Hence, they are not respected as eminent by their [social] environment, and they themselves consider [their activities] merely a means to earn their livelihood. If someone calls them for the most trifling matter, they follow his call immediately. Do they not practice a most inferior occupation?

A heavy responsibility can be shouldered only by persons with extraordinary faculties. [On the other hand,] an inferior occupation will never be adopted by any eminent scholar.

There exists a severe contradiction here, allowing for an easy deterioration of the profession.

When I was young, I had set my mind on studying the classics, but almost all my relatives died from illnesses in consecutive years. As a result I read widely in prescription literature. For many years, I neglected sleep and food, and even though I was unable to find a formula to bring my deceased relatives back to life, I truly acquired a learning that brought me the foundations and allowed me to trace the origins [of medicine. The old saying:] "Break your arm nine times and you will be a physician yourself" still holds true today. I myself consider it most regrettable that since the T'ang and Sung, scholars have no longer contributed to a [continued] prospering [of medicine]. Rather, they regarded [the practice of medicine] as a lower occupation. Hence step by step the [ancient] traditions were lost. Once the true principles [of medicine] had been lost, reliable patterns [of therapeutic intervention] were no longer available either. This is so sad!

I fear that the art of keeping the people alive will never exist again. Its words are still applied, but the incompetence and the errors associated with them are beyond any guesses. To repair it, or even to bring it back to completion, this would require more than one person, [and it would take longer than] one generation.

Written in the twenty-second year of Ch'ien-lung, autumn, seventh month, by Hui-hsi Hsü Ta-ch'un in the Split Pine Library on Mount Wu.

I. [Main] Conduits and
and
Network [Vessels],
Viscera and Bowels

元氣存亡論

養生者之言曰天下之人皆可以無死斯言妄也何則

人生自免乳哺以後始而孩既而長既而壯日勝一日

何以四十以後飲食奉養如昔而日且就衰或者曰嗜

慾戕之也則絕嗜慾可以無死乎或者曰勞動賊之

則戒勞動可以無死乎或者曰思慮擾之也則屏思慮

可以無死乎果能絕嗜慾戒勞動減思慮免于疾病夭

札則有之其老而眊眊而死猶然也況乎四十以前未

嘗無嗜慾勞苦思慮然而日生日長四十以後雖無嗜

慾勞苦思慮然而日減此其故何歟蓋人之生也

顧夏蟲而却笑以為是物之生死何其促也而不知我

實猶是耳當其受生之時已有定分焉所謂定分者元

氣也視之不見求之不得附于氣血之內宰乎氣血之

先其成形之時已有定數譬如置薪於火始燃尚微漸

久則烈薪力既盡而火熄矣其有久暫之殊者則薪之

堅脆異質也故終身無病者待元氣之自盡而死此所

謂終其天年者也至于疾病之人若元氣不傷雖病甚

不死元氣或傷雖病輕亦死而其中又有辨焉有先傷

元氣而病者此不可治者也有因病而傷元氣者此不

可不預防者也亦有因誤治而傷及元氣者亦有元氣

雖傷未甚尚可保全之者其等不一故診病決死生者

不視病之輕重而視元氣之存亡則百不失一矣至所

謂元氣者何所寄耶五藏有五藏之真精此元氣之分

體者也而其根本所在即道經所謂丹田難經所謂命

門內經所謂七節之旁中有小心陰陽闔闢存乎此呼

吸出入係乎此無火而能令百體皆溫無水而能令五

藏皆潤比中一線未絕則生氣一線未亡皆賴此也若

夫有疾病而保全之法何如益元氣雖自有所在然實

54

與藏腑相連屬者也寒熱攻補不得其道則實其實而

虛其虛必有一藏大受其害邪入於中而精不能續則

元氣無所附而傷矣故人之一身無處不宜謹護而藥

不可輕試也若夫預防之道惟上工能慮在病前不使

其勢巳橫而莫救使元氣克全則自能托邪于外若邪

盛為害則乘元氣未動與之背城而一決勿使後事生

悔此神而明之之術也若欲與造化爭權而令天下之

人終不死則無是理矣

1. On the Presence and Loss of Original Influences

The [basic] doctrine of those who [strive to] nourish their lives is: Everyone on earth has the possibility to escape death. That is just nonsense! Why so? Once the [age of] suckling is over, human life passes through [the stages of] childhood, of growing up, and of strong [adulthood], and [its quality] increases each day over each previous day. For what reason, now, does it weaken day by day, once the age of forty is passed, even though it is nourished with the same drinks and food as before?

Some say [man's life] is brought to an end by his addiction to lust, and hence [they imply that] it is possible to escape death by eliminating one's lustful desires! Others say [man's life] is destroyed through toil and labor, and hence [they imply that] it is possible to escape death when one avoids toil and labor! Still others say [man's life] is jeopardized through thoughts and pondering, and hence [they imply that] it is possible to escape death by refraining from thoughts and pondering!

No doubt, occasionally it is possible to prevent illness and early death if one eliminates one's lustful desires, if one avoids toil and labor, and if one refrains from thoughts and pondering. Nevertheless [the people who achieve this] grow old and their eyes turn dim, and after their eyes have turned dim they die — just as anyone else! Also, before one has reached the age of forty, everyone has lustful desires, everyone toils and labors, and everyone thinks and ponders, and still he grows day by day. After the age of forty, even though there are no more lustful desires, toil and suffering, as well as thoughts and pondering, one deteriorates day by day. What, then, is the reason behind all of this?

[People] compare human life with [the life span of] summer insects and laugh; how can it be that birth and death of these beings follow each other so quickly? But [these same people] do not know that we, in fact, are not different from these [little beings]. At the moment we get our lives, we have already received a fixed share. This so-called fixed share is the original influences. If one were to look for them, one would not see them. If one were to search for them, one would not find them. They are attached to the interior of the influences and the blood, but they already govern [life] prior to [the existence of] influences and blood.

When [influences and blood] assume shape, the duration [of one's life] has already been determined. One may compare this with firewood that is placed on the fire. At first, the fire is still quite weak. After a while, [the fire] turns violent. Once the strength of the firewood is exhausted, the fire will go out. The difference between [fires that burn] longer and [others that burn] shorter results from differences in the quality of the firewood — it may be solid or brittle. Hence those who do not fall ill for their entire life will die once their original influences have exhausted themselves. They are those who may be said to have gone through all the years allotted to them by heaven. Those who fall ill will survive if their original influences are not harmed, even if their illness is quite severe. Those, however, whose original influences have been harmed will die, even if their illness is only minor. Within these [two categories] there are further variations.

If the original influences were harmed prior to the illness, the latter will not be curable. Harm to one's original influences as a result of an illness, that is to be prevented. It may also be that the original influences are harmed because of a mistaken medical treatment. Sometimes the original influences are harmed, but not seriously, and can be fully restored. The degree of harm varies, and those who, in diagnosing an illness, attempt to determine whether [the patient] will die or survive, they should not investigate whether an illness is minor or serious; they should examine whether the [patient's] original influences are [sufficiently] present or not! [If this course is followed], one will not lose one patient in one hundred [cases]!

Now, where do these so-called original influences reside]? Each of the five viscera[1] has its genuine essence; these [essences] are separate materializations of the original influences. Their basic location, though, is [the place] called the "cinnabar field" in the Taoist classics, called the "gate of life" in the *Nan-ching,* and said to be the "small heart" between the [kidneys, which are located on both] sides of the seventh vertebra in the *Nei-ching.*

This is where the interchange of yin and yang takes place. The exit and the entrance of exhalation and of inhalation connect with each other there. [This place] has no fire and yet it may keep all parts of the body warm; it has no water and yet it may keep the five viscera moist. As long as one last thread remains uncut in there, one thread of vital influences will continue [to maintain a person's life]. Everything depends on [the condition of] these [influences].

What, then, are the methods to protect [the original influences] in case of illness? The original influences may have a location by themselves; nevertheless, they are closely associated with the body's viscera and bowels.[2] If [in case of an illness] cold or hot [drugs, or efforts to] attack or supplement, are not appropriately applied, one may replenish a repletion, or deplete a depletion, and the body's viscera will suffer great harm from this. Evil [influences] will penetrate the [body's] center, and the essential [influences] will not be able to stay. As a result, the original influences will have nothing to remain attached to, and will suffer harm. Hence man's entire body must be carefully protected, and no drug should be tested lightly!

Only superior practitioners, though, are able to consider appropriate methods of prevention prior to the onset of an illness; only they can prevent [an illness] from becoming so strong that no effort can save [the patient]. [Superior practitioners] see to it that the original influences are complete and remain in control, so that [the original influences] themselves may keep the evil [influences] outside. If, however, evil influences gain the upper hand and cause harm, the [superior practitioners] activate original influences that remained untouched so far; they have them fight with their back toward the city wall and enter a decisive struggle, and thus they avoid the shame that follows the death [of a patient].

This is an intelligent procedure. To assume one could compete with creation, and keep all the people on earth away from death, is completely unreasonable.

Notes

1.   "Five viscera" refers to the five major functional units in the organism and includes the tangible organs lung, heart, spleen, liver, and kidneys, and their functions. The Chinese term *tsang* suggests the notion of "storage."

2.   "[Six] bowels" refers to a second set of functional units in the organism including the stomach, the gallbladder, the urinary bladder, the large intestine, and the small intestine, as well as an anatomically non-verifiable entity, the triple burner. The functions of the bowels are closely associated with those of the viscera. The Chinese term *fu* suggests the notion of "processing."

軀殼經絡藏府論

凡致病必有因而受病之處則各有部位今之醫者曰
病必分經絡而後治之似矣然亦知病固非經絡之所
能盡者乎夫人有皮肉筋骨以成形所謂軀殼也而虛
其中則有藏府以實之其連續貫通者則有經有絡貫
乎藏府之內運乎軀殼之中為之道路以傳變周流者
也故邪之傷人或在皮肉或在筋骨或在藏府或在經
絡有相傳者有不相傳者有久而相傳者有久而終不
傳者其大端則中於經絡則易傳其初不在經絡或病
甚而流於經絡者亦易傳經絡之病深入藏府則以生
尅相傳惟皮肉筋骨之病不歸經絡者則不傳所謂軀
殼之病也故識病之人當直指其病在何藏何府何筋
何骨何經何絡或傳或不傳其傳以何經始以何經終
其言歷歷可驗則醫之明者矣今人不問何病謬舉一

經以藉口以見其煩識內經實與內經全然不解也至
治之難易則在經絡者易治在藏府者難治且多死在
皮肉筋骨者難治亦不易死其大端如此至於軀殼藏
府之屬于某經絡以審其針灸用藥之法則內經明言
之深求自得也

59

2. On One's Physical Shell, the Conduits and Network [Vessels], the Viscera and Bowels

Whenever an illness emerges, it must have a cause, and the locations affected by an illness can always be specified in terms of body sections. Today's physicians say: In case of an illness one must distinguish [which] conduits and network [vessels are affected], and then start the treatment. That is quite correct. However, do they also know that the location of illness is by no means restricted to the conduits and network [vessels]?

Man's physical appearance consists of skin, flesh, sinews, and bone; these form the so-called physical shell. The empty space inside [this shell] is filled by the viscera and bowels. The [viscera and bowels] are interconnected and communicate with each other through the conduits and network [vessels], and transport [influences] within the physical shell. They are the pathways of transmission, transformation and circulation. Hence, when evil influences harm man, they may settle in his skin and flesh, or they may settle in his sinews and bones, or they may settle in his viscera and bowels, or they may settle in his conduits and network [vessels].

In some cases [evil influences] are transmitted further from one [location] to another, in other cases not. Sometimes, it takes a long time for further transmission [to occur]; sometimes a long period passes and no transmission occurs at all. Generally speaking, those [evil influences] that settle in the conduits and network [vessels] tend to be more easily transmitted [to other locations].

It may be that [evil influences] have initially settled outside of the conduits and network [vessels]. Then the illness [becomes more] serious, and the [evil influences] flow into the [main] conduits and network [vessels] whence they are easily transmitted further. When illnesses that are located in the conduits and network [vessels] penetrate deeply into the viscera and bowels, they are transmitted among [the viscera and bowels] according to the [patterns of mutual] generation and destruction [in the relationships among the five phases]. Only such illnesses that have settled in the skin, the flesh, the sinews, and the bones, and that do not find their way into the [main] conduits and network [vessels], will not be transmitted further. These are the so-called illnesses of the physical shell.

Therefore, those who know about illnesses should [be able] to point out directly in which of the viscera or in which of the bowels, in which of the sinews or in which of the bones, in which of the conduits or in which of the network [vessels] an illness is located; whether it will be transmitted further or whether it will not be transmitted further; where in the conduits its transmission begins, and where in the conduits its transmission ends. What these [knowledgeable people] say can be verified in each and every case — they are the enlightened among physicians. Today, no one inquires about [the nature and location] of an illness; [people] erroneously pick one particular conduit to have a pretext [for their treatment], and to demonstrate how very much they know of the *Nei-ching*, while, in fact, they know nothing at all of the *Nei-ching*.

Now, as to whether [an illness] is difficult or easy to cure: those that have settled in the conduits and network [vessels] are easy to cure, while those that have settled in the body's viscera and bowels are difficult to cure, resulting in many deaths. Those [illnesses] that are located in the skin, in the flesh, in the sinews, and in the bones are difficult to cure [too], but at the same time, one does not easily die from them. These are, at least, the general principles. As to how the physical shell and the viscera and bowels are tied to specific conduits — [these connections are important] to determine the [appropriate] patterns of needling, of cauterization, and of drug application — all of that is clearly outlined in the *Nei-ching*; those who look seriously for it will find it on their own.

表裏上下論

欲知病之難易先知病之淺深欲知病之淺深先知病之部位夫人身一也實有表裏上下之別焉何謂表皮肉筋骨是也何謂裏藏府精神是也而經絡則貫乎其間表之病易治而難死裏之病難治而易死此其大畧也而在裏在表者又各有難易此不可執一而論也若夫病本在表而傳於裏病本在裏而并及於表是為內外無病尤不易治身半已上之病往往近於熱身半已下之病往往近於寒此其大畧也而在上在下又各有寒熱此亦不可執一而論也若夫病本在上而傳于下病本在下而傳于上是之謂上下兼病亦不易治所以然者無病之處多有病之處少則精力猶可維持使正氣漸充而邪氣亦去若夫一人之身無處不病則以何者為驅病之本而復其元氣乎故善醫者知病勢之盛而必傳也豫為之防無使結聚無使泛溢無使併合此上工治未病之說也若其已至于傳而必先求其本後求其標相其緩急而施治之此又参榆之收也以此決病之生死難易思過半矣

3. On Exterior and Interior, Upper and Lower [Locations of Illnesses in the Body]

If one wants to know whether an illness is difficult or easy [to cure], one should first know whether this illness is located near the [body's] surface or in its depth. And, if one wants to know whether an illness is near the [body's] surface or in its depth, one should first know which section [of the body] it occupies. The human body constitutes one single unit, but it has, nevertheless, different [sections that may be categorized as] exterior and interior, or upper and lower.

What is meant by "exterior"? ["Exterior" refers to] the skin, the flesh, the sinews, and the bones. What is meant by "interior"? ["Interior" refers to] the viscera, the bowels, essence, and the spirit. The conduits and network [vessels] serve to connect [all these regions of the body]. Illnesses in the exterior [sections of the body] are easy to cure, and one hardly ever dies of them. Illnesses in the interior [sections of the body] are difficult to cure, and one easily dies of them. But, that is only a general rule because [illnesses] in both the exterior and the interior [sections of the body] may be difficult or easy [to cure and to die of]. One cannot treat them all alike!

If an illness was located originally in the exterior [sections of the body] whence it has spread into the [body's] interior, or if an illness was located originally in the interior, whence it has affected also the [body's] exterior [regions], [such cases] are called combined illnesses of the inside and outside. They are particularly difficult to cure.

Illnesses in the upper half of the body are often accompanied by heat, while illnesses in the lower half are often accompanied by cold. But, that is only a general rule because cold and heat may occur [together with illnesses affecting] the upper as well as the lower [half of the body]. If an illness was originally located in the upper [half of the body], whence it was transmitted to the lower [half], or if an illness was originally located in the lower [half], whence it was transmitted to the upper [half, such cases] are called combined illnesses of the upper and lower [half of the body]. They, too, are not easy to cure.

The reason is that if [the patient's body] has many areas that have not been affected by illness, while those areas that have been affected are few, it will be quite possible to maintain [the patient's] essence and strength, and to cause his regular influences to gradually reach their fullest extent again. The evil influences [that had invaded his body] will leave at the same time.

If someone's body has been affected by an illness everywhere, from where should one start to expel his illness and to restore his original influences? Medical experts know, therefore, that if an illness reaches its full strength, it will inevitably be transmitted [throughout the body]. Such [a transmission] is to be prevented beforehand, so that there may not be any clottings [of evil influences], any overflow [of an illness into neighboring areas], or any unions [between hitherto separate problems]. That is [what is meant by] the statement: The superior practitioner treats those who are not yet sick.[1]

If an [illness] has reached a state of transmission already, one must search first for its origin [and start a cure here] and one must search then for its secondary location [to complete the cure there]. One must observe whether it travels slowly or with great speed, and carry out one's treatment accordingly. This way, old age will be reached. If one applies [these principles] to decide whether an illness will result in [the patient's] survival or death, and whether it is difficult or easy [to cure], the major part [of the problem at hand] will have already been considered.

Note

1.   See *Su-wen*, treatise 2, "Ssu ch'i t'iao shen ta lun," where it says, "The Sages did not treat the sick, they treated those who were not yet sick." The *Nan-ching* 77th difficult issue states, "The superior practitioner treats what is not yet ill; the mediocre practitioner treats what is already ill." While the author of the *Su-wen* statement may have had a general concept of preventive versus curative health care in mind, the meaning of the *Nan-ching* statement is more subtle. Here "ill" and "not yet ill" refer to functional units in the body, and the prevention of the transmission of illness from one such unit to another. The concept of "treating what is not ill" was redefined by several authors in later centuries.

陰陽升降論

人身象天地天之陽藏于地之中者謂之元陽元陽之
外布者謂之浮陽浮陽則與時升降若人之陽氣則藏
於腎中而四不于周身惟元陽則固守于中而不離其
位故太極圖中心白圈即元陽也始終不動其分陰分
陽皆在白圈之外故發汗之藥皆鼓動其浮陽出于營
衛之中以洩其氣耳若元陽一動則元氣漓矣是以發
汗太甚動其元陽即有亡陽之悲病深之人發喘呃逆
即有陽越之虞其危皆在頃刻必用參附及重鎮之藥
以墜安之所以治元氣虛弱之人用升提發散之藥最
防陽氣散越此第一關也至于陰氣則不患其升而患
其竭竭則精液不布乾枯燥烈廉泉玉英毫無滋潤舌
燥唇焦皮膚粗槁所謂天氣不降地氣不升孤陽無附
害不旋踵內經云陰精所奉其人壽故陰氣有餘則上

溉陽氣有餘則下固其人無病病亦易愈反此則危故
醫人者慎毋發其陽而竭其陰也

65

4. On the Ascension and Descension of Yin and Yang [Influences]

The human body reflects heaven and earth. Those yang [influences] of heaven that are stored inside the earth are called original yang, and those [influences] that are the outer protection of the original yang, they are called surface yang. Surface yang [influences] ascend and descend following the [course of the] seasons. Similarly, man's yang influences are stored inside the kidneys, and they spread throughout the entire body. Only the original yang [influences] are kept firmly inside [the kidneys] and never leave their location.

The white dot in the center of the *t'ai-chi* symbol refers, therefore, to the original yang. It never moves. Its separation into yin and yang lies outside the white dot.[1]

Consequently, drugs that stimulate normal sweating excite [only] the surface yang [influences; that is to say] they leave from the [body's surface regions, of the] constructive and protective [influences,] and drain influences from there. Once the original yang [influences] are caused to move, the original influences will flow off. That is, if one has stimulated excessive sweating, exciting the [patient's] original yang, he may suffer from a loss of yang.

When someone is seriously ill and pants and coughs, the risk of excessively rising yang [influences] emerges, and a critical situation may appear quite rapidly. [If such a situation occurs], one must use *shen* and *fu* as well as heavy and settling drugs in order to push down and calm these [yang influences]. Hence when treating weak persons who suffer from a depletion of their original yang influences by means of drugs causing [influences] to ascend and disperse, it is imperative to take every precaution against an excessive dispersion of these [patients' yang] influences. That is the first thing to consider [in treatment].

With the yin influences, [it is different. Here] one does not suffer from their [inappropriate] ascension, but from their exhaustion. If [one's yin influences] are exhausted, one's essence and [body] liquids cannot be spread [throughout the body]. This results in desiccation and scorching; throat and saliva will dry up completely. The tongue is dry, and the lips burn up, and the skin turns rough and brittle. [All of this is summarized] in the expression: When the influences of heaven do not descend, and when the influences of earth do not ascend, the solitary yang [influences] have nothing to attach themselves to, and harm follows at once.

The *Nei-ching* says, "Those people who are [sufficiently] endowed with yin essence will reach longevity."[2] A surplus of yin influences results in irrigation (of one's throat, tongue, and lips) above; a surplus of yang influences guarantees a firm [storage of original influences in the kidneys] below. People [with such surpluses] have no illness, and if they have an illness, it will be cured easily. The opposite [to such surplus] means danger. Therefore, in treating people, one must be very cautious not to let their yang [influences disperse] excessively, and not to have their yin [influences] become exhausted.

Notes

1.   The *t'ai-chi* symbol with the white dot in the center, and the "separation into yin and yang outside the white dot," is as follows:

2.   See *Su-wen,* "Wu ch'ang cheng ta lun."

治病必分經絡藏府論

病之從內出者必由于藏府病之從外入者必由于經
絡其病之情狀必有鑒鑒可徵者如怔忡驚悸為心之
病洩瀉臌脹為腸胃之病此易知者又有同一寒熱而
六經各殊同一疼痛而筋骨皮肉各別又有藏府有病
而反現于肢節肢節有病而反現于藏府若不究其病
根所在而漫然治之則此之寒熱非彼之寒熱此之痛
癢非彼之痛癢病之所在全不關着焉病之處反以藥
攻之內經所謂誅伐無過則故病未已新病復起醫者
以其反增他病又復治其所增之病復不知病之所從
來雜藥亂投愈治而病愈深矣故治病者必先分經絡
藏府之所在而又知其七情六淫所受何因然後擇何
經何藏對病之藥本於古聖何方之法分毫不爽而後
治之自然一劑而即見效矣今之治病不效者不咎已

藥之不當而反咎病之不應藥此理終身不悟也

68

5. On the Necessity of Distinguishing between the [Various] Conduits and Network [Vessels] as well as between the [Various] Viscera and Bowels in the Treatment of an Illness

When an illness emerges from inside [of the body] it must start [its course] from the viscera and bowels. When an illness enters [the body] from the outside, it must start its course from the conduits and network [vessels]. Among illnesses there are those whose nature is quite obvious. For instance, if [a person] is agitated, or frightened and perturbed, that is an illness of the heart. Diarrhea and swelling of the abdomen are illnesses of the intestines and stomach. That is easy to know.

But, then there may be identical cases of cold or heat, and yet there may be differences as to which of the six conduits [is affected]. There may be identical cases of pain, and yet there may be differences as to whether the sinews or bones, the skin or the flesh [are affected]. Furthermore, it may well be that the viscera and bowels have an illness — while, contrary [to what one might expect], the illness appears in the [patient's] limbs and joints. Or one's limbs and joints may have an illness, and, contrary [to what one might expect, the illness] appears in the viscera and bowels.

If one does not carefully investigate where the roots of an illness are located, and if one carries out thoughtless treatments, [one will fail to notice that] one person's cold and heat are not the same as another person's cold and heat, and that one person's pain and itching are not the same as another person's pain and itching. If one disregards the location of an illness entirely and employs drugs to attack, contrary [to what would be correct], a place that is absolutely free of illness, this is what the *Nei-ching* calls "punishing the innocent."[1]

As a result, a new illness arises before an original illness has been cured, and the physician who has, contrary [to his intentions], strengthened a secondary illness, will direct his treatment against this secondary illness, which he had strengthened himself. Again, he is unaware of the origins of this [secondary] illness, and he tosses, in utter confusion, various drugs [into the patient]. The longer the treatment continues, the deeper the illness [penetrates the viscera and bowels].

Therefore, if one sets out to treat an illness, one must first distinguish in which of the conduits and network [vessels], viscera and bowels it is located, and one must know, in addition, through which of the seven emotions[2] or six excesses[3] it was caused. And, if one then selects drugs against an illness in this or that conduit, or in this or that viscus, and if one bases [one's therapy] on a pattern underlying this or that prescription created by the Sages of antiquity and does not commit the slightest mistake, then the subsequent treatment will prove a success after only one dose.

When today's [physicians] have no success in their treatment of illness, they do not blame themselves because their drugs were inappropriate; on the contrary, they blame the illness because it did not respond to the drugs! Never in their entire lives do they understand the logic at work here.

Notes

1.   See *Su-wen* "Li ho chen hsieh lun."

2.   The "seven emotions" are joy, anger, grief, pondering, hate, fear, fright.

3.   The "six excesses" refer to the following environmental factors that turn harmful if they enter the human organism in excessive, or unbalanced, amounts: wind, cold, heat, dampness, dryness, fire.

治病不必分經絡藏府論

病之分經絡藏府夫人知之於是天下遂有因經絡藏
府之說而拘泥附會又或誤認穿鑿并有借此神其說
以欺人者葢治病之法多端有必求經絡藏府者有不
必求經絡藏府者葢人之氣血無所不通而藥性之寒
熱溫涼有毒無毒其性亦一定不移入于人身其功能
亦無所不到豈有其藥止入某經之理即如參茋之類
無所不補砒鴆之類無所不毒並不常于一處也所以
古人有現成通治之方如紫金錠至寶丹之類所治之
病甚多皆有奇效葢通氣者無氣不通解毒者無毒不
解消痰者無痰不消其中不過畧有專宜耳至張潔古
輩則每藥注定云獨入某經皆屬附會之談不足憑也
曰然則用藥竟不必分經絡藏腑耶曰此不然也葢人
之病各有所現之處而藥之治病必有專長之功如柴

胡治寒熱往來能愈少陽之病桂枝治畏寒發熱能愈
太陽之病葛根治肢體大熱能愈陽明之病葢其止寒
熱已畏寒除大熱此乃柴胡桂枝葛根專長之事因其
能治何經之病後人即指為何經之藥孰知其功能實
不僅入少陽太陽陽明也顯然者尚如此餘則更無影
響矣故以某藥為能治某經之病則可以某藥為獨治
某經則不可故不知經絡而用藥其失也泛必無捷
入他經則不可故不知經絡而用藥其失也泥反能致害總之變化不一
效執經絡而用藥其失也泥反能致害總之變化不一
神而明之存乎其人也

6. On [Situations] Where It Is Not Necessary to Distinguish between the Conduits and Network [Vessels], the Viscera and the Bowels, in the Treatment of an Illness

Everyone knows that in the case of an illness one distinguishes [whether it is located in one of] the conduits or network [vessels], viscera or bowels. Consequently, there is a doctrine [to treat illness] in accordance with the [condition of the] conduits and network [vessels], or viscera and bowels, but any bigoted adherence [to this doctrine] may lead to wrong ideas and forced interpretations. Also, there are those who intend only to cheat the people by mystifying this doctrine.

The treatment of an illness may follow many principles. It may well be that one has to take the conduits and the network [vessels], as well as the viscera and bowels, into account. But, it may also be that one does not have to take the conduits and the network [vessels], the viscera and bowels, into account. Man's influences and his blood penetrate every [region of his body]. Similarly, whether the nature of a drug is cold or hot, warm or cool, and whether [a substance] is toxic or not, that is firmly determined and does not change; and when [a drug] enters the human body, its effects will reach every [region]. How could it be that a particular drug enters only a particular conduit?

[Drugs] like *shen* and *ch'i* exert their [ability to] supplement everywhere [in the body], and [drugs] like arsenic and the *chen* [bird] distribute their poison everywhere [in the body] — certainly not only at one single location! It is for this reason that the people of ancient times had ready-made cure-all prescriptions, such as the "dark-red golden ingot" or the "extremely valuable pills," [prescriptions] that cured very many illnesses and that achieved miraculous successes in all cases. The fact is, [drugs] that cause influences to move cause all influences to move; [drugs] that dissolve poison dissolve all poisons; and [drugs] that diminish phlegm diminish all phlegm — and among them there is only a small number [of drugs] that are appropriate [to treat only very] specific [problems].

However, beginning with people like Chang Chieh-ku,[1] each drug was given a commentary specifying that it would enter a particular conduit. All of that was farfetched rhetoric, and there is not enough evidence [to support it. Now, someone might] say: If that is so, is it absolutely unnecessary to distinguish between conduits and network [vessels], and between viscera and bowels, in the application of drugs? [My] answer would be: That is not the case.

The fact is, all human illnesses appear at specific locations [in the body], and drugs, when they are used in the treatment of an illness, do, of course, show effects that are based on their specific abilities. For instance, *ch'ai-hu* [is used to] treat alternating fits of cold and heat; it cures illnesses in the minor-yang [region]. *Kuei-chih* [is used to] treat aversion to cold and the development of heat. It cures illnesses in the great-yang [region]. *Ke-ken* [is used] to treat great heat in one's limbs and body. It cures illnesses in the yang-brilliance [region]. That is to say, the halting of fits of cold and heat, the ending of an aversion to cold, and the elimination of great heat are all the workings of the specific abilities of *ch'ai-hu, kuei-chih,* and *ke-ken.*

Because these [drugs] are able to cure illnesses in specific conduits, the people in later times pointed to them as drugs of specific conduits. Who would know that the effects of these [drugs] in reality do not enter exactly into the minor-yang, the great-yang, or the yang-brilliance [conduit, respectively]? If this applies to obvious cases like these, then all the remaining drugs leave even less trace [of their paths of action]. Hence it is quite possible to assume that a particular drug is capable of treating an illness in a particular conduit, but it is not possible to take a particular drug and think [that] it [can be used] solely to treat [illnesses] in a particular conduit. To say [that for the treatment of] an illness in a particular conduit one must use a particular drug, that is quite possible. But, to say [that] a particular drug does not also enter into other conduits, that is impossible.

Hence, if someone does not know about the conduits and network [vessels, his treatments] will definitely fail to have any good results. [On the other hand, those] who cling only to the conduits and network [vessels] in their use of drugs, their mistake lies in their narrowmindedness. Contrary [to their intentions], they may even cause harm.

To sum up, there are many variations [in the effects of drugs, and in the locations of their effects]. To [employ one's] spirit to reach an understanding of all this is up to capable individuals.

Note

1.   Chang Chieh-ku, i.e. Chang Yüan-su (fl. 1180), was closely associated with the beginning of so-called Sung-Chin-Yüan medicine, linking the theories of yinyang and the five phases with hitherto largely pragmatic pharmaceutics. See also below VII, 3, and P.U. Unschuld, *Medicine in China: A History of Ideas,* Berkeley, Los Angeles, London: University of California Press, 1985, 181 ff.

腎藏精論

精藏于腎人盡知之至精何以生何以藏何以出則人

不知也夫精即腎中之脂膏也有長存者有日生者腎

中有藏精之處充滿不缺如井中之水日夜充盈此長

存者也其慾動交媾所出之精及有病而滑脫之精乃

日生者也其精旋去旋生不去亦不生猶井中之水日

日汲之不見其虧終年不汲不見其溢易云井道不可

不草故受之以革其理然也曰然則縱慾可無害乎曰

是又不然蓋天下之理總歸自然有腎氣盛者多慾無

傷腎氣衰者自當節養左傳云女不可近乎對曰節之

若縱慾不節如淺狹之井汲之無度則枯竭矣曰然則

強壯之人而絕慾則何如曰此亦無咎無譽惟腎氣畏

堅實耳但必浮火不動陰陽相守則可耳若浮火日動

而強制之則反有害蓋精因火動而離其位則必有頭

眩目赤身痒腰疼遺洩偏墜等症甚者癃癰疽此強

制之害也故慾動則生不動則不生能自然

不動則有益強制則有害過用則衰竭任其自然而無

所勉強則保精之法也老子云天法道道法自然自然

之道乃長生之訣也

7. On the Storage of Essence in the Kidneys

Everyone knows that the essence[1] is stored in the kidneys, but no one knows how this essence is generated, how it is stored, and how it leaves [the kidneys. The] essence is a fatty paste [stored] inside the kidneys. Some of it stays there for a long [time], some of it is generated daily anew. Inside the kidneys is a location where the essence is stored; it is [always] filled and never empty in the same way as a well is filled with water day and night. This is [the essence] that stays [in the kidneys] for a long time.

Essence leaving [the kidneys] as a result of sexual agitation or intercourse, as well as essence that is lost [at night] as a result of illness, are both created daily anew. As soon as the essence leaves [the kidneys], it is generated anew. If it does not leave [the kidneys], nothing is generated anew.

Again, this is similar to the water in a well. It may be drawn day by day, and yet, the [well] would never appear empty; and if no [water] is drawn for an entire year, [the water in the well] would still not overflow. The [Book of] Changes states, "The Way of the well is continuous renewal. Hence [the hexagram of the well] is followed by [that of] renewal."[2] This principle applies [to the essence and the kidneys] too.

[Someone might] ask: Is it, then, at all possible that one can [always] follow one's lustful desires without suffering any harm as a result? [I would] answer: No, this is not the case. The principle of [an adequate functioning of all things] under heaven lies entirely in their being as they are. If someone is rich in renal influences, he may engage in frequent sexual activities and still suffer no harm. Those, however, whose renal influences are weak, of course, must curb [their passions] and nourish [their essence].

In the Tso-chuan, [the Marquis of Chin] asked, "May women not be approached at all?" [And the physician from Ch'in] answered, "One should be moderate [in one's intercourse with them]."[3] If one follows one's passions without any moderation, this is as if one drew [water] from a shallow, narrow well without any restraint. It would dry up and be exhausted.

[Someone might] say: Why, now, should anyone who is strong and vigorous curb his passions? [I would] answer: Here, too, no [single alternative] is to be warned against or to be recommended! If the influences of one's kidneys are rather weak, it is still possible for yin and yang to meet as long as the floating fire is not agitated. If, however, the floating fire is activated daily, and is suppressed by force, that causes harm. The reason is that the essence leaves its position because of the agitation of the fire. As a result, one's head turns dizzy, and one's eyes become red. The body will itch and one's loins will start to ache. [Nocturnal] emissions occur, and unilateral descent of the testicles. In severe cases, welling abscesses may develop. These are the types of harm resulting from forcefully suppressing [one's passion].

One's essence is a substance that is generated if one's passions are agitated. If no agitation occurs, no [essence] is generated. If [someone] is able to to avoid agitation without active interference, that will be beneficial [for his health]. If, however, one forcefully suppresses [one's passions], that means harm. Excessive use leads to weakness and exhaustion. To follow one's being as one is, and to refrain from forced [activities], that is the [correct] method to preserve one's essence.

Lao-tzu has said, "Heaven follows the law of the Way. The law of the Way is its being as it is."[4] The Way of being as one is — that is the secret of longevity.

Notes

1.   The Chinese term *ching* refers to "essence" in general, and here specifically to male semen.

2.   See *I Ching*, hexagram 49, *ko.*

3.   See *Tso chuan*, Book X, first year.

4.   See Lao-tzu, *Tao te ching*, ch. 25.

一藏一腑先絕論

人之死大約因元氣存亡而決故患病者元氣已傷即
變危殆蓋元氣脫則五藏六腑皆無氣矣竟有元氣深
固其根不搖而內中有一藏一腑先絕者如心絕則昏
昧不知世事肝絕則喜怒無節腎絕則陽道痿縮胖絕
則食入不化肺絕則氣促聲啞六腑之絕而失其所司
亦然其絕之象亦必有顯然可見之處大約其氣尚存
而神志精華不用事耳必明醫乃能決之又諸藏腑之
中惟肺絕則死期尤促蓋肺為藏腑之華蓋藏腑賴其
氣以養故此藏絕則藏腑皆無稟受矣其餘則視其絕
之甚與不甚又觀其別藏之盛衰何如更觀其後天之
飲食何如以此定其吉凶則脩短之期可決矣然火段
亦無過一年者此皆得之目觀非臆說也

8. On [Situations Where] at First One Single Viscus or One Single Bowel Was Cut Off [from the Circulation of Influences]

In general, whether a person will die [or not] is determined by the presence or loss of his original influences. If, therefore, someone's original influences have received harm in the course of an illness, [his situation] may become quite dangerous. The reason is [that] as soon as one's original influences are lost, none of the five viscera and six bowels is supplied with influences any longer.

Still, even if someone's original influences are stored deeply and secure, that is, if [their] basis is undisturbed, it may be that, at first, just one single viscus or bowel is cut off [from the circulation of influences in the body].

If, for instance, the heart has been cut off [from the circulation of influences], that person is benighted and will not recognize anything.

If the liver has been cut off, one's joy and anger are immoderate.

If the kidneys have been cut off, one's male organ is weakened and shrinks.

If the spleen has been cut off, the food that enters [the body] is not digested.

If the lung has been cut off, one's [breathing] influences move rapidly and one's voice fails.

In the same way, the six bowels lose their functions once they have been cut off [from the circulation of the influences], and there are [specific] locations where [the fact that] any of them has been cut off is reflected quite clearly [in specific symptoms].

Generally speaking, as long as some influences are still present, a knowledgeable physician will be able to determine [the patient's imminent death or chance of survival], even if [the patient's] mind and senses have already ceased to function. Also, among all the viscera and bowels, only when the lung has been cut off [from the circulation of influences] will the moment of death very soon follow. This is because the lung covers all the other viscera and bowels like a canopy. [All the other] viscera and bowels depend on the [lung's] influences for nourishment. If, therefore, this particular viscus is cut off [from the circulation of influences], none of the remaining viscera and bowels will receive any further supplies.

In all cases besides [the lung], one should see whether the [respective viscus or bowel] is severely cut off or not [from the circulation of influences]. Also, one should investigate to what extent the remaining viscera still flourish. Finally, one should investigate [the patient's intake] of later dependencies,[1] [i.e., of] beverages and food. On the basis of all these [data], one determines the auspicious and inauspicious outcome [of the patient's illness] and one will be able to determine the length [of his survival]. Usually, though, [such predictions] cannot exceed a period of one year.

I have witnessed all [the situations outlined above] with my own eyes. These are by no means statements without foundation.

Note

1.   Traditional Chinese medical theory distinguishes between "earlier dependencies," *hsien t'ien* 先天 and "later dependencies," *hou t'ien* 後天. The former are influences determining one's life that are active prior to one's birth, i.e., influences transmitted to offspring by their parents. "Later dependencies" are those influences one's survival depends on after birth, i.e., mainly food and drink.

君火相火論

近世之論心火謂之君火腎火謂之相火此說未安蓋

心屬火而位居于上又純陽而為一身之主名曰君火

無異議也若腎中之火則與心相遠乃為水中之火也與

心火不類名為相火似屬非宜益陰陽互藏其宅心固

有火而腎中亦有火心火中之火腎火為水中之

火腎火守於下心火守于上而三焦為火之道路能引

二火相交心火動而腎中之浮火亦隨之腎火動而心

中之浮火亦隨之亦有心火動而腎火不動其患獨在

心亦有腎火動而心火不動其害獨在腎故治火之法

必先審其何火而後用藥有定品治心火以苦寒治腎

火以鹹寒若二藏之陰不足以配火則又宜取二藏之

陰藥補之若腎火飛越又有回陽之法反宜用溫熱與

治心火迥然不同故五藏皆有火而心腎二藏為易動

故治法宜詳究也若夫相火之說則心胞之火能令人

怔忡而赤煩燥眩暈此則在君火之旁名為相火似為

確切試以內經炎之自有真見也

9. On the [Designations] Ruler Fire and Minister Fire

In discourses of recent times, the fire of the heart is called ruler fire, and the fire of the kidneys is called minister fire. This [latter] designation is problematic.

The heart is associated with the [phase of] fire, and it is located in the upper [part of the body]; also, it represents the pure yang and governs the entire body. To speak here of a ruler fire seems quite agreeable [to the facts]. The fire in the kidneys, though, is located at quite a distance from the heart. Also, it is a fire amidst water and is, therefore, different from the fire of the heart. To call it minister fire appears to be inappropriate.

The fact is that yin and yang [influences] are both stored in each other's location. The heart, of course, has a fire, but inside the kidneys there is a fire too. The fire of the heart is a fire inside the fire; the fire of the kidneys is a fire inside the water. The fire of the kidneys is kept in the lower [part of the body]; the fire of the heart is kept in the upper [part of the body]. And, the triple burner is a pathway of fire; it allows the two fires [of the heart and the kidneys] to interact.

Once the fire of the heart has been agitated, the floating fire inside the kidneys will follow it. If the fire of the kidneys was agitated [first], the floating fire inside the heart will follow it too. It may also be that the fire of the heart is agitated without the fire of the kidneys being agitated as a consequence. In this case, only the heart suffers. Also, the fire of the kidneys may have been agitated without the fire of the heart being agitated subsequently. In this case, only the kidneys suffer. Hence in treating a fire, one must first investigate what kind of a fire is at issue.

The drugs to be used after [the nature of the fire has been determined] are clearly defined substances. A fire of the heart is to be treated with [substances of] bitter [flavor] and cold [thermo-influence]; a fire of the kidneys is to be treated with [substances of] salty [flavor] and cold [thermo-influence]. If the yin [influences] of neither of [these two] viscera suffice to match the fire, one should employ drugs that supplement the yin [influences] of the two viscera concerned. If [only] the fire of the kidneys flares up excessively, patterns exist to return the yang [influences], and, contrary [to what was outlined above], one should use warm or hot [substances]. That is, of course, quite different from treating a fire of the heart.

Now, all the five viscera have a fire, but [those of] the heart and kidneys are easily agitated. Hence one should carefully consider an appropriate treatment pattern. The designation "minister fire," though, applies [in fact] to the fire of the heart-enclosing [network]. It is responsible if one feels uneasy, has a red [face], is perplexed, and suffers from vertigo. It is at the side of the ruler fire, and to call it minister fire appears to be very fitting indeed. One need only check the *Nei-ching* to get the right view.

II. The [Movement in the] Vessels

診脈決死生論

生死于人大矣而能于兩手方寸之地微末之動即能決其生死何其近于誣也然古人往往百不失一者何哉其大要則以胃氣為本葢人之所以生本乎飲食靈樞云穀入于胃乃傳之肺五臟六腑皆以受氣寸口屬肺經為百脈之所會故其來也有生氣以行乎其間融和調暢得中土之精英此為有胃氣得者生失者死其大較也其次則推天運之順逆人氣與天氣相應如春氣屬木脈宜弦夏氣屬火脈宜洪之類反是則與天氣不應又其次則審臟氣之生尅如脾病畏弦木尅土也肺病畏洪火尅金也反是則與臟氣無害又其次則辨病脈之從違病之與脈各有宜與不宜如脫血之後脈宜靜細而反洪大則氣亦外脫矣寒熱之症脈宜洪數而反細弱則真元將陷矣至于真臟之脈乃因胃氣已

絕不營五臟所以何臟有病則何臟之脈獨現凡此皆內經難經等書言之明白詳盡學者苟潛心觀玩洞然易曉此其可決者也至云診脈即可以知何病又云人之死生無不能先知則又非也葢脈之變遷無定或有卒中之邪未即通于經絡而脈一時未變者或病輕而不能現于脈者或有沉痼之疾久而與氣血相併一時難辨其輕重者或有依經傳變流動無常不可執一時之脈而定其是非者況病之名有萬而脈之象不過數十種且一病而數十種之脈無不見何能診脈而即知其何病此皆推測偶中以此欺人也若夫真臟之脈臨死而終不現者則何以決之是必以望聞問三者合而參觀之亦百不失一矣故以脈為可憑而脈亦有時不足憑以脈為不可憑而又鑿鑿乎其可憑總在醫者熟通經學更深思自得則無所不驗矣若世俗無稽之

説皆不足聽也

1. On [the Possibility of] Determining [a Patient's] Death or Survival Through Investigating the [Movement in His] Vessels

Life and death are important for man, and [to state that] one is able to determine at locations on both hands, of the size of a square inch, and on the basis of some weak movements, whether [a patient] will die or survive, does this not border on false claims?

In ancient times, the people [who treated patients] generally did not lose one in a hundred. How could that be? The most important [principles of predicting a patient's death or survival are the following].

One considers the influences of the stomach as the basis [of life]. Human life is based on beverages and food. The *Ling-shu* states, "The grains enter the stomach, whence they are transmitted to the lung. From there all the five viscera and six bowels are supplied with influences."[1]

The inch opening belongs to the conduit [associated with the] lung. It is a meeting point of [the movement through] all the vessels. Hence, among [all the influences] arriving there, there are also vital influences [sent out by the stomach]. If the influences arriving [at the inch opening] are mild and unimpeded, and if they contain the essence of the center[2] and of the [phase of] soil, that is a sign that stomach influences are present. As long as they are present, [the patient] will survive. If they are lost, [the patient] will die. That is a general rule.

Second, one investigates whether [the movement in the vessels] follows or contradicts the course of heaven. The influences in man and the influences of heaven reflect each other. For example, the influences of spring are associated with [the phase of] wood. [During spring, the movement in] the vessels should be stringy. The influences of summer are associated with [the phase of] fire. [During summer, the movement in] the vessels should be surging — and so on. If the [movement in the] vessels is contrary [to what it should be], then it does not reflect the influences of heaven.

Thirdly, the [successful healers of ancient times] examined the influences [emitted by the] viscera in terms of the [relationships of] mutual generation and destruction [among the phases]. For instance, in case of an illness in the spleen, they feared a stringy [movement in the vessels because] wood overcomes soil; and in case of an illness in the lung, they feared a surging [movement in the vessels, because] fire overcomes metal. However, when [they diagnosed movements] contrary [to those they feared], no harm [was to be expected] for the influences of the viscera.

Fourthly, one differentiates among those [movements in the] vessels that fit the illness [of the patient], and others that do not. For instance, after one has lost blood, [the movement in the] vessels should be calm and fine. If it is, in contrast, surging and large, this [indicates that not only blood, but] also influences have been lost to the outside. In case of a cold-hot condition, the [appropriate movement in the] vessels is surging and rapid. If it is, by contrast, fine and weak, one's true and original [influences may also have been affected].

[Movements in the] vessels [indicating the presence of] the true influences of a viscus occur when the [flow of the] influences of the stomach has already been cut off, and hence fails to circulate through all the five viscera. Consequently, only a [movement in the] vessels related to the particular viscus that is affected by an illness appears.

All [that I have outlined now] is treated clearly and in great detail in such books as the *Nei-ching* and *Nan-ching*. Anyone who studies [these works] with diligence and joy will acquire a good knowledge [of all this]. This, then, is what can be determined [with respect to whether a patient will die or survive]. When it is said, though, that through investigating the [movements in the] vessels one can diagnose [in all instances] what kind of an illness [someone has], and when it is said, furthermore, that it is always possible to know beforehand whether a person will die or survive, then this is just not true.

The fact is that the variations of [the movement in the] vessels are not regular. Someone may suddenly have been struck by evil [influences], but these [influences] may have not yet penetrated into his conduits and network [vessels]. Hence, the [movement in the] vessels will show no change for the time being.

Or an illness may be minor to a degree that it does not appear in the [movement in the] vessels.

Or an illness may be located in the depth [of the body], where it has become chronic. After a long time has passed, [the influences associated with the illness] may have merged with the [normal] influences and the blood [circulating in the body. In this case,] it will be difficult, for the time being, to distinguish whether [the problem] is minor or severe.

Or [an illness] may be transmitted through, and undergo transformations in, the [different] conduits, moving here and there, without any [location to settle in] for good. Hence it is impossible to grasp [a specific movement in] the vessels at a specific moment and to identify it in a correct way.

Finally, the designations for illnesses are innumerable, yet they are reflected in merely a few dozens of [movements in the] vessels; and in the course of one single illness, those few dozens of [movements in the] vessels may all appear.

How could anyone know what kind of an illness [affects a patient] just by investigating [his movement in the] vessels? This would be entirely guesswork, with only accidental success — employed to cheat people! If, for example, even shortly prior to death, the true [influences of a] viscus do not yet appear, how could one determine [that that person will die]?

It is, therefore, essential to employ [also the other three diagnostic methods of] looking [for changes in the patient's complexion, of] listening [to his voice and of smelling his odors, and of] asking [him for his preferences for specific flavors of his food]. If these three [methods] are taken into account together [with an investigation of the movement in the vessels, contemporary healers, too,] will not lose one patient in a hundred.

Hence one may assume that one can rely on the [movement in the] vessels, but at times it is just insufficient to rely on the [movement in the] vessels. And, there may be situations where one assumes that one should not rely on [movement in the] vessels, while in fact [the movement in the] vessels is very clear and reliable. It is always such that those physicians who have thoroughly studied the doctrines of the [ancient] classics, and who have, through [their own] deep thoughts, perfected themselves, will be successful in all [cases they treat].

The unfounded statements now in fashion are not worth listening to.

Notes

1.   See *Ling-shu*, treatise 18, "Ying wei shen hui."

2.   The term *chung* refers to the stomach.

症脈輕重論

人之患病不外七情六淫其輕重死生之別醫者何由
知之皆必問其症切其脈而後知之然症脈各有不同
有現症極明而脈中不見者有脈中甚明而症中不見
者其中有宜從症者有宜從脈者必有一定之故審之
既真則病情不能逃否則不為症所誤必為脈所誤矣
故宜從症者雖脈極順而症危亦斷其必死宜從脈者
雖症極險而脈和亦決其必生如脫血之人形如死狀
危在頃刻而六脈有根則不死此宜從脈不從症也如
痰厥之人六脈或促或絕痰降則愈此宜從症不從脈
也陰虛咳嗽飲食起居如常而六脈細數久則必死此
宜從脈不宜從症也噎膈反胃脈如常人久則胃絕而
脈驟變百無一生此又宜從症不從脈也如此之類甚
多不可枚舉總之脈與症分觀之則吉凶兩不可憑合

觀之則某症忌某脈某症忌某脈其吉凶乃可定矣又
如肺病忌脈數肺屬金數為火火刑金也餘可類推皆
不外五行生尅之理今人不按其症而徒講乎脈則講
之愈密失之愈遠若脈之全體則內經諸書詳言之矣

2. On the Minor and Serious [Nature of Movements in the] Vessels and of Pathoconditions

All the illnesses man may suffer from [are related either to the] seven emotions or to the six excesses. How, then, does a physician know how to distinguish whether [an illness] is minor or serious, and whether [the patient will] die or survive?

He must ask for pathoconditions, and he must press the vessels, and then he will know all this. But, there are many variations in the [appearances and mutual relationships of] pathoconditions and [movements in the] vessels. It may be that [in the case of an illness the resulting] pathoconditions are quite clear, while the illness fails to appear in the [movement in the] vessels. Or [an illness] may appear quite distinctly in the [movement in the] vessels, but fails to manifest itself in any pathocondition.

Among [the illnesses] are those where [one's judgement concerning the patient's impending death or survival] should follow the pathoconditions, and others where one should follow the [movement in the] vessels. [Any such judgement] must have a definite cause. If [a physician] is able to decide correctly [whether to follow the movement in the vessels or the pathoconditions], the nature [of the patient's illness] will not escape him either. Otherwise, if one is not misled by the pathoconditions, one will be misled by the [movement in the] vessels.

Hence in cases where one should follow the pathoconditions, the [movement in the] vessels may be quite favorable. If the pathoconditions signal danger, one must conclude that [the patient] will die. And, in cases where one should follow [in one's judgement and treatment,] the movement [in the vessels], the pathoconditions [exhibited] may be highly alarming. If the [movement in the] vessels is balanced, one should decide that [the patient] will survive.

For instance, when someone has lost blood his body may be [as pale] as a corpse, and [he may appear to] approach a very critical moment. As long, though, as the [movement in his] six vessels has a root,[1] he will not die. That is [an example of a situation where] one should follow the [movement in the] vessels, not the pathoconditions.

Or take, for instance, a person suffering from phlegm [blocking his conduits with the effect of] ceasing [influences in his extremities. The movement in his] six vessels is sometimes hasty, sometimes interrupted. Once the phlegm descends, [the patient] is cured. That is [a case when] one should follow the pathoconditions, not the [movement in the] vessels.

If [a person suffers from] a depletion of yin [influences, accompanied by] cough, his consumption of beverages and food, as well as his daily routine of rising and resting may continue as usual. If the [movement in his] six vessels is fine and rapid for an extended period of time, he must die. That is [another example of a situation where] one should follow [the movement in the] vessels, not the pathoconditions.

If [a person is] unable to swallow food, and vomits instead, the [movement in this person's] vessels may be similar to that of a healthy person. If, however, this goes on for long, his stomach will be cut off [from supplies] and the [movement in his] vessels will undergo a violent change. Not one [person] in a hundred will survive this. That, again, is [an example of a situation where] one should follow the pathoconditions, not the [movement in the] vessels.

There are more [examples] like these — too many to enumerate here. In general, though, if one investigates only the [movement in the] vessels or [only] the pathoconditions, any prediction concerning the auspicious or inauspicious [outcome of an illness] must remain unreliable. If both [the movement in the vessels and the pathoconditions] are taken into account, and if [one knows] which pathocondition must not occur together with which [movement in the] vessels, and which [movement in the] vessels must not occur together with which pathocondition, the auspicious or inauspicious [outcome of an illness] can be determined.

For example, an illness in the lung must not be accompanied by a rapid [movement in the] vessels. The lung is [associated with the phase of] metal. A rapid [movement in the vessels] is [associated with the phase of] fire. Fire kills metal. Other [examples] can be deduced from this one; no situation stands outside the principles of the [mutual] generation and destruction of the five phases.

Today, people do not examine the pathoconditions; all they do is discuss the [movement in the] vessels. The closer their discussions focus on the [movement in the vessels, though,] the further it escapes them. The essentials of the [movement in the] vessels are delineated in detail in the various books of the *Nei-ching*.

Note

1.   The kidneys are for man what roots are for a tree, namely, sources of continuous nourishment. Hence if no movement associated with the kidneys, i.e., with the "root" of human life, can be felt in the vessels, the patient will soon die.

脈症與病相反論

症者病之發現者也病熱則症熱病寒則症寒此一定
之理然症竟有與病相反者最易誤治此不可不知者
也如冒寒之病反身熱而惡熱傷暑之病反身寒而惡
寒本傷食也而反易飢能食本傷飲也而反大渴口乾
此等之病尤當細考一或有誤而從症用藥即死生判
矣此其中益有故焉或一時病勢未定如傷寒本當發
熱其時尚未發熱將來必至於發熱此先後之不同也
或內外異情如外雖寒而內仍熱是也或有名無實如
欲食好飲及至少進即止飲食之後又不易化是也或
有別症相雜誤認此症為彼症是也或此人舊有他病
新病方發舊病亦現是也至于脈之相反亦各不同或
其人本體之脈與常人不同或輕病未現于脈或痰氣
阻塞營氣不利脈象乖其所之或一時為邪所閉脈似

危險氣通即復或其人本有他症仍其舊症之脈凡此
之類非一端所能盡總宜潛心體認審其真實然後不
為脈症所惑否則徒執一端之見用藥愈真而愈誤矣
然苟非辨症極精脈理素明鮮有不惑者也

3. On Contradictions between the [Movement in the] Vessels and Pathoconditions [on the One Side], and the Illness [Itself on the Other Side]

Pathoconditions are manifestations of an illness. If the illness is heat, the pathocondition is heat; if the illness is cold, the pathocondition is cold. That is a definite principle. But one should also know that pathoconditions and illnesses may contradict each other — a fact that may very easily lead to a mistaken treatment, and that should be known to everyone.

For instance, the illness is "affliction by cold," but the body, contrary [to what one might expect], is hot, and one has an aversion to heat. Or, the illness is "harm caused by heat," but the body, contrary [to what one might expect], is cold and one has an aversion to cold. If one was harmed, originally, by [too much] food, but, contrary [to what one might expect], easily gets hungry and is quite able to eat, or if one was harmed, originally, by drinking [too much], but has, contrary [to what one might expect], great thirst and a dry mouth, such illnesses must be analysed with particular care.

If someone commits a mistake [in treating such illnesses], and follows the pathoconditions in his application of drugs, he will have decided the [question of] death and life. In all these cases there must be a reason [for a contradiction between the nature of an illness and its pathoconditions].

Sometimes, the strength of an illness remains undetermined for some time. For instance, a harm caused by cold should generate heat. At the moment [of the examination] it may not yet have caused heat, but it will definitely reach a state later where it generates heat. Here, now, the earlier and later [stages of the illness] differ.

Or, the internal and external nature [of an illness may] differ. For instance, someone may be cold outside and hot inside.

Or, [an illness] may be such that it has a name but is not accompanied by any tangible reality. For instance, someone longs for food, or would like to drink, but [his thirst or hunger] stop as soon as he consumes even the smallest [portion of food]. And, after he has consumed beverage or food, there follows no digestion.

Or, [the pathoconditions of one illness] are mixed with pathoconditions related to another [illness], and one may mistakenly confuse the pathocondition of one [illness] with that of the other.

Or, someone has had one illness for a long time already, and just at the moment when his new illness breaks out, his old illness manifests itself [through pathoconditions again].

Similarly, there are many different discrepancies between the [movements in the] vessels [and a person's illness]. For instance, a person's [movement in the] vessels may [in the absence of any illness, solely] because of its natural condition, already differ from that of a normal [person].

Or, a minor illness may not appear in the [movement in the] vessels.

Or, phlegm influences may have caused blockages with the result that constructive influences cannot flow freely, while the [movement in the] vessels causes the mistaken image of [constructive influences] proceeding [as usual].

Or, it may be that, at one time, [the passage of one's normal influences] is blocked by evil influences, with the [movement in the] vessels giving an impression of great danger. Then the influences [suddenly] pass freely again, and [the patient] recovers.

Or, a person may display pathoconditions of one [illness], and, yet, his [movement in the] vessels is related to the pathoconditions of a former [illness].

All these [discrepancies] cannot be subsumed under one rule. In general, one should conduct diligent studies and take great pains to gain a thorough understanding. One should examine what is real; then one will not be misled by pathoconditions and the [movement in the] vessels. If one does not [conduct diligent studies, and if one fails to gain a thorough understanding], one will stick to but a partial view, and the more [one thinks one's] use of drugs is correct, the more mistaken it will be. If one does not very clearly distinguish between different pathoconditions, and if one is not perfectly familiar with the principles of the [movement in the] vessels, it will be rare that one is not misled [in one's diagnosis and treatment].

III. Illnesses

中風論

今之患中風偏癱等病者百無一愈十死其九非其症俱不治皆醫者誤之也凡古聖定病之名必指其實名曰中風則其病屬風可知既為風病則主病之方必以治風為本故仲景侯氏黑散風引湯防巳地黃湯及唐人大小續命等方皆多用風藥而因症增減益以風入經絡則內風與外風相煽以致痰火一時壅塞惟宜先驅其風繼清痰火而後調其氣血則經脉可以漸通今人一見中風等症即用人參熟地附于肉桂等純補溫熱之品將風火痰氣盡行補住輕者變重重者即死或有元氣未傷而感邪淺者亦必遷延時日以成偏枯永廢之人此非醫者誤之耶或云邪之所湊其氣必虛故補正即所以驅邪此大謬也惟其正虛而邪湊尤當急驅其邪以衛其正若更補其邪氣則正氣益不能支矣

即使正氣全虛不能托邪於外亦宜於驅風藥中少加扶正之品以助驅邪之力從未有純用溫補者譬之盜賊入室定當先驅盜賊而後固其牆垣未有盜賊未去而先固其牆垣者或云補藥托邪猶之增家人以禦盜也是又不然蓋服純補之藥斷無專補正不補邪之理非若家人之專於禦盜賊也是不但不驅盜并助盜矣況治病之法凡久病屬虛驟病屬實所謂虛者謂正虛也所謂實者謂邪實也中風乃急暴之症其為實邪無疑天下未有行動如常忽然大虛而昏仆者豈可不以實邪治之哉其中或有屬陰虛陽虛感濕感寒之別則於治風方中隨所現之症加減之漢唐諸法具在可取而觀也故凡中風之類苟無中藏之絕症未有不可治者余友人患此症者遵余治法病一二十年而今尚無恙者甚多惟服熱補者無一存者矣

1. On Being Struck by Wind

Today, not one in a hundred of those who suffer from illnesses such as "struck by wind" and "unilateral obturation" is cured. Of ten [patients], nine die. However, it would be wrong [to assume that] the pathoconditions [related to these illnesses] are incurable. [The high mortality mentioned is] always the result of mistaken [treatments applied] by physicians.

Whenever the Sages in ancient times determined the designation of an illness, they made sure that the name [of an illness] corresponded to the facts. Hence one knows that the illness named "struck by wind" is related to wind. Since it is a wind illness, the prescriptions employed to master this illness must be based on [drugs] curing wind. Thus, "Mr. Hou's Black Powder" recorded by [Chang] Chung-ching, the "Wind-Guiding Decoction," the *"Fang-chi ti-huang* Decoction,"[1] as well as the "Comprehensive Decoction for the Continuation of Life" and the "Small [Decoction for the Continuation of Life," both recorded] by the man who lived during the T'ang,[2] all these prescriptions rely heavily on wind-drugs, with [their respective ingredients being] increased or decreased in accordance with the pathoconditions [exhibited by the patient].

When wind enters the conduits and the network [vessels], internal winds and the wind [intruding] from outside excite each other until suddenly phlegm-fire[3] [emerges] and causes obstructions. In such a situation there is no other way but to, first, expel the wind [from the body], then cool the phlegm-fire, and finally, harmonize the [body's regular] influences and the blood. As a result, the conduits and the vessels will gradually become passable again.

When today's people see such pathoconditions as "struck by wind," they use only *jen-shen, shou-ti, fu-tzu,* and *jou-kuei* — substances that do nothing but supplement with warmth or heat. This way, the wind-fire and the phlegm influences move everywhere and are caused to settle. Minor [problems] turn serious; serious [illnesses] end in death.

Or, someone's original influences may not have been harmed yet, and so far, the effects of the evil influences may have remained near the surface — [the drugs mentioned above] will but protract [the illness] for hours and days, until the patient is paralyzed unilaterally, and disabled forever. Is not this the fault of the physician?

Some say, when evil [influences] accumulate, there must [first] be a depletion of [proper] influences. Hence [those who say so] supplement the proper [influences] to expel the evil [influences]. That, however, is a great mistake! When the proper [influences] are depleted, and evil [influences] accumulate, one must [first] expel the evil [influences] as fast as possible to protect the [remaining] proper [influences]. If, however, the evil influences are supplemented even further, the proper influences will be even less able to withstand [the attempted takeover by the evil influences]. The proper influences are entirely delpleted, it will be impossible to push the evil [influences] out.

Hence, one should add, to the drugs employed to expel wind, some substances supporting [the patient's] proper influences to assist their ability to expel the evil [influences. But] it has never been [appropriate] to use only drugs that supplement [the patient] with warmth [or heat]. One may compare this with a situation where thieves enter a house. One must, of course, expel the robber first, and strengthen the walls only afterwards. It is just impossible to start strengthening the walls before the robber has left!

Someone might respond to this: To push out evil [influences] by employing drugs that supplement [the body with heat] is the same as to increase one's servants to ward off the robbers. This, again, is not the case, because if one consumes drugs that do nothing but supplement [heat], one does, by no means, supplement only the proper [influences] without supplementing the evil [influences]. This is different from the specific defense by one's servants against a robber. [By employing drugs that supplement] one not only fails to expel the robbers, the robbers are even supported!

Also, in terms of treatment patterns, all long-term illnesses are associated with a depletion; sudden illnesses are associated with a repletion. What is called depletion is a depletion of proper [influences]. What is called repletion is a repletion with evil [influences]. [The illness] "struck by wind" is a very sudden and violent condition. It is, without any doubt, a repletion with evil [influences]. It has never been such that one carried on his daily activities as usual, and all of a sudden, was dizzy and fell down because of a severe depletion. One would, of course, have to treat such [a patient] for a repletion with evil [influences].

It is necessary that one distinguish between depletions of yin [influences] and depletions of yang [influences], as well as between affections by dampness and affections by cold. And, as far as the prescriptions employed to treat wind are concerned, one must add or take away [some ingredients] according to the respective pathoconditions that become apparent.

All the [therapeutic] patterns of the Han and T'ang eras are still available, and it is quite possible to examine them. Hence all these "struck by wind" [illnesses] that are not accompanied by [extreme] pathoconditions indicating that one of the viscera has been cut off [from circulation], can be successfully [treated]. Those of my friends who suffer from this pathocondition, and who followed my therapeutic pattern during illness episodes [already] lasting ten to twenty years, and who have no complaint, are very many. Of those, however, who took [drugs] supplementing heat, none is still around.

Notes

1.   These three prescriptions were recorded in Chang Chung-ching's (142-220) *Chin-kuei Yao lüeh*.

2.   "The man who lived during the T'ang" is Sun Ssu-mo (581-682); the two prescriptions for the "Continuation of Life" were recorded in his work *Pei-chi Ch'ien Chin Yao Fang*.

3.   "Phlegm-fire" is a condition where internal processes generate material phlegm and immaterial fire.

臟腑論

臟腑同為極大之病然臟可治而腑不可治益臟者有
物積中其症屬實腑者不能納物其症屬虛實者可治
虛者不可治此其常也臟之為病因腸胃衰弱不能運
化或痰或血或氣凝結於中以致膨脝脹滿治之
當先下其結聚然後補養其中氣則腸胃漸能尅化矣
內經有雞矢醴方即治法也後世治臟之方亦多見效
惟藏氣已絕臍凸手心及背平滿青筋繞腹腫種
惡症齊現則不治若腑症乃肝火犯胃木來侮土謂之
賊邪胃脘枯槁不復用事惟留一線細竅又為痰涎瘀
血閉塞飲食不能下達即勉強納食仍復吐出益人生
全在飲食經云穀入於胃以傳於肺五臟六腑皆以受
氣令食既不入則五藏六腑皆竭矣所以得此症者能
少納穀則不出一年而死全不納穀則不出半年而死

凡春得病者死於秋秋得病者死于春益金木相尅之
時也又有卒然嘔吐或嘔吐而時止時發又或平常少
壯是名反胃非腑也此亦可治至於類臟之症如浮腫
水腫之類或宜針灸或宜洩瀉病象各殊治亦萬變醫
者亦宜廣求諸法而隨宜施用也

2. On Bloating and Blockage

Bloating and blockage are both very serious illnesses. And yet, bloating can be cured while blockage cannot be cured. In a case of bloating, substances accumulate in [one's body] center. This [illness is accompanied by a] pathocondition belonging to [the category of] repletions. In a case of blockage, one is unable to ingest any substances. This [illness is accompanied by] a pathocondition belonging to the [category of] depletions. Repletions can be cured; depletions cannot be cured. That is the rule.

The illness of bloating results from a weakness of the intestines and of the stomach which [therefore] are unable to pass on and transform [any substances they may receive]. It may be phlegm or blood, or [certain] influences or food that agglomerate in the center [of the body], causing bloating and swelling.

To treat this [illness], one must first purge these accumulations, and after that supplement and nourish the central influences. As a result, the intestines and the stomach will slowly recover their ability to digest. The *Nei-ching* has a wine made from chicken droppings as a prescription [against this illness].[1] That is an [appropriate] method for curing [this illness]. The prescriptions used in later generations to treat bloating have often shown [positive] effects too. Only when the viscera are already cut off from [the flow of] influences, when the arms are emaciated and when the navel protrudes, when the palms and the back of one's hands are both swollen, and when greenish-blue sinews wind around the abdomen, if all these bad pathoconditions appear, only in that case [is] no cure [possible].

As for the pathoconditions of a blockage: here the fire of the liver has offended the stomach; the wood has come to insult the soil. That is called a "destroyer evil."[2] The stomach duct dries out and can no longer perform its functions. Only a hole as fine as a thread remains, and that is blocked by phlegm, saliva, or stagnating blood. Neither food nor drink can pass downward. One forces oneself to consume food, but this is thrown up again.

Man's life depends entirely on food and beverages. The Classic states, "The grains enter the stomach, whence they are transmitted to the lung. [From the lung] all the five viscera and the six bowels receive their influences."[3] Here, now, the food no longer enters [into the stomach]. As a result, the five viscera and six bowels are all exhausted.

Those who get this illness and are able to consume a small amount of grains [per day], they will die before one year has passed. Those who are unable to consume any grains, they will die before half a year has passed.

Whenever one is affected by this illness in spring, death will occur in autumn. If one gets this illness during autumn, death will occur in spring. The reason is that these seasons are related to the mutual destruction of [the phases] metal and wood.[4]

Then there are cases where suddenly one vomits, or the vomiting stops at times and erupts at times, and it may well be that [someone who suffers from such signs] is young of age and strong. That is called "a stomach that turns back [the food it receives]"; it is not a blockage. Such [an illness] can be cured.

As for complaints similar to bloating, such as surface swellings or water swellings: in some cases it is advisable to needle or cauterize; in others one should drain. The images of the illnesses are all different, and their treatment [follows] ten thousand variations. A physician must search extensively for all possible patterns, and apply them in accordance with what is suitable.

Notes

1.   This prescription is recorded in the *Su-wen*, treatise 40, "Fu chung lun." The use of roasted chicken droppings in the treatment of children's digestive problems has persisted in Chinese folk medicine to the present time, and is praised as effective in modern literature. See *Su-wen Chu Shih Hui Ts'ui*, Ch'eng Shih-te et al., eds. Peking 1982, p. 564.

2.   A "destroyer evil" is sent out by a viscus or bowel associated, in order of mutual control or destruction of the five phases, with a phase that controls or destroys the phase associated with the viscus or bowel receiving the evil. Wood, for instance, as a spade, controls [i.e, moves] soil. Hence evil influences sent out from the liver [which is associated with the phase of wood] to the stomach [which is associated with the phase of soil] are very destructive.

3.   See *Ling-shu*, treatise 18, "Ying wei sheng hui."

4.   Spring is associated with the phase of wood; autumn with the phase of metal.

寒熱虛實真假論

病之大端不外乎寒熱虛實然必辨其真假而後治之
無誤假寒者寒在外而熱在內也雖大寒而惡熱飲假
熱者熱在外而寒在內也雖大熱而惡寒飲此其大較
也假實者形實而神衰其脈浮洪扎散也假虛者形衰
而神全其脈靜小堅實也其中又有人之虛實症之虛
實如怯弱之人而傷寒傷食此人虛而症實也強壯之
人而失血勞倦此人實而症虛也或宜正治或宜從治
或宜分治或宜合治或宜從本或宜從標寒因熱用熱
因寒用上下異方煎丸異法補中兼攻攻中兼補精思
妙術隨變生機病勢千端立法萬變則真假不能惑我
之心亦不能窮我之術是在博求古法而神明之稍執
已見或學力不至其不為病所惑者幾希矣

3. On True and False [Cases of] Cold or Heat, Depletion or Repletion

Basically, all illnesses fall within [one of these four] categories: cold, heat, depletion, or repletion. Still, [before treating a patient,] it is essential to determine whether [one is confronted with a case of] true or false [cold or heat, depletion or repletion], so that one's subsequent therapy will not be marred by mistakes.

False cold [is diagnosed when the patient] is cold outside while his inside is hot. Although he [feels] quite cold, he has an aversion to hot beverages. [In case of] false heat, [the patient is] hot outside but cold inside. Although he [feels] very hot, he has an aversion to cold beverages. This is the general principle [of false cold and of false heat].

False repletion [must be diagnosed if someone's] physical form manifests repletion, while his spirit is weak, and if the [movement in that person's] vessels is floating, surging, hollow, and dissipate. [A case of] false depletion [is diagnosed when someone's] physical form shows weakness while his spirit is in perfect shape, and if the [movement in this person's] vessels is calm, small in shape, firm, and replete.

Also [one should be aware of the fact that] there are [different relationships between] a person's [actual] depletion or repletion [on the one hand, and] a depletion or repletion [as it appears in the patient's] pathocondition. For instance, if someone is fearful and weak, and has now been harmed by cold or [inadequate] food, this is [a case of] a person [actually suffering from a] depletion with a pathocondition of repletion. If a strong and vigorous person has lost blood, suffers from fatigue, and is tired, this is [a case of] a person [basically characterized by] repletion [to which is now added] a pathocondition of depletion.

Sometimes it may be suitable to carry out a treatment directly [opposed to the nature of the illness, and] sometimes it may be suitable to treat [with drugs whose nature] follows [the nature of the illness]. Sometimes it is advisable to treat [different pathoconditions] separately; sometimes it is advisable to treat them jointly.

In some cases, one starts [one's treatment] beginning from the primary location [of the illness]. In other cases, one starts [one's treatment] beginning from the secondary location [of an illness].

Cold [drugs] are employed because of a hot [nature of an illness, and] hot [drugs] are employed because of a cold [nature of an illness].

Different prescriptions [are needed to treat illnesses in the] upper and lower [regions of the body respectively].

There are various ways to boil [drugs and prepare] pills, [and there are therapeutic patterns] linking supplementation with attack, or linking attack with supplementation. If [a physician] is brilliant in his considerations and perfect in his skills, he will adapt his [treatment] to the [individual] circumstances [of each illness]. And, since the circumstances of an illness may vary one thousandfold, he will establish ten thousand different [therapeutic] patterns. [To proceed this way] means that true or false [cases of cold or heat, depletion or repletion] will not confuse my heart, and will not overtax my skills.

It is most important [in this regard] to search widely through the [therapeutic] patterns [employed by the people] in ancient times, and to gain a perfect understanding [of their underlying principles]. Of those, however, who cling but to their own views and whose drive to learn is insufficient, only very few will not be misled when they are confronted with an illness.

内傷外感論

七情所病謂之內傷六淫所侵謂之外感自內經難經

以及唐宋諸書無不言之深切著明矣二者之病有病

形同而病因異者亦有病因同而病形異者又有全乎

外感全乎內傷者更有內傷無外感無內傷者則

因與病又互相出入參錯雜亂治法迥殊蓋內傷由於

神志外感起於經絡輕重淺深先後緩急或分或合一

或有誤為害非輕能熟于內經及仲景諸書細心體認

則雖其病萬殊其中條理井然毫無疑似出入變化無

有不效否則徬徨疑慮雜藥亂投全無法紀屢試不驗

更無把握不咎已之審病不明反咎藥之治病不應如

此死者醫殺之耳

4. On Harm from Inside, and on Affections from Outside

Illnesses related to the seven emotions[1] are called "harm from inside." [Illnesses caused by] an intrusion of any of the six excesses[2] are called "affection from outside." Beginning with the *Nei-ching* and the *Nan-ching*, and throughout the T'ang and Sung, all books contained detailed and lucid discourses on these [two etiological categories].

If two [persons suffer from] such illnesses, it may be that the physical manifestations of their illnesses are identical, while the causes of their [respective] illnesses are different. Or, it may be that the causes were identical, while the physical manifestations of the [resulting] illnesses are different.

Also, there are those [illnesses] that [were caused] entirely by an affection from outside, and there are others that [were caused] entirely by harm from inside. Furthermore, there are cases where harm from inside is accompanied by an affection from outside, or where an affection from outside is joined by harm from inside. Causes and illnesses condition each other; they are intertwined in many ways, and the therapeutic patterns [to be employed must] vary [from case to case].

Harm from inside originates from one's spirit and mind; affections from outside emerge from the conduits and network [vessels]. [The resulting illnesses] may be minor or serious, they may be near the surface or in the depth, they may manifest themselves immediately or later. They may develop slowly or fast, and they may have [to be treated] individually or together.

If even one mistake is committed, serious harm [will be inevitable]. To anyone who is familiar with the *Nei-ching*, and the books written by [Chang] Chung-ching, and who strives carefully for a thorough understanding, the central principles within all illnesses will appear straightforward, even though [these illnesses] may manifest themselves in countless variations. No doubt whatsoever will remain, and no matter which direction [an illness takes], and what kind of changes it undergoes, [one's therapies] will always be successful.

If one fails [to gain a thorough understanding], though, one will be confused and hesitant [in one's therapeutic efforts]. One will toss various drugs without following any rule, and since not a single one of one's attempts will show any effects, one will even less be able to gain security. And still, one will not seek the reason [for all these failures] in one's own insufficient understanding of these illnesses. On the contrary, one blames the drugs for not responding to [one's intentions in the] treatment of the illnesses! [Patients] who die as a result of such [misguided approaches] were killed by their physician.

Notes

1.   The seven emotions include: joy, anger, pondering, fear, fright, grief, and sadness.

2.   The six excesses include: [excessive] wind, fire, summerheat, cold, dampness, and dryness.

病情傳變論

病有一定之傳變有無定之傳變一定之傳變如傷寒

太陽傳陽明及金匱見肝之病如肝傳脾之類又如痞

病變臟血虛變浮腫之類醫者可豫知而防之也無定

之傳變或其人本體先有受傷之處或天時不和又感

時行之氣或調理失宜更生他病則無病不可變醫者

不能豫知而為防者也總之人有一病皆當加意謹慎

否則病後增病則正虛而感益重病亦變危矣至于

既傳之後則標本緩急先後分合用藥必兩處兼顧而

又不雜不亂則諸病亦可漸次平復否則新病日增無

所底止矣至於藥誤之傳變又復多端或過於攻伐

成寒中之病或過服溫燥而成熱中之病或過於寒涼而

而元氣大虛或過于滋潤而脾氣不實不可勝舉近日

害人最深者大病之後邪未全退又不察病氣所傷何

處即用附子肉桂熟地參冬人參白术五味萸肉之類

將邪火盡行補澁始若相安久之氣逆痰升脹滿昏沉

如中風之狀邪氣與元氣相併諸藥無效而死醫家病

家猶以為病後大虛所致而不知乃邪氣固結而然也

余見甚多不可不深戒

5. On Transformations of the Nature of an Illness during its Transmission [through the Organism]

Sometimes illnesses are transmitted [from one location in the body to another], and undergo transformations, following definite rules. In other cases, [illnesses] are transmitted and transformed [without] following any fixed rule.

A transmission and transformation according to fixed rules occurs, for instance, in the case of harm caused by cold. [Such an illness] is [always] transmitted from the great-yang [conduit] into the yang-brilliance [conduit]. Also, if one reads, in the *Chin-kuei* [*yao-lüeh*], on illnesses of the liver, there are those [illnesses] that are transmitted from the liver to the spleen. Or, as further examples, obstruction illnesses [always] transform themselves into bloating, and depletion of one's blood [always] transforms itself into surface swellings. A physician should know of these [transmissions and transformations according to fixed rules] in advance, and prevent them.

Transmissions and transformations that do not follow definite, clear rules occur, for instance, if someone's body has already been harmed at some location [prior to the current illness], or if weather and season do not correspond to each other [while one suffers from an illness]. Also, if one is affected by seasonally prevalent [irregular] influences, or if a therapy was inappropriate and has generated secondary illnesses — in all such cases illnesses will change [their character] and physicians have no way of knowing these [changes] in advance and of preventing them accordingly. To conclude, as soon as someone has an illness, [the physician called to give treatment] must always be most careful and diligent.

If he fails [to be careful and diligent], a [second] illness will be added to the [first] illness. The proper [influences] will be depleted, and the affection will turn increasingly serious. Even minor illnesses change into critical situations. As soon as a transmission has occurred [one should examine the illness's] secondary and primary locations, whether it proceeds slowly or fast, [which of its pathoconditions are to be treated] first and [which are to be treated] later, and whether [its different pathoconditions should be treated] separately or jointly. One's application of drugs must take both [the primary and the secondary] locations into account, and [one's prescription] should be neither confused nor chaotic.

As a result [of such careful therapies], all illnesses will gradually give way to a condition of normalcy. Otherwise, new illnesses will join [the original illness] day by day without end.

There are, furthermore, many possibilities as to how a transmission and a transformation [of an illness] may result from [therapies using] the wrong drugs. For instance, if [the thermo-influences of the drugs employed] were too cold or too cool, a [secondary] illness of "cooled center" is generated. Or, if [the thermo-influences of the drugs employed against a primary illness] are too warm or too fiery, a [secondary] illness of "heated center" is generated.

Or, if [one has employed] attacking [drugs] too strongly, [the patient's] original influences will suffer from severe depletion. Or, if [one has employed] too many nourishing [drugs], the influences of the [patient's] spleen will suffer from severe repletion.

I cannot enumerate all such possibilities here one by one. However, the greatest harm caused to people in recent times [is the following]. If, after a severe illness, before the evil [influences] have been eliminated completely, one fails to investigate carefully exactly which locations have been harmed by the influences of that [original] illness, and if one offers [the recovering patients drugs such] as *fu-tzu, jou-kuei, shou-ti*[*-huang*], *mai-*[*men*]*-tung, jen-shen, pai-chu, wu-wei*[*-tzu*], or *yü-jou,* the evil fire will be effectively stimulated [again].

At first, [the situation may] appear peaceful, but after a while the influences [in the body] will move contrary to their proper direction, and phlegm will rise. Swelling and a feeling of fullness emerge, and [the patient] will fall into deep unconsciousness, as if he had been struck by wind. [At that time,] the evil influences have merged with the [patient's] original influences. No drug could be of help here, and death [is inevitable].

Physicians and patients believe that a severe depletion has followed the illness. But they do not know that [this depletion] resulted from the fact that the evil influences have merely consolidated themselves. I have seen very many [such situations], and one should be extremely careful about them.

病同人異論

天下有同此一病而治此則效治彼則不效且不惟無

效而反有大害者何也則以病同而人異也夫七情六

淫之感不殊而受感之人各殊或氣體有強弱質性有

陰陽生長有南北性情有剛柔筋骨有堅脆肢體有勞

逸年力有老少奉養有膏粱藜藿之殊心境有憂勞和

樂之別更加天時有寒暖之不同受病有深淺之各異

一概施治則病情雖中而於人之氣體適乎相反則利

害亦相反矣故醫者必細審其人之種種不同而後輕

重緩急大小先後之法因之而定內經言之極詳即針

灸及外科之治法盡然故凡治病者皆當如是審察也

6. On Identical Illnesses in Different Persons

When [two patients suffer from] an identical illness, it may happen that [the same] treatment is effective in one of these patients, but remains without effect in the other. Or, it may be that not only does it remain without [positive] effects, [but] contrary [to one's expectations], it may even cause great harm! How is that?

Well, illnesses may be identical, but the persons [suffering from them] are different. The seven emotions and the six excesses affecting [the people are the same], but the people who are affected by them are not the same. Some may be strong and others may be weak as far as [their resources of] influences, or as far as [the condition of their] body is concerned. One's personal constitution may [be characterized by a domination of] either yin or yang [influences]. Some have grown up in the South, others in the North. One's nature may be tough or soft. One's sinews and bone may be firm or brittle. One's extremities and one's body may be worn by toil, or may enjoy an easy life. One may be old, and one's strength may have declined in the course of the years, or one may be young. There are those whose food is rich, and others whose [food] is coarse. There are [patients] who suffer, in their heart, from grief, and there are others who enjoy happiness. There are also differences between the seasons in that they may be cold or mild. Also, illnesses may enter [the body] in its depth, or they may stay near the surface.

If one treats [all those patients who appear to suffer from one identical illness] with one and the same therapy, one may hit the nature of the illness, but [one's approach] may still be exactly contraindicated by the [condition of a] patient's influences and body. Hence the [intended] benefit and the [resulting] harm are in complete contrast to each other, as well. Physicians, therefore, must carefully take into account the differences between people, and only then can they determine whether the [therapeutic] method [they are going to employ] should suit a minor or a serious [case, or an illness spreading] slowly or fast, and whether an encompassing [prescription is needed] or only a small one, and whether the earlier [locations of an illness should be treated first] or the later ones.

The *Nei-ching* discusses all [these issues] in great detail, and such therapeutic patterns that are based on needling, cauterization, and [other] external methods [may be applied in differentiating treatments] in much the same way [as drugs]. Whenever one treats a patient, one should examine [his personal constitution], therefore, on the basis of the criteria mentioned above.

113

病症不同論

凡病之總者謂之病而一病必有數症如太陽傷風是
病也其惡風身熱自汗頭痛是症也合之而成其為太
陽病此乃太陽病之本症也若太陽病而又無泄瀉不
嘔心煩痞悶則又為太陽病之無症矣如瘧病也往來
寒熱嘔吐畏風口苦是症也合之而成為瘧之
本症也若瘧而無頭痛脹滿噯逆便閉則又為瘧疾之
兼症矣若瘧而又下痢數十行則又不得謂之無症謂
之無病益瘧為一病痢又為一病而二病又各有本症
各有無症不可勝舉以此類推則病之與症何分併何
當千萬不可不求其端而分其緒也而治之法或當合
治或當分治或當先治或當後治或當專治或當不治
尤在視其輕重緩急而次第奏功一或倒行逆施雜亂
無紀則病變百出雖良工不能挽回矣

7. On The Differences between Illness and Pathoconditions

Any illness in its entirety is called "illness," but one single illness is inevitably accompanied by several pathoconditions. For instance, when the great-yang [conduit and viscus] have been harmed by wind, that is the illness. An aversion against wind, a hot body, sweating without external reason, and headache are pathoconditions [accompanying this illness]. Together, these [pathoconditions] constitute a great-yang illness; they are the basic pathoconditions of a great-yang illness.

If [someone suffers from] a great-yang illness, and in addition, [suffers from] diarrhea and inability to sleep; if he has an uneasy feeling in his heart, combined with pressure in his chest due to [influences] blocked there, these then are concomitant pathoconditions of the great-yang illness. Or take, as another example, the *yao* illness.[1] Alternating fits of cold and heat, vomiting, fear of wind, and bitter taste in the mouth, these are the pathoconditions that together constitute the *yao* illness. They are the basic pathoconditions of *yao*. If a *yao* [illness] is accompanied by headache and swellings, together with [a feeling of] fullness, by coughing and retention of stools and urine, these, then, are concomitant pathoconditions of the *yao* illness.

If, however, a *yao* illness occurs simultaneously with *li* diarrhea of such a severity that it passes dozens of times [a day], then this cannot be called a concomitant pathocondition. It must be called a concomitant illness. *Yao* is one illness, and *li* diarrhea is an illness too, and both these illnesses have their respective basic pathoconditions and also their respective concomitant pathoconditions.

I cannot list all possibilities here one by one. [Further examples] can be inferred from [the two listed above]. Illnesses and pathoconditions may appear separate or combined in innumerable variations. Hence, it is essential to search for the beginning and to sort out the different ends.

And as far as therapeutic patterns are concerned, in some cases [different illnesses or pathoconditions] are to be treated jointly, while in others they are to be treated separately. Some must be treated first, and others must be treated later. Some must be treated alone [without any attention to others existing simultaneously], others should not be treated at all. And, if one takes care to investigate whether [an illness] is minor or whether it is serious, whether it is slow or whether it is fast, [one will be able to devise] successful [treatments] for each single [problem].

If, however, one acts contrary [to the requirements of the illness], and applies therapies that are confused and follow no rules, then the illness [treated] will appear in many new variations, and even a good practitioner will, in the end, not be able to restore [the patient's] health.

Note

1.   This term appears to have referred to illnesses that included malaria. See also V.13.

病同因別論

凡人之所苦謂之病所以致此病者謂之因如同一身

熱也有風有寒有痰有食有陰虛火升有鬱怒憂思勞

怯蟲疰此謂之因知其因則不得專以寒涼治熱病矣

益熱同而所以致熱者不同則藥亦迴異凡病之因不

同而治各別者蓋然則一病而治法多端矣而病又非

止一症必有兼症焉如身熱而腹痛則腹又為一症而

腹痛之因又復不同有與身熱相合者有與身熱各別

者如感寒而身熱其腹亦因寒而痛此相合者也如身

熱為寒其腹痛又為傷食則各別者也又必審其食為

何食則以何藥消之其立方之法必切中二者之病源

而後定方則一藥而兩病俱安矣若不問其本病之何

因及兼病之何因而徒曰某病以某方治之其偶中者

則投之或愈再以治他人則不但不愈而反增病必自

疑曰何以治彼效而治此不效并前此之何以愈亦不

知之則倖中者甚少而誤治者甚多終身治病而終身

不悟歷症愈多而愈惑矣

8. On Identical Illnesses Resulting from Different Causes

When a person suffers from [an ailment] this is called "illness." The reasons why this illness has emerged is called "cause." Now, identical body heat may be associated with wind or cold, with phlegm or food, with rising fire due to yin depletion, with depression and grief, with fatigue and fear, and with worms occupying [one's body]. All these are to be called causes. Once the cause [of the illness] is known, it will be inappropriate to merely use drugs with a cold or cool [thermo-influence] to treat [all] heat illnesses.

[Various patients may suffer from] identical heat but the reasons why this heat emerged are different. Hence, the drugs [employed to treat these patients must be] very different too. Whenever the causes of illness are different, the treatments employed must differ also. Therefore, one and the same illness may have to be treated in many different ways.

Also, an illness is accompanied not only by one [basic] pathocondition, it must be accompanied by concomitant pathoconditions too. Take, for example, the two pathoconditions hot body and abdominal pain. The abdominal [pain] is a pathocondition by itself, and may be the result of various causes. These [causes] may be identical with those responsible for the hot body, but it may also be that they have no relationship with those that caused the hot body. For example, if the body is hot because it was affected by cold, and if the abdomen aches because of this same cold, then this [is an example of one] identical [cause]. If, however, a hot body has resulted from cold, while the abdominal pain has resulted from harm caused by food, then this [is an example of] unrelated [causes].

Also, one must investigate, in the case of [harm caused by] food, which food [was responsible], and hence with which drugs it may be dissolved. The pattern underlying the prescription to be composed must be such that it hits both sources of [the patient's entire] illness. That is, the prescription must be composed in such a way that one single drug cures both illnesses.

If someone fails to inquire about the cause of the original illness, and about the cause of a concomitant illness, and if he simply states, "Such and such an illness is to be treated with such and such drugs," his [therapy] may hit [the illness] by chance, and the drugs tossed [into the patient] may indeed sometimes effect a cure. But, if he uses them again to treat people [seemingly suffering from an identical illness], it may well be that he not only fails to effect a cure but, contrary [to his expectations], adds to [the severity of] the illness.

Then he will become confused himself and ask: "How is it that a treatment of one [patient] was successful while the treatment [of the same illness with the same drugs] in another [patient] remained without success?" And, since he does not really know why the earlier case was cured in the first place, such lucky hits will remain few but mistaken therapies will occur often. That is, one treats illnesses for one's entire life without ever realizing [how to conduct a proper therapy], and the more pathoconditions one encounters, the more one will be confused.

亡陰亡陽論

經云奪血者無汗奪汗者無血血屬陰是汗多乃亡陰也故止汗之法必用涼心斂肺之藥何也心主血汗為心之液故當清心火汗必從皮毛出肺主皮毛故又當斂肺氣此正治也惟汗出太甚則陰氣上竭而腎中龍雷之火隨水而上若以寒涼折之其火愈熾惟用大劑參附佐以鹹降之品如童便牡礪之類冷飲一碗直達下焦引其真陽下降則龍雷之火反乎其位而汗隨止此與亡陰之汗真大相懸絕故亡陰亡陽其治法截然而轉機在頃刻當陽氣之未動也以陰藥止汗及陽氣之既動也以陽藥止汗而龍骨牡礪黃芪五味收澁之藥則兩方皆可隨宜用之醫者能於亡陰亡陽之交分其界限則用藥無誤矣其亡陰亡陽之辨法何如亡陰之汗身畏熱手足溫肌熱汗亦熱而味鹹口渴喜涼飲氣粗脈洪實此其驗也亡陽之汗身反惡寒手足冷肌涼汗冷而味淡微粘口不渴而喜熱飲氣微脈浮數而空此其驗也至于尋常之正汗熱汗邪汗自汗又不在二者之列此理知者絕少即此汗之一端而聚訟紛紛毫無定見誤治甚多也

9. On Losses of Yin and on Losses of Yang [Influences]

The Classic states, "When the blood is gone, there can be no sweat; when the sweat is gone, there can be no blood."[1] The blood belongs to the yin. If one sweats a lot, one loses yin [influences]. Consequently, any [therapeutic] method [employed] to stop sweating must make use of drugs that cool the heart and control the lung.

How is that? The heart masters the blood. Sweat is the liquid [produced by the] heart. Hence one should cool the fire of the heart. Sweat leaves [the body] through the skin and its hair. The lung masters the skin and its hair. Hence one must control the influences of the lung. That is a direct treatment.

However, [when] the sweat leaves [the body] profusely, the yin influences move upward [in the body] until they are exhausted. Accordingly, the fire of dragon and thunder[2] in the kidneys will follow the water, and move upward too. If one were to attempt to interrupt [this movement and the sweating] with cold or cooling [drugs], that [treatment] would only fan the fire. There is only [one possibility to treat such an illness correctly], and that is to employ large doses of *shen* and *fu,* and to add salty and descending substances for assistance — as, for instance, boy's urine or oyster shells. If one drinks one bowl [of these substances] — cold — they will proceed directly into the lower [section of the triple] burner and, thus, draw genuine yang [influences] to descend downward too. As a result, the fire of dragon and thunder will return to its [proper] position, and the sweating will come to an end.

This, though, is quite different from sweating accompanied by a loss of yin [influences]. Both in case of a loss of yin and in case of a loss of yang [influences], the therapeutic patterns [to be employed are] quite obvious, and [once they have been employed], the turning point [of such an illness follows] immediately. As long as no yang influences have been set in motion yet, one relies on yin drugs to stop the sweating. As soon as the yang influences move, one uses yang drugs to stop the sweating. Astringent and roughening drugs like dragon bones, oyster shells, *huang-ch'i,* or *wu-wei*[*-tzu*] may be added to both prescriptions, if called for.

A physician who is able to determine the borderline between a loss of yin [influences] and a loss of yang [influences] will not commit any errors in his application of the drugs. How, now, is it possible to distinguish between a loss of yin and loss of yang [influences]?

Sweating [that] is accompanied by a loss of yin [influences] can be verified as follows: the body fears heat, hands and feet are warm, the flesh is hot, and the sweat is hot too, and tastes salty. [The patient] is thirsty, and he longs for cooling drinks. His breathing goes rough; and the [movement in his] vessels is surging and replete.

Sweating accompanied by a loss of yang [influences] can be verified as follows: contrary [to a loss of yin influences], the body now hates cold. Hands and feet are cold. The flesh is cool, and the sweat is cold — it tastes neutral to slightly sticky. The [patient] is not thirsty and longs for hot drinks. His breathing is weak, and the [movement in his] vessels is at the surface, frequent, and empty.

Such common [phenomena] as ordinary sweating, sweating due to heat, sweating resulting from evil [influences], or sweating without apparent cause, have nothing to do with the two [conditions outlined above]. Only very few people, though, are aware of these principles, and all the discussions of the particular types of sweating [mentioned here] are quite confused. Nowhere does one find a definite [explanation. Not surprisingly,] many [patients suffering from sweating accompanied by a loss of yin or yang influences] are treated incorrectly.

Notes

1.   See *Ling-shu*, treatise 18, "Ying wei shen hui." Since blood and sweat originate from the same source, it is not advisable to induce sweating in a person who has already lost blood, and similarly it is not advisable to let blood from someone who has already been sweating.

2.   "The fire of dragon and thunder" refers to the fire of the kidneys, and also of the gate of life (said to be one of the two kidneys by some writers).

病有不愈不死雖愈必死論

能愈病之非難知病之必愈必不愈為難夫人之得病

非皆死症也庸醫治之非必皆與病相反也外感內傷

皆有現症約畧治之自能向愈況病情輕者雖不服藥

亦能漸痊即病勢危迫醫者苟無大誤邪氣漸退亦自

能向安故愈病非醫者之能事也惟不論輕重之疾一

見即能決其死生難易百無一失此則學問之極功而

非淺嘗者所能知也夫病輕而預知其愈病重而預知

其死此猶為易知者惟病象甚輕而能決其必死病勢

甚重而能斷其必生乃為難耳更有病已愈而不久必

死者益邪氣雖去而其人之元氣與病俱亡一時雖若

粗安真氣不可復續如兩虎相角其一雖勝而力已脫

盡雖良工亦不能救也又有病必不愈而人亦不死者

益邪氣盛而元氣堅固邪氣與元氣相併大攻則恐傷

其正小攻則病不為動如油入麪一合則不可復分而

又不至于傷生此二者皆人之所不知者也其大端則

病氣入藏府者病與人俱盡者為多病在經絡骨脈者

病與人俱存者為多此乃內外輕重之別也斯二者方

其病之始形必有可微之端良工知之自有防微之法

既不使之與病俱亡亦不使之終身不愈此非深通經

義之人必不能窮源極流挽回于人所不見之地也

10. On Illnesses That Do Not Lead to Death Even Though They Do Not Heal, and On Those That Lead to Death Even Though They Do Heal

It is by no means difficult to acquire an ability to cure illnesses, but it is difficult to know whether an illness will end in a cure or not. Not each and every illness befalling man is associated with fatal pathoconditions, and it is not so that common physicians[1] in their treatment always act contrary to [the requirements of] an illness.

When pathoconditions emerge as a result of affections from outside, or of harm from inside, they heal by themselves, even though one devotes [only] little attention to their treatment. This is even more true for minor illnesses; they may heal gradually even without any intake of drugs. Even in cases [where] the strength of the illness is quite dangerous, the evil influences will recede gradually, and a state of normalcy will return by itself, if the physician in charge does not commit too great a mistake. That is to say, whether [such] illnesses are cured has nothing to do with the competence of a physician.

However, if [a physician] is able to determine instantaneously — no matter whether an illness is minor or serious — whether [the patient] will die or survive, and whether [a cure is] difficult or easy, and if [his judgement] is correct in each single case, that is [to be considered] a great success of his learning. Those whose [scholarship] is but superficial, they will never have such knowledge.

For, if an illness is minor and one knows beforehand that it will heal, or if an illness is serious, and one knows beforehand that [the patient] will die, such knowledge is easy [to acquire]. However, when the appearance of an illness indicates that it is only a minor [problem], and if one is still able to determine that it must end in death, or when the strength of an illness is critical, and if one is still able to determine that [the patient] will survive, that is difficult.

Furthermore, there are illnesses that have been cured already and, nevertheless, before long will end in death, because the evil influences have left together with the illness. For a time everything appears normal, but the true influences cannot recover — just as in a fight between two tigers, one wins but has exhausted all his strength. Even a good practitioner could not be of help here. Also there are illnesses that cannot be cured, and, still, the patient will not die.

When evil influences are present in abundance, and when the original influences are strong, the evil influences and the original influences will merge with each other. If one were to carry out a major attack, it might well be that the [patient's] proper [influences] would be harmed too. If one were to carry out but a minor attack, the illness would remain unmoved. It is like oil poured into flour; once [the oil and flour] have merged, they cannot be separated again, but [the patient's] life will remain unharmed anyway. Nobody, however, knows of these two [possibilities].

Generally speaking, when the influences of an illness enter into the viscera and bowels, it often happens that the illness ends, and the [affected] person's [life] ends too. When the illness is in the conduits or the network [vessels] or in the bones or [blood] vessels, the illness will continue for long [periods], and the [affected] person's [life] will continue too. This, then, is the difference between [illness in the] interior and exterior [sections of the body and, hence, between those that are] minor and others that are serious.

At the very beginning, when an illness takes shape, there are definite clues [to its nature] that must be known to a good practitioner. Since he has methods at hand to ward off that which is as yet only weak, he does not allow [the patient] to perish together with his illness, and he is able to prevent [the illness] from remaining uncured for the rest of the [patient's] life. Only someone who has deeply penetrated the meaning of the Classics will be in a position to search the stream [of an illness] (all along) to its sources, and save [the patient] from death.

Notes

1.   "Common physician" is a derogatory term, sometimes translated as "quack." For the genesis of this term, see Paul U. Unschuld, *Medical Ethics in Imperial China,* Berkeley, Los Angeles, London: University of California Press, 1975.

2.   Lit.: "to save [him] from a land that man has not yet seen."

卒死論

天下卒死之人甚多其故不一內中可救者十之七八

不可救者僅十之二三惟一時不得良醫故皆枉死耳

夫人內外無病飲食行動如常而忽然死者其藏府經

絡本無受病之處卒然感犯外邪如惡風穢氣鬼邪毒

厲等物閉塞氣道一時不能轉動則大氣阻絕昏悶迷

惑久而不通則氣愈聚愈塞如繫繩于頸氣絕則死矣

若醫者能知其所犯何故以法治之通其氣驅其邪則

立愈矣又有痰涎壅盛阻遏氣道而卒死者通氣降痰

則甦所謂痰厥之類是也以前諸項良醫皆能治之惟

藏絕之症則不治其人或勞心思慮或酒食不節或房

慾過度或惱怒不常五藏之內精竭神衰惟一線真元

未斷行動如常偶有感觸其元氣一時斷絕氣脫神離

頃刻而死既不可救又不及救此則卒死之最急而不

可治者也至於暴遇神鬼適逢寃譴此又怪異之非不

在疾病之類矣

126

11. On Sudden Death

Many people on earth succumb to sudden death, and there are various reasons for this. Seven or eight out of ten could be saved; only two or three cannot be saved. However, [those who could be saved] die a needless death when they are not immediately attended by a good physician.

[Consider the following situation.] A person with neither an internal nor an external illness, who drinks and eats and carries out his daily activies as normal, dies suddenly. His viscera and bowels, and his conduits and network [vessels], may not have harbored an illness anywhere, and suddenly he is affected by some external evil, as for instance, malign wind, foul influences, demonic evil, or [some other] terrible poison that closes the passageways of his influences. At this moment [the influences] cannot move [through the body], and the vital influences are blocked [in their flow]. The patient feels dizzy and experiences pressure on his chest, and is confused. When the influences are blocked for a long time, the more they stagnate, the more they block [their own passageways]. It is as if a rope were tied around the [patient's] neck. When [the flow of his] breath is cut off, he dies.

If a physician discovers what has caused the attack, and if he treats the [patient] according to a [proper] method, letting [the patient's] influences pass through [the body again], and expelling the evil, then [the patient] will be cured immediately.

It may also be that people die a sudden death because accumulations of phlegm and saliva block the passageways of their influences. They will be brought back to life only if the phlegm is made to descend, and if the passage of their influences can be opened once again. Such cases belong to [the category of] so-called "ceasing [influences due to blockages caused by] phlegm."

All the cases [of sudden death] listed above can be treated successfully by a good physician. Only when the pathocondition of "cut off viscera" emerges is no cure possible. In persons [manifesting this pathocondition] the essence is exhausted and the spirit is weakened in their five viscera because they have tired their heart with excessive pondering, or because of intemperate consumption of alcohol and food, or because of unrestrained sexual intercourse, or because of extreme anger. Only one [last] thread of original influences has not yet been cut.

[These people] continue their daily activities as usual until, suddenly, they are struck. The [remaining thread of their] original influences is cut off immediately. They lose their influences, and their spirit departs. Within but a short moment they die. They cannot be helped, and no help could come in time — these are the fastest cases of sudden death. They cannot be treated successfully.

As for sudden encounters with spirits and demons, or when someone is unexpectedly scolded [by a ghost] suffering from a wrong that has not been righted, these are occurrences of a strange nature. They do not belong to the categories of illness and disease.

病有鬼神論

人之受邪也必有受之之處有以名之則應者斯至矣
夫人精神完固則外邪不敢犯惟其所以禦之之具有
虧則侮之者斯集凡疾病有為鬼神所憑者其愚魯者
以為鬼神實能禍人其明理者以為病情如此必無鬼
神二者皆非也夫鬼神猶風寒暑濕之邪耳衛氣虛則
受寒營氣虛則受熱神氣虛則受鬼益人之神屬陽陽
衰則鬼憑之內經有五藏之病則現五色之鬼難經云
脫陽者見鬼故經穴中有鬼床鬼室等穴此諸穴者皆
賴神氣以充塞之若神氣有虧則鬼神得而憑之猶之
風寒之能傷人也故治寒者壯其陽治熱者養其陰治
鬼者充其神而已其或有因痰因驚者則當求其
本而治之故明理之士必事事窮其故乃能無所惑而
有據否則執一端之見而昧事理之實均屬憒憒矣其

外更有觸犯鬼神之病則祈禱可愈至於冤譴之鬼則
有數端有自作之孽深仇不可解者有祖宗貽累者有
過誤害人者其事皆鑿鑿可徵似儒者所不道然見于
經史如公子彭生伯有之類甚多目覩者亦不少此則
非藥石祈禱所能免矣

12. On the Causation of Illness by Demon-Spirits

When a person has evil [influences in his body], there must be a place where they are granted entrance. [These evil influences] have gone there because they responded to a summons! As long as a person's essence and spirits are complete and strong, no external evil will dare to offend [that person]. If, however, those agents that are responsible for warding off [evil intruders] fail to do so, those [intruders] attacking them will gather in their place. Whenever demon-spirits have taken advantage of an illness, ignorant [people] believe that demon-spirits are actually able to harm man, while those who understand the principles [of nature] believe that such illnesses have definitely nothing to do with demon-spirits. Both are equally wrong.

Demon-spirits are comparable to such evils as wind, cold, heat and dampness. When the protective influences are depleted, one absorbs cold. When the constructive influences are depleted, one absorbs heat. When one's spirit-influences are depleted, one absorbs demons. Man's spirits belong to [the category of] yang. When one's yang [influences] are weak, demons avail themselves of [their place].

The *Nei-ching* has [a passage stating that] in case of illness in the five viscera, demons appear in the [respective] five colors.[1] The *Nan-ching* states, "When the yang [influences] have left, one sees demons."[2] Hence among the holes[3] on the conduits there are some bearing such [names as]: "demons' bed" and "demons' dwelling." All these holes depend on [man's] spirit influences to be closed and filled.

Once there is a deficiency of spirit influences, the demon-spirits will be able to avail themselves [of the position of the spirit influences]. That may be compared to the harm caused to man by wind or cold. In treating cases of cold, one strengthens the respective [patient's] yang [influences]. In treating cases of heat, one nourishes the respective [patient's] yin [influences]. In treating cases of demon [intrusion], one simply has to fill the respective [patient's] spirits.

In cases where [an illness] is caused by phlegm or by pondering or by someone's being terrified, one must search for the origin [of the affliction] and then treat it. Hence those scholars who understand the principles [of life] will take all circumstances into account and conduct a thorough investigation of the cause of a particular [illness]. Only then can they eliminate all doubt and have evidence [at hand]. To those who fail to [conduct such thorough investigations], and who stick to a one-sided perspective, the reality of the facts and principles involved will remain obscure. Their [efforts] will end in confusion in every respect.

In addition [to what I have presented so far], there are illnesses [resulting from one's having] offended demon-spirits. [Such illnesses] can be cured by prayers. Furthermore, there are numerous reasons for demons [to seek revenge for] some wrong [they had been subjected to while they were still humans.] Patients succumbing to illnesses caused by these demons may have brought their misfortune upon themselves [by creating a] hatred so deep [in someone who is a demon now] that it cannot be dissolved. In other cases, [the original offense] may have been tied to [the patient's] ancestors, and it may also be that one has inadvertently caused harm to someone else [who now seeks revenge as a demon]. For all such occurrences indisputable proof exists.

It seems, though, as if the Confucians did not speak about this! However, both in the [Confucian] classics and in historic records one can see very many examples, such as those of Kung-tzu P'eng-sheng[4] and Po Yu.[5] Also, [I myself have] witnessed not a few such [occurrences] with [my own] eyes. These [demons are out for nothing but revenge]; they can be expelled neither by [herbal] drugs and mineral [drugs], nor by prayers.

Notes

1.   In chapter 12 of his *Lei-ching,* commenting on the concept of *chu-yu* ("exorcising the cause"), Chang Chieh-pin (fl. 1624) refers to a *Su-wen* treatise entitled "Tz'u fa lun" ("On Methods of Needling") as a source of the statement quoted here by Hsü Ta-ch'un. The "Tz'u fa lun" is no longer extant.

2.   See Paul U. Unschuld, *Nan-ching: The Classic of Difficult Issues,* Berkeley, Los Angeles, London: University of California Press, 1978, p. 268 ("The Twentieth Difficult Issue").

3.   "Hole" is a literal translation of the term used for points to be needled in acupuncture; it is mostly translated as "insertion point" today. Here, though, the ancient meaning appears more suitable.

4.   Kung-tzu P'eng-sheng refers to a pig-shaped demon whose appearance was described in the *Annals of the Spring and Autumn Period (Ch'un ch'iu Tso-shi Chuan).*

5.   Po Yu is another name of Liang Hsiao who was killed by Ssu Tai and returned as a demon to take revenge. This story is also recounted in the *Annals of the Spring and Autumn Period.*

腎虛非陰症論

今之醫者以其人房勞之後或遺精之後感冒風寒而
發熱者謂之陰症病者遇此亦自謂之陰症不問其現
症何如總用參术附桂乾姜地黃等溫熱峻補之藥此
可稱絕倒者也夫所謂陰症者寒邪中於三陰經也房
後感風豈風寒必中腎經即使中之亦不過散少陰之
風寒如傷寒論中少陰發熱仍用麻黃細辛發表而已
豈有用辛熱溫補之法耶若用溫補則補其風寒于腎
中矣況陰虛之人而感風寒亦必由太陽入仍屬陽邪
其熱必甚焦以燥悶煩渴尤宜清熱散邪豈可反用熱
藥若果直中三陰則斷無壯熱之理必有惡寒倦卧厥
冷喜熱等症方可用溫散然亦終無用滋補之法即如
傷寒差後房事不慎又發寒熱謂之女勞復此乃久虛
之人復患大症依今人之見尤宜峻補者也而古人治

之用竹皮一升煎湯服然則無病而房後感風更不宜
用熱補矣故凡治病之法總視目前之現證現脈如果
六脈沉遲表裏皆畏寒的係三陰之寒證即使其本領
強壯又絕慾十年亦從陰治若使所現脈證的係陽邪
發熱煩渴並無三陰之症即使其人本體虛弱又復房
勞過度亦從陽治如傷寒論中陽明大熱之證宜用葛
根白虎等方者瞬息之間轉入三陰即改用溫補若陰
症轉陽症亦即用涼散此一定之法也近世唯喻嘉言
先生能知此義有寓意草中黃長人之傷寒案可見餘
人皆不知之其殺人可勝道哉

13. On Depletions in the Kidneys That Are Not Associated with Yin Pathoconditions

When someone who has exhausted himself sexually, or who has lost [seminal] essence [through nocturnal emissions], is then struck by wind or cold and develops heat, today's physicians speak of a yin pathocondition. Even patients themselves, when being confronted with such [a problem], speak of a yin pathocondition; and no matter what kind of pathocondition appears, they always use warm or hot drugs with rapidly supplementing [abilities], such as *shen, shu, fu, kuei,* or dried ginger, or *ti huang*. One may well say that [such treatments] are completely wrong.

Now, the term yin pathocondition [refers to the situation that results] when any of the three yin conduits was struck by a cold evil. But, if someone is affected by wind subsequent to sexual intercourse, why should this wind, or cold, have no choice but to strike [that person's] renal conduit? And if [the renal conduit] were struck, indeed, then [this could only be the result of] wind and/or cold spreading through the minor-yin [conduit].

Take, for example, the *Shang-han Lun,* which in case of heat developing from the minor-yin (region) nevertheless recommends only *ma-huang* and *hsi-hsin* to disperse [the evil]. How could a pattern [be correct that] uses acrid, hot, warm, and supplementing [drugs]? If one were to use warm and supplementing [drugs in such a case], one would merely supplement the wind and cold in the kidneys. Also, when someone who already suffers from a depletion of yin [influences] is then affected by wind and cold, [this wind and cold] must enter through the great-yang [conduit], and, therefore, is a yang evil. The [resulting] heat will be extreme, and will be accompanied by dryness and chest-pressure, by a feeling of uneasiness, and by thirst. Here in particular the only suitable [therapy] is to cool the heat and to dissipate the evil [influences]. How could anyone use hot drugs here — that would be contrary [to what is required]!

Even if [the evil] had struck [any of] the three yin [conduits] directly, there would still be no reason for excessive heat. Only if such pathoconditions as aversion to cold, tiredness, and [a desire to] lie down, ceasing [yin influences with] cold [extremities], and a longing for heat emerge, is it appropriate to use warming and dissipating therapeutic patterns — but never nourishing and supplementing [drugs]!

If someone who was only recently cured of a harm caused by cold is not cautious about his sexual activities and develops fits of cold and heat, this is called "recurrence due to fatigue [through sexual intercourse] with females." In this case, someone who had already experienced a depletion for a long time, again suffers from a severe pathocondition. In the view of people of today, it is advisable to apply rapidly supplementing drugs [in such situations]. In ancient times, though, the people treated [such a condition] with one pint of bamboo bark, which was consumed as a decoction.

However, if someone had not been ill before and was affected by wind following sexual intercourse, it is even less justified to employ anything hot or supplementing. Hence, whenever [one is about to employ] a therapeutic pattern against an illness, one should always [carefully] inspect currently apparent symptoms and the current [movement in the] vessels.

If the six vessels [are filled by a movement that is] deep and slow, and if both one's exterior and interior regions fear cold, these are definitely symptoms of cold [affecting the] three yin [regions]. And even if [such a patient] has a strong and vigorous constitution, and even if he has already refrained from sexual intercourse for ten years, his treatment must still focus on his yin [conduits and viscera].

If, however, the [movement in the] vessels and [other] apparent symptoms [signal that] it is a genuine yang evil with heat developing, with a feeling of uneasiness, as well as with thirst — that is, he has definitely no pathoconditions related to the three yin [conduits and viscera] — then the treatment must focus on the yang [conduits and viscera] even if the [patient's] body is depleted and weak, and even though he may have exhausted himself with excessive sexual intercourse.

Take, for instance, [the therapy recommended] in the *Shang-han Lun* for great heat in the yang-brilliance [region]. Here it is advisable to employ prescriptions containing *ke* root or *pai-hu*. But in the twinkling of an eye, [such an illness] may be transmitted into the three yin [conduits and viscera], and [become] different [from before]. [Now] one must use warming and supplementing [drugs].

Similarly, if yin pathoconditions turn into yang pathoconditions, one uses cooling and dissipating [drugs]. These are firmly established patterns. Nowadays, only Mr. Yü Chia-yen[1] knows that this is the only correct way [to treat such problems], as one may well see from the case of an adult named Huang, who suffered from harm caused by cold, [that is recorded in his book] *Yü I Ts'ao*. No one else knows of this, and the [number of] people who have been killed [this way] is beyond the power of expression.

Note

1.   Yü Ch'ang, style-name Chia-yen, was a famous physician, as well as medical writer and teacher, in the middle of the 17th century. Among other books, he published in 1643 a collection and discussion of difficult cases under the title of *Yü I Ts'ao*.

吐血不死咳嗽必死論

今之醫者謂吐血為虛勞之病此大謬也夫吐血有數種大概咳者成勞不咳者不成勞間有吐時偶咳者當其吐血之時猖獗頗甚吐血止即痊皆不成勞何也其吐血一止則週身無病飲食如故而精神生矣即使亡血之後或陰虛內熱或筋骨疼痛皆可服藥而痊若咳嗽則血止而病仍在日嗽夜嗽痰壅氣升多則三年少則一年而死矣益咳嗽不止則腎中之元氣震盪不寧肺為腎之母母病則子亦病故也又肺為五藏之華蓋經云穀氣入胃以傳于肺五藏六府皆以受氣其清者為營濁者為衛是則藏府皆取精于肺肺病則不能輸精于藏府一年而藏府皆枯三年而藏府竭矣故咳嗽為真勞不治之疾也然亦有咳嗽而不死者其嗽亦有時稍緩其飲食起居不甚變又其人善于調攝延至三年之後起居如舊間或一發靜養即愈此乃百中難得一者也更有不咳之人血症屢發肝竭肺傷亦變咳嗽久而亦死此則不善調攝以輕變重也執此以決血症之死生百不一失矣

14. On Blood Spitting That Does Not Result in Death and on Coughing That Must End in Death

Today's physicians call blood spitting an illness associated with depletion and fatigue. That is a great error! There are many types of blood spitting, and in general, it is such that [if blood spitting is accompanied by] coughing, it will generate fatigue, but if it is not accompanied by coughing, no fatigue will result.

In some cases it is just accidental that one coughs while one spits [blood]. At the moment one spits blood, one tends to panic, but once the [blood] spitting stops the patient feels well, and there is no fatigue. How can that be? As soon as the blood spitting stops, the body is entirely free of any illness. One's consumption of beverages and food is normal, and one's essence and spirit grow again.

If, after a loss of blood [through spitting], a depletion of yin [influences] occurs together with internal heat, or if one's sinews and bones ache, that can be cured by means of drugs. [In contrast, when someone suffers from] coughing, his blood [spitting] may stop, but the illness nevertheless remains. The coughing continues day and night; phlegm blockages emerge and influences rise. Most [patients] die within one to three years.

The reason [for these deaths] is that when the coughing does not stop, the original influences in the kidneys are severely shaken and cannot calm down. The lung is the mother of the kidneys, and when a mother is sick, the child will also be sick. Also, the lung covers the five viscera like a canopy. The Classic states, "The influences of the grains enter into the stomach, whence they are transmitted into the lung; and all the five viscera and six bowels are supplied with influences from the [lung]. The clear portions of the [influences of the grains] turn into constructive [influences], the turbid portions turn into protective [influences]."[1] That is to say, all the viscera and bowels get their essence from the lung. When the lung has an illness, it is unable to transport essence to the [other] viscera and bowels. Within one year, all viscera and bowels are dried up. Within three years all the viscera and bowels are exhausted. Coughing, therefore, is an illness associated with genuine fatigue; it cannot be treated.

There are some cases of coughing, though, which do not result in death. Sometimes, a [patient's] coughing may be rather weak, and his eating and drinking, as well as his daily activities and his periods of rest, may not be too different from normal. And, if this person knows well how to care for his recovery, after three years his daily activities will be as before [his illness]. If [the coughing] breaks out again, once in a while, he must only rest and nourish [his body], and [the illness] will be healed. Such [cases], though, are one in one hundred.

Also, there are persons who do not cough, but who have frequent outbreaks of blood [spitting] pathoconditions. When their liver is exhausted, and when their lung is harmed, their [illness] will also turn into [permanent] coughing, and after a while, they too will die. These are cases where [the patients or their physicians] do not know well how to care for a recovery, and, as a result, minor [problems] turn into serious [crises].

If one keeps all this [in mind], one will not be lose one out of a hundred [patients], when one has to determine whether [a patient with a] blood [spitting] pathocondition must die or will survive.

Note

1.   See *Ling-shu,* treatise 18, "Ying wei sheng hui."

胎產論

婦科之最重者二端墮胎與難產耳世之治墮胎者往往純用滋補治難產者往往專於攻下二者皆非也蓋半產之故非一端由于虛滑者十之一二由于內熱者十之八九蓋胎惟賴血以養故得胎之後經事不行者因衝任之血皆為胎所吸無餘血下行也苟由內熱火則胎枯竭而下墮矣其血所以不足之故皆由內熱火盛陽旺而陰虧也故古人養胎之方專以黃芩為主又血之生必由于脾胃經云營衛之道納穀為寶故又以白朮佐之乃世之人專以參芪補氣熟地滯胃氣旺則火盛胃濕則不運生化之源衰而血益少矣至于產育之事乃天地化育之常本無危險之理險者千不得一世之遭厄難者乃人事之未工也其法在乎產婦不可令早用力蓋胎必轉而後下早用力則胎先下墜斷難舒轉于是橫生倒產之害生又用力則胞漿驟下胎已枯澀何由能產此病不但產子之家不知即收生穩婆亦有不知者至于用藥之法則交骨不開胎元不轉種種諸症各有專方其外或宜潤或宜降或宜溫或宜涼亦當隨症施治其大端以養血為主蓋血足則諸症自退也至于易產強健之產婦最多卒死蓋大脫血之後衝任空虛經脉嬌脆健婦不以為意輕舉妄動用力稍重衝脉斷裂氣冒血崩死在頃刻先忌舉手上頭如是死者吾見極多不知者以為奇異實理之常生產之家不可不知也

15. On [the] Fetus and Birth

The two major concerns of gynecology are miscarriage and difficult birth. Today, mostly nourishing and supplementing [drugs] are used to treat [women who are about to have a] miscarriage, while attacking and downward pushing [drugs are given] to treat difficult births. Both of these [approaches] are wrong. The reason is that premature births may have various causes. One or two [such cases] out of ten may [indeed] be such that [the fetus] slides down because of some depletion [of influences in its mother]. Eight or nine [miscarriages out of ten, however], result from internal heat.

A fetus depends entirely on [maternal] blood for nourishment. When, therefore, menstruation stops during pregnancy, that is because all the blood from the throughway and controller [vessels] is absorbed by the fetus, and there is no surplus of blood that could pass down. If the available blood is insufficient, the fetus will dry out and be lost.

Insufficiencies of blood always result from internal heat and blazing fire, [that is to say, from] a prospering of yang and a dearth of yin [influences]. Hence in ancient times the people relied most of all on *huang-ch'in* in their prescriptions designed to nourish the fetus. Also, the generation of [additional] blood must start from the spleen and stomach. The Classic states, "For the passage of the constructive and of the protective [influences], the intake of grains is most valuable."[1] Hence [they gave the drug] *pai-chu* to assist [*huang-ch'in*]. Today, however, the people supplement the [patient's yang] influences with *shen* and *ch'i*, and they moisten the [patient's] stomach with *shou-ti*. When the [yang] influences prosper, the fire [in the body] will blaze; and when the stomach is moist, it cannot move [its influences] further on. Given this weakening of the source of all life and transformation, the amount of blood [available in the body] decreases continuously.

Births are part of the normal processes of transformation and creation in heaven and on earth. There is no reason why [births] should be dangerous. Not even one [delivery] in a thousand is critical. When people today are confronted with critical and difficult [births], it is because they do not know how to handle [deliveries].

The correct way to behave for a woman giving birth [to a child] is to not use force too early. The fetus must turn around first before it moves down. If [the woman] uses force too early, and the fetus is pushed down prior [to the proper moment], it will have great difficulty stretching and turning around, and the danger arises that it will be a transverse or inverted presentation. Also, if [the woman] uses force [too early], the uterine liquid rushes down, and the fetus dries up. How could it [be] delivered?

These [possibilities of] illness are unknown not only to the households of those who give birth to children, but also to some of the midwives. As for patterns of an [appropriate] drug therapy, special prescriptions exist for all pathoconditions such as failure of the interlocking bones[2] to part, or failure of the fetus to turn around. Furthermore, one must design one's treatment in accordance with whatever pathoconditions are present. Sometimes it is advisable to moisten, or it may be advisable to push down, or it may be advisable to supply warmth, or it may be advisable to cool. Generally speaking, it is most important to nourish the blood. When enough blood is available, all pathoconditions will recede by themselves.

Women who are strong and healthy and give birth [to children] easily often die a sudden death, because, after having lost large amounts of blood, when the throughway and controller vessels are depleted, and when the [movement in the] conduit-vessels is but frail and delicate, healthy women do not pay any attention [to their condition]. They move around at will, but when they overtax their strength only a little, their throughway vessel will rupture. They faint, and blood will rush down. Death follows instantaneously.

[Women] should particularly avoid raising their hands above their head. I have seen very many who died for this reason. Those who do not know of this consider [such deaths] to be strange, while in fact, [they result but from] normal principles. Anybody who is about to give birth must be aware of this.

Notes

1.   This is the opening line of treatise 16, "Ying ch'i," of the *Ling-shu*. The original text, though, speaks only of constructive, not protective, influences.

2.   The pubic bone was called *chiao-ku*, "interlocking bones," in ancient Chinese medicine, and it was believed that these "interlocking bones" would part at the moment of delivery to allow the fetus to pass.

病有不必服藥論

天下之病竟有不宜服藥者如黃疸之類是也黃疸之
症仲景原有煎方然輕者用之俱效而重者俱不效何
也蓋疸之重者其脇中有囊以裹黃水其囊並無出路
藥祇在囊外不入囊中所服之藥非補邪即傷正故反
有害若輕病則囊尚未成服藥有效至囊成之後則百
無一效必須用輕透之方或破其囊或消其水另有秘
方傳授非泛然煎丸之所能治也痰飲之病亦有囊常
藥亦不能愈外此如吐血久痞等疾得藥之益者甚少
受藥誤者甚多如無至穩必效之方不過以身試藥則
寧以不服藥為中醫矣

16. On Illnesses that do not Require an Intake of Drugs

Among the illnesses are indeed some where the intake of drugs is contraindicated. One example is jaundice. Decoction recipes against the pathoconditions of jaundice were already recorded by [Chang] Chung-ching. However, even though [prescriptions] are always effective when used against minor cases, they remain without effect when used against serious cases. How is that?

Well, in the case of serious jaundice, a bag containing yellow water is located in one's flanks. This bag has absolutely no opening. Drugs can reach only the outside of this bag, but they cannot enter it. Therefore, if the drugs that [one consumes for a serious case of jaundice] do not add to the evil [influences already present], they will [at least] harm [the patient's] proper [influences], and contrary [to one's intentions, the treatment will result in further] injury.

In minor cases of this illness, the bag is not yet complete, and an intake of drugs shows positive effects. Once the bag is complete, not a single [prescription] in a hundred will be effective. [In such cases] one must make use of light and penetrating prescriptions that either break the bag or drain the water from it. For this purpose secret prescriptions exist in addtion [to normal formulas] that have been handed down [through generations] and are able to cure what ordinary decoctions and pills are not able to [cure].

The illness of phlegm-fluid[1] is related to a bag too, and, like [jaundice], cannot be cured by ordinary drugs. Furthermore, only a few [people who suffer from] such illnesses as blood spitting and long-term constipation receive benefits from an intake of drugs, but many [are harmed because a] mistaken pharmacotherapy was applied to them.

If no very secure and definitely effective prescriptions exist, and if one is but to test drugs with one's own body, then one should rather [recall the fact that] taking no drugs at all is [at least as effective as a treatment conducted by a] mediocre physician.

Note

1.   "Phlegm-fluid" refers to the pathological stagnation of fluids.

IV. Prescriptions and Drugs

方藥合論

方之與藥似合而實離也得天地之氣成一物之性各
有功能可以變易血氣以除疾病此藥之力也然草木
之性與人殊體人人腸胃何以能如人之所欲以致其
效聖人為之製方以調劑之或用以專攻或用以兼治
或相輔者或相反者或相用者或相制者故方之既成
能使藥各全其性亦能使藥各失其性操縱之法有大
權焉此方之妙也若夫按病用藥藥雖切中而立方無
法謂之有藥無方或守一方以治病方雖良善而其藥
有一二味與病不相關者謂之有方無藥譬之作書之
法用筆已工而配合顛倒與夫字形俱備而點畫不成
者皆不得謂之能書故善醫者分觀之而無藥弗切于
病情合觀之而無方不本于古法然後用而弗效則病
之故也非醫之罪也而不然者即偶或取效隱害必多

則亦同于殺人而已矣至于方之大小奇偶之法則内
經詳言之兹不復贅云

1. On the Separation and Combination of Drugs in Prescriptions

It looks as if prescriptions and drugs form an entity, while, in fact, they [should be seen] separately! Any substance that is endowed with the influences of heaven and earth has a particular nature and, hence, a particular ability. It may be able to transform and change the blood or the influences to eliminate illness. This, then, is the strength of a drug. However, the natures of herbs and trees are different from [the nature of] man. How, then, is it possible to have them act according to human will, and manifest their effects when they enter man's intestines and stomach?

The Sages composed [individual drugs] into prescriptions to moderate [their specific effects in accordance with specific therapeutic goals]. Some [of these prescriptions] were used to carry out specific attacks. Others were used to treat various [illnesses or pathoconditions] simultaneously.

Some [drugs] supported each other, others were directly opposed to each other. Some [drugs] made use of each other, others restrained each other. Hence, when they composed a prescription, [the Sages] were able to assure that each drug could fully realize its nature, and they were also able to create a situation where each drug lost its [original] nature. The patterns of controlling [drug effects] were of great importance in those times, hence the prescriptions [in ancient times] were so effective.

If one uses drugs in accordance with [the requirements of] an illness, it may be that the drugs [are well suited to] hit the illness directly. If, however, the composition of the prescription did not follow a [proper] method, this is called "drugs without a prescription." Or, one may hold on to a prescription in one's treatment of an illness. The prescription may be quite good. If, however, it contains but one or two drugs that have nothing to do with the [particular illness to be treated], that is called "a prescription without drugs."

One may compare this to calligraphy. Someone may already be quite an expert in using the brush, but his composition [of characters] is unbalanced; or the form of the characters is complete, but the individual strokes are not accomplished. In all these cases one could not state that [this person] was an able calligrapher.

An expert in medicine, therefore, considers all the drugs individually and [makes sure that] all drugs correspond to the nature of the illness [to be treated]; and he considers [the drugs] in combination [to make sure that] all his prescriptions are based on ancient patterns. If their subsequent application remains without positive results, the illness is the reason and

147

not some wrong committed by the physician. Otherwise one may still produce some accidental successes, but in many cases hidden harm results — and this is nothing but homicide!

The patterns of large and small prescriptions, and those of odd and even [number of ingredients], are outlined in the *Nei-ching* in great detail, and need not be repeated here.

古方加減論

古人製方之義微妙精詳不可思議益其審察病情辨

別經絡終考藥性斟酌輕重其於所治之病不爽毫髮

故不必有奇品異術而沈痼艱險之疾病不輒有神效

此漢以前之方也但生民之疾病不可勝窮若必每病

製一方是曷有盡期乎故古人即有加減之法其病大

端相同而所現之症或不同則不必更立一方即於是

方之內因其現症之異而為之加減如傷寒論中治太

陽病用桂枝湯若見項背強者則用桂枝加葛根湯喘

者則用桂枝加厚朴杏子湯下後脈促胸滿者桂枝去

白芍湯更惡寒者去白芍加附子湯此猶以藥為加減

者也若桂枝麻黃各半湯則以兩方為加減矣若發奔

豚者用桂枝為加桂枝湯則又以藥之輕重為加減矣

然一二味加減雖不易本方之名而必名著其加減之

藥若桂枝湯倍用芍藥而加飴糖則又不名桂枝加飴

糖湯而為建中湯其藥雖同而義已別則立名亦異古

法之嚴如此後之醫者不識此義而又欲托名用古取

古方中一二味則即以某方目之如用柴胡則即曰小

柴胡湯不知小柴胡之力全在人參也用豬苓澤瀉即

曰五苓散不知五苓之妙專在桂枝也去其要藥雜以

他藥而仍以某方目之用而不效不知自咎或則歸咎

於病或則歸咎於藥以為古方不可治今病嗟乎即使

果識其病而用古方支離零亂豈有效乎遂相戒以為

古方難用不知全失古方之精義故與病毫無益而反

有害也然則當何如曰能識病情與古方合者則全用

之有別症則據古法加減之如不盡合則依古方之法

將古方所用之藥而去取損益之必使無一藥之不對

症自然不倍於古人之法而所投必有神效矣

2.   On Increasing and Reducing [the Number of Drugs in] Ancient Prescriptions

When the people in ancient times composed a prescription, the underlying rationale was both sophisticated and subtle to a degree that is inconceiveable [today]. The way they examined the nature of an illness, differentiated between the conduits and network vessels, took the special characteristics of each drug into account, and calculated the amount [of each drug in a prescription] prevented them, in their treatment of illnesses, from committing even the slightest mistake.

Hence there was no need whatsoever to have recourse to strange substances and to weird techniques, and yet, by taking their [drugs] the [people in ancient times] achieved immediate and miraculous successes even in cases of deep-seated and chronic [illness], as well as difficult and dangerous illnesses.

Such were the prescriptions during Han times and earlier. However, the illnesses befalling mankind are innumerable, and how could anyone have sufficient time to compose a [specific] prescription for each single illness? It is for this reason that the people of ancient times resorted to the method of increasing and reducing [the ingredients of certain standard prescriptions].

Illnesses may be basically identical, but the pathoconditions accompanying them may vary. In such cases, it is not necessary to compose separate prescriptions. Rather, one increases or reduces [the number of drugs] in a particular prescription in accordance with the different pathoconditions that have become apparent. For example, the *Shang-han Lun* [suggests] using a [prescription called] "Decoction with *kuei-chih*" for treatment of illnesses affecting the great-yang [regions]. If it appears [that in the course of such an illness the patient's] neck and back are stiff, [the *Shang-han Lun* suggests the] use of a [prescription called] "Decoction with *kuei-chih* amended by *ke* root."

In case [someone who suffers from an illness affecting the great-yang regions] pants, [the *Shang-han Lun* suggests the] use of a [prescription called] "Decoction with *kuei-chih* amended by *hou-p'u* and *hsing-tzu*."

In case the [movement in the patient's] vessels is urgent and [a feeling of] fullness occurs in the chest after [the patient] has passed [stools, the *Shang-han Lun* recommends the use of a prescription called] "Decoction with *kuei-chih* without *pai-shao*[-*yao*]." If, in addition, [the patient] has an aversion to cold, [the *Shang-han Lun* recommends the] use [of a prescription called] "Decoction with *kuei-chih*] without *pai-shao*[-*yao*] but amended by *fu-tzu.*" These are [examples of how the] drugs [in a prescription were] increased or reduced [in the *Shang-han Lun*].

The "Decoction with half-half *kuei-chih* and *ma-huang*" [of the *Shang-han Lun* is, on the other hand, an example of how drugs were] increased or reduced by combining two prescriptions.

If [a patient] develops the running piglet [pathocondition,[1] the *Shang-han Lun* recommends] an application of the "Decoction with *kuei-chih* amended by *kuei-chih*." This is [an example of how] the amount of one particular drug was increased or reduced [in a prescription].

Now, as long as but one or two substances are added or taken away from [a prescription], the name of the basic prescription does not change, but one must specify, in the name, which drugs were added and which were taken away. A *kuei-chih* decoction, though, which makes use of a doubled amount of *shao-yao* and to which was added *i-t'ang*, is no longer called "Decoction with *kuei-chih* amended by *i-t'ang*." It is [called] "Decoction to fortify the center" because, even though the drugs are [mostly] identical, the [therapeutic] rationale is different, and, hence, a different name has to be established as well. The ancient patterns were that strict! Since then, though, physicians are no longer aware of such principles, and yet they prefer to infringe on the names of the ancients and make use of their [prescriptions]. They take one or two substances from an ancient prescription, and retain the name of that prescription. For instance, when they apply [just] *ch'ai-hu,* they still call this "Minor decoction with *chai-hu*" without realizing that the strength of "Minor decoction with *ch'ai-hu*" [as composed in the *Shang-han Lun*] is entirely dependent on [the fact that this prescription also contains] *jen-shen.*

Or, they apply *chu-ling* and *tse-hsieh,* and call this "Powder with *wu-ling,*" not knowing that the surprising effects of the "Powder with *wu-ling*" [recommended in the *Shang-han lun*, result] in particular from [the fact that it includes] *kuei-chih* [too. In recent times, physicians] discarded the important drugs, added some other drugs, and still named [these compositions] after a specific [ancient] prescription.

When an application shows no positive effects, they fail to realize that they only have themselves to blame. Sometimes they blame the illness, sometimes they blame the drugs, and they conclude that ancient prescriptions are inappropriate for today's illnesses.[2] Alas! Even though they know the illness, how could they achieve any therapeutic success given their heterodox and unsystematic application of ancient prescriptions?

As a result, [physicians of recent times] warn each other and believe that the application of ancient prescriptions is difficult, while, in fact, they simply do not know that they no longer have access to the subtle rationale underlying these ancient prescriptions. Hence [when they apply such prescriptions], they not only fail to benefit the patient, they even cause harm!

How, then, should one proceed?! If one concludes that the nature of an illness and an ancient prescription correspond to one another, then one should use [this ancient prescription] unchanged. If secondary pathoconditions appear, one increases or reduces [the number of drugs in the prescription] in accordance with ancient patterns. If [the illness and prescription] do not correspond to each other entirely, one takes drugs that were already used in ancient prescriptions, and exchanges, again according to the methods underlying the ancient prescriptions, one for another. This will result [in a situation where] not a single drug remains that is not directly opposed to any of the pathoconditions [exhibited by the patient]. One will automatically conform with the patterns developed by the people of antiquity, and any [combination of drugs] given [to the patients] must have miraculous effects.

Notes

1.   "Running piglet" is an ancient term; it appears in the *Ling-shu,* the *Nan-ching,* and the *Shen-nung Pen-ts'ao.* It refers to a feeling of meteorism moving upwards in the body as unsteady as a herd of piglets.

2.   Chang Yüan-su (fl. 1180) justified his contribution to a theoretical reorientation of medicine with the words "ancient prescriptions cannot be applied to the ills of today." Hsü Ta-ch'un, a conservative and adherent of the Han medical doctrines, regarded the ideas of Chang Yüan-su and other Sung-Chin-Yüan theoreticians as responsible for the decline of medicine he observed. (see P. U. Unschuld, *Medicine in China: A History of Ideas.* p. 210).

方劑古今論

後世之方已不知幾億萬矣此皆不足以名方者也昔者聖人之製方也推藥理之本原識藥性之專能察氣味之從逆審臟腑之好惡合君臣之配耦而又探索病源推求經絡其思邃其義精味不過三四而其用變化不窮聖人之智真與天地同體非人之心思所能及也上古至今千聖相傳無敢失墜至張仲景先生復申明用法設為問難註明主治之症其傷寒論金匱要畧集千聖之大成以承先而啓後萬世不能出其範圍此之謂古方與內經並垂不朽者其前後名家如倉公扁鵲華佗孫思邈諸人各有師承而淵源又與仲景微別然猶自成一家但不能與靈素本草一線相傳為宗枝正脉耳既而積習相仍每著一書必自撰方千百唐諸公用藥雖博已乏化機至于宋人并不知藥其方亦板

實膚淺元時號稱極盛各立門庭徒騁私見迫乎有明蹈襲元人緒餘而已今之醫者動云古方不知古方之稱其指不一若謂上古之方則自仲景先生流傳以外無幾也如謂宋元所製之方則其可法可傳者絶少不合法而荒謬者甚多豈可奉為典章若謂自明人以前皆稱古方則其方不下數百萬夫常用之藥不過數百品而為方數百萬隨拈幾味皆已成方何必定云某方也嗟嗟古之方何其嚴今之方何其易其間亦有奇巧之法用藥之妙未必不能補古人之所未及可備叅考者然其大經大法則萬不能及其中更有違經背法之方反足貽害安得有學之士為之擇而存之集其大成刪其無當實千古之盛舉余益有志而未遑矣

153

3. On the Composition of Prescriptions in Ancient Times and Today

No one knows how many millions of prescriptions [have been introduced] in recent generations, but not a single one of them is worth calling a prescription. When the Sages of antiquity composed prescriptions, they searched for the origins of pharmaceutic principles. They were familiar with the special abilities associated with the characteristics of drugs. They examined whether the [thermo-]influence and the flavor [of a drug] corresponded to or contradicted [an illness]. They investigated what the body's viscera and bowels preferred and disliked, they combined ruler and minister [drugs] to form appropriate teams, and, furthermore, they searched for the origins of illnesses, and they examined the conduits and the network [vessels].

Their thoughts went far, and their deliberations were subtle. Although [they employed] not more than three or four substances [in their prescriptions], their effects appeared in countless variations. The wisdom of the Sages [of antiquity] was truly identical with the essentials of heaven and earth; it cannot be reached by the mind and by the thoughts of [ordinary] men. From high antiquity until today, there were a thousand Sages who transmitted [this ancient wisdom among themselves], and no one dared to fail in observing this [wisdom].

Then, Mr. Chang Chung-ching provided clear instructions about using [the ancient prescriptions]. He clarified various difficult issues, and he offered instructions on the main pathoconditions cured [by these prescriptions]. His [works,] Shang-han Lun and Chin-kuei Yao-lüeh, combine the great achievement of thousands of Sages [preceding him]. They carry on what was before, to instruct those who come later. Their scope [is so encompassing that] even ten thousand generations will not be able to transcend it. They are the so-called ancient prescriptions; together with the Nei-ching they will never cease to flourish.

All those famous authors prior to and following [Chang Chung-ching], like Ts'ang-kung, Pien Ch'io, Hua T'o, and Sun Ssu-mo, all received [their knowledge from respectable] teachers, but the origins [of their knowledge] were slightly different from [the origins of the knowledge inherited by] Chang Chung-ching. Still, each [of these famous authors] established himself as an authority. None of them, though, can be handed on in one line with the Ling[-shu], Su[-wen], and the Pen-ts'ao as if they represented direct descendants [of the teachings of these works].

Later, certain customs developed in that everyone who wrote a book invented countless prescriptions himself. All the masters of the T'ang era used drugs extensively, but they lacked adaptive ingenuity. The people of the Sung, then, did not know anything about drugs. Their prescriptions were stiff like boards and superficial like skin. The Yüan era is said to have been extremely flourishing. Everyone established his personal school, vainly hastening to put forward his private views. And the Ming, finally, did nothing but plagiarize the leftovers of the Yüan people.

Today's physicians take every opportunity to use the term "ancient prescriptions," but they fail to realize that the term "ancient prescriptions" carries several meanings. If one speaks of the prescriptions of high antiquity, there are almost none except those transmitted by Mr. Chang Chung-ching. If one speaks of the prescriptions designed during the Sung and Yüan era, there are very few that could be accepted as standard and that are worth handing on, while the majority do not correspond to any [ancient] method and rest on nothing but errors. How could anyone accept [these Sung and Yüan prescriptions] as mandatory rules [to be followed in one's treatment of illness]?

If one were to call all prescriptions [designed] by Ming and earlier people "ancient prescriptions," one would have [to include] no less than millions of prescriptions [in this definition]. Now, the number of frequently employed drugs does not exceed several hundred substances, and when [I stated that] there are several million prescriptions, this is because [in later generations], as soon as someone had picked a few substances, he had already created a prescription. Why, though, did they need to define these [unsystematic combinations of a few substances] as fixed prescriptions with a fixed name?

Alas! How rigid were the [rules for composing] prescriptions in antiquity, and how easy it is [to compose a prescription] today! Still, even among [the prescriptions composed in later times] are some [that display] extraordinary patterns, and a subtle use of drugs, and that may well be suitable to supplement what the ancients had not yet achieved, and that may serve as additional data. And yet, they will never reach the major classics, and the major methods [introduced by the ancients]. And among these [prescriptions composed in later times] there are some that contradict the classics, and turn their backs on the patterns [introduced by the ancients], and that are, therefore, suited to cause harm to posterity!

How is it possible that educated scholars pick one of these and keep it [in use]? To collect the great achievements [of the ancients], and to eliminate what is unsuited [for further transmission], is truly a great undertaking. I have focussed my mind on this task, but I have not found the necessary time!

單方論

單方者藥不過一二味治不過一二症而其効則甚捷

用而不中亦能害人即世所謂海上方者是也其原起

於本草蓋古之聖人辨藥物之性則必著其功用如逐

風逐寒解毒定痛之類凡人所患之症止一二端則以

一藥治之藥專則力厚自有奇效若病兼數症則必合

數藥而成方至後世藥品日增單方日多有效有不效

矣若夫內外之感其中自有傳變之道虛實之殊久暫

之別深淺之分及夫人性各殊天時各異此非守經達

權者不能治若皆以單方治之則藥性專而無製偏而

不醇有利必有害故醫者不可以此嘗試此經方之所

以為貴也然參考以廣識見且為急救之備或為專攻

之法是亦不可不知者也

4. On Single[-Substance] Prescriptions

Single[-substance] prescriptions are composed of no more than one or two substances. They cure no more than one or two pathoconditions, and their effects are very swift. If their application fails to hit [the illness, single-substance prescriptions] may cause harm to the person [treated]. Single-substance prescriptions] are so-called "prescriptions by the sea,"[1] and they have originated from [the drug descriptions in] the *pen-ts'ao* literature.

That is to say, in ancient times the Sages distinguished among the characteristics of drugs, and they wrote down their specific abilities and applications, such as "drives off wind," "drives off cold," "dissolves poison," and "settles pain." When a person suffered from no more than one or two pathoconditions, the [ancient Sages] treated [that person] with but one drug.

Since such drugs had special [therapeutic abilities], their power was rather strong, and they produced, therefore, extraordinary effects. However, when an illness resulted in several simultaneous pathoconditions, [the ancients] always combined several drugs and created a [complex] prescription.

In later times, the number of [available] drugs increased day by day, and [the number of] single[-substance] prescriptions increased day by day too, with some of them showing positive effects, others not. Because internal and external affections may be transmitted to [different areas throughout the body], and may change [their nature], and because differences exist between [states of] depletion and those of repletion, and because one has to distinguish between long-term and short-term [illnesses], as well as between those that are located in the depth and others that are located near the surface, and because no one's nature is alike and the seasons differ too, successful therapies can be conducted only by those who cherish the [contents of the] classics and who are, at the same time, able to adapt themselves to the circumstances confronting them.

If one were to use single[-substance] prescriptions in all instances, the nature of the [individual] drugs would be specific, but it would not be modified [according to the requirements of an illness]. It would be one-sided but it would not be mild, and any benefit [resulting from such an application] would definitely be accompanied by harm, as well. Consequently, physicians should not test [such single-substance prescriptions on their patients], and it is for this reason that the prescriptions of the classics are to be valued so highly. Still, one must study [single-substance] prescriptions in order to broaden one's knowledge, and one must be familiar with their usage in urgent crises, as well as with patterns for employing them in specific attacks.

157

Notes

1. "By the sea" is an expression referring to unorthodoxy, in this case to the prescriptions that are not documented in standard literature.

禁方論

天地有好生之德聖人有大公之心立方以治病使天下共知之豈非天地聖人之至願哉然而方之有禁則何也其故有二一則懼天下之輕視夫道也夫經方之治病視其人學問之高下以為效驗故或用之而愈或用之而反害變化無定此大公之法也若禁方者義有所不解機有所莫測其傳也往往出於奇人隱士仙佛鬼神其過之也甚難則其愛護之必至若輕以授人必生輕易之心所以方家往往愛惜此乃人之情也一則恐燮天地之機也禁方之藥其製法必奇其配合必巧竊陰陽之柄窺造化之機其修合必虔誠敬慎少犯禁忌則藥無驗若輕以示人則氣洩而用不神此又陰陽之理也靈樞禁服篇黃帝謂雷公曰此先師之所禁割臂歃血之盟也故黃帝有蘭臺之藏長桑君有無洩之戒

古聖皆然若夫詭詐之人專欲圖利托名禁方欺世惑眾更有修煉熱藥長慾道淫名為養生實速其死此乃江河惡習聖人之所必誅也又有古之禁方傳之已廣載入醫書中與經方並垂有識者自能擇之也

5.   On Prescriptions that are Kept Secret

The virtue of heaven and earth lies in their appreciation of life. The mind of the Sages is characterized by [their devotion to the interests of] the public. When [the latter] established prescriptions to cure an illness, they saw to it that [these prescriptions] became known to everyone throughout the world. [To spread their knowledge] has been the utmost desire of heaven and earth and of the Sages, and yet, how is it that prescriptions exist that are kept secret?

Two reasons account for this. The first is that those [who keep prescriptions secret] fear that the ways of the Sages are treated without the necessary respect. The treatment of illnesses with prescriptions publicized in the classics depends — in the results achieved — on the degree of knowledge of the person [applying them]. Sometimes their application achieves a cure; sometimes, by contrast, they may cause harm. All types of different situations may arise, and nothing is predetermined. Such is the pattern of the widely publicized [prescriptions].

On the other hand, the prescriptions that are kept secret have a meaning that cannot be explained, and their working mechanism is not entirely accessible. Their transmission, often enough, originated from strange persons, scholars living in seclusion, hermits in the mountains, boddhisatvas, demons, or spirits. To meet such [a person] is quite difficult, and therefore, these [prescriptions] are extremely well guarded [by those who have gained access to them]. If they are handed on to others carelessly, they will only generate a disrespectful attitude. Hence most prescription masters guard them as a most precious belonging.

That is to say, [the first reason why certain prescriptions are kept secret is based on] human nature. The second [reason for the existence of secret prescriptions] is a hesitation to lay open the workings of heaven and earth.

In secret prescriptions the drugs are composed in accordance with extraordinary patterns. The way [drugs] are combined [in such prescriptions] is ingenious. [Such prescriptions] usurp all the authority of yin and yang, and they look deeply into the workings of creation. It is utterly imperative to be sincere and devout. Even the slightest violation [of any prohibitions and taboos] renders the drugs [employed] ineffective. If, therefore, someone lightheartedly teaches [such prescriptions] to others, the influences [of these prescriptions] leak away, and their application no longer yields miraculous [results].

That is to say, [the second reason why certain prescriptions are kept secret is based on] the principles of yin and yang. In the treatise

"Prohibitions [against passing on what one has] memorized" of the *Ling-shu* [it is stated], "The Yellow Emperor told Lei-kung, [that passing this knowledge on to others carelessly] was prohibited by the teachers in former times. [Students, before they were instructed in this knowledge,] had to take an oath by cutting an arm and smearing their mouth with their blood." Hence the Yellow Emperor stored [his secret prescription] in the Orchid Tower, and Ch'ang sang chün was warned not to transmit [the knowledge he was about to pass on to Shun-yü I any] further. All the ancient Sages acted this way.

Dishonest persons, who have nothing but profit in mind, falsely claim [to possess] secret prescriptions. They cheat the world and delude the masses. Furthermore, there are drugs that are prepared through melting procedures; they increase one's passions and support obscenities. They are designated as prolonging life while, in fact, they hasten death. Such are the malicious practices of itinerant ["healers"]. The Sages, naturally, would have eliminated them. Also, some prescriptions that had been secret in antiquity have since been transmitted widely, and they have found entrance into medical literature where they are kept together with prescriptions based on the classics. Knowledgeable people can pick them from there.

161

古今方劑大小論

今人以古人氣體充實。故方劑分兩甚重。此無稽之說也。自三代至漢晉。升斗權衡。雖有異同。以今較之。不過十分之二。如桂枝湯。傷寒大劑也。桂枝芍藥各三兩。甘草二兩。共八兩。爲一劑。在今只一兩六錢。又分三服。則一服不過五錢三分零。他方有藥品多者。亦不過倍之而已。況古時之藥。醫者自備。俱用鮮者。分兩以鮮者爲準。乾則折算。如半夏麥冬之類。皆生大而乾小。至附子。則野生者甚小。後人種之。乃肥大。皆有確證。今人每方必十餘味。每味三四錢。則一劑重二三兩矣。更有熟地用至四兩一劑者。尤屬可怪。古丸藥如烏梅丸。每服如桐子大十丸。今秤不過二三分。今則用三四錢。至七八錢矣。古末藥用方寸七。不過今之

六七分。今服三四錢矣。古人用藥分兩未嘗從重。二十年來。時醫誤閱古方。增重分兩。此風日熾。即使對病。元氣不勝藥力。亦必有害。況更與病相反。害不尤速乎。既不考古。又無師授。無怪乎其動成笑柄也。

162

6. On the Dosage of Prescriptions in Antiquity and Today

When today's people hold that the people in ancient times enjoyed a sturdy constitution, and that, therefore, their prescriptions were [characterized by] heavy [doses of drugs], then this is unfounded. Some differences already existed between the weights and measures of the Three [Ancient] Dynasties and those of the Han and Chin, but if the [weights and measures of antiquity] are compared with those of today, they correspond to but twenty per cent [of the weight that the same term refers to now]. For example, the "Decoction with *kuei-chih*" is a large dosage decoction against harm caused by cold. [It contains] three *liang*[1] of both *kuei-chih* and *shao-yao*, and two *liang* of *kan-ts'ao*, adding up to eight *liang* as the dosage [of one preparation]. In today's terms, this amounts to only one *liang* and six *ch'ien*. With this [total] dosage, [the decoction] is divided into three doses, each of which amounts to no more than five *ch'ien* and three *fen*.

Other prescriptions with more drugs may have doses twice this amount, but not more. Also, in ancient times, drugs were prepared by physicians themselves. They always used fresh [drugs], and the weights [given in the literature] always refer to fresh [drugs]. If one uses dried [substances], the amounts to be taken have to be decreased accordingly. For example, [drugs] like *pan-hsia* or *mai-tung* are large when raw and small when dried. Or *fu-tzu*, it is very small when it grows in the wilderness, but later it was cultivated by man, and grew very large. All of this is clearly evident.

With the people of today, each prescription combines definitely ten or more substances, and each substance comes in amounts of three or four *ch'ien*. Hence the weight one preparation amounts to is two or three *liang*. And when, as happens, as much as four *liang* of *shou-ti* are included per preparation, then this is truly absurd!

In ancient times, about ten pills of the size of *t'ung* seeds were consumed per dose — "Pills with *wu-mei*" are an example. Today, that corresponds to a weight of no more than two or three fen. Today, though, three or four *ch'ien* up to seven or eight *ch'ien* [of pills] are taken [per individual dose]. As for powdered drugs, the ancients used a square spoon corresponding to no more than six or seven of today's *fen*. Nowadays, though, three to four *ch'ien* are consumed [per individual dose].

When the ancients employed drugs, they never applied extreme doses. But during the past twenty years, those physicians who but follow the fashions of their own times have — wrongly interpreting ancient

163

prescriptions — heavily increased the weights [of individual drugs in a prescription], and this custom appears to spread day by day. Even if their [prescriptions] are directed against an illness, the [patient's] original influences cannot withstand the force of the drugs, and harm is unavoidable. And when [the drugs] fail to correspond to the illness [treated], will harm not result even faster? Hence it is no wonder when those who fail to study antiquity, and who do not receive [their instructions] from a teacher, always give rise to laughter.[2]

Notes

1.   A *liang* is a Chinese ounce, or tael. It corresponds to ten *ch'ien,* or one hundred *fen.*

2.   This paragraph was significantly shortened and altered in its contents in the 1778 *Ssu K'u Ch'üan-shu* version of the text. It is reproduced here in its original length from the Wu chou Publishing Co. edition, Taipei, 1969.

藥誤不即死論

古人治法無一方不對病無一藥不對症如是而病猶
不愈此乃病本不可愈非醫之咎也後世醫失其傳病
之名亦不能知宜其胸中毫無所主也凡一病有一病
之名如中風總名也其類有偏枯痿痺風痱歷節之殊
而諸症之中又各有數症各有定名各有主方又如水
腫總名也其類有皮水正水石水風水之殊而諸症又
各有數症各有定名各有主方凡病盡然醫者必能實
指其何名遵古人所主何方加減何藥自有法度可循
乃不論何病總以陰虛陽虛等籠統之談概之而試以
籠統不切之藥然亦竟有愈者或其病本輕適欲自愈
或偶有一二對症之藥亦奏小效皆屬誤治其得免於
殺人之名者何也蓋殺人之藥必大毒如砒鴆之類或
大熱大寒峻厲之品又適與病相反服後立見其危若

尋常之品不過不能愈病或反增他病耳不即死也久
而病氣自退正氣自復無不愈者間有遷延日久或隱
受其害而死更或屢換庸醫偏試諸藥久而病氣益深
元氣竭亦死又有初因誤治變成他病輾轉而死又有
始服有小效久服太過反增他病而死益日日診視小
效則以為可愈小劇又以為難治並無誤治之形確有
誤治之實病家以為病久不痊自然不起非醫之咎因
其不即死而不之罪其實則真殺之而不覺也若夫誤
按峻厲相反之藥服後顯然為害此其殺人人人能知
之矣惟誤服參附峻補之藥而即死者則病家之所甘
心必不歸咎於醫故醫者雖自知其誤必不以此為戒
而易其術也

7. On [Situations Where] a Mistaken [Therapy with] Drugs Does Not Result in Immediate Death

The therapeutic patterns of the ancients were such that each prescription was directly focused on the illness [to be treated], and that each drug was directly focused on the [individual] pathoconditions [accompanying this illness]. If any illness could not be cured despite [the application of such careful methods], this meant that the illness itself was incurable, and the physician was not to be blamed. Since then, physicians have lost this tradition, they no longer know even the names of the illnesses. No wonder they have absolutely no guidelines!

Each single illness has a name characterizing this specific illness. For instance, "struck-by-wind" is an encompassing designation. It includes [pathoconditions] such as "partial paralysis," "[limb] paralysis," "wind[-induced] heat," and "[pain] pervading all joints." All these pathoconditions are, in turn, accompanied by numerous [individual] pathoconditions, each of which bears a specific name, and each of which has a master prescription.

Or, as another example, "swelling from water" is [also] an encompassing designation. It includes different [pathoconditions] such as "skin water," "regular water," "stone[-hard swellings from] water," and "water [rising in the body due to] wind." All these pathoconditions are, in turn, accompanied by numerous [individual] pathoconditions, each of which bears a specific name, and each of which is mastered by a [specific] prescription. This applies to all other illnesses as well, and a physician must be able to point out their [specific] names, and to obey whatever prescription the ancient [Sages] developed to master [a specific illness. A physician must be able] to add [to a prescription] any drug [required by an individual case], or to leave out [those drugs that may not be necessary. If a physician has this knowledge,] he has rules on hand that he can follow.

Those who merely apply such general concepts as "yin depletion" or "yang depletion," and try merely general, non-specific drugs, regardless of the illness [they are confronted with], they may still achieve some cures. But the reason [for such successes] must be sought in facts such as that the illness was basically minor anyway, and had a tendency towards healing by itself, or that one or two drugs that were focused on some pathocondition did indeed exert some small effect.

Still, all of this is malpractice. Why, now, can those [who apply such malpractices] avoid being called killers? Well, drugs that kill people must be strong poisons, such as arsenic and the *chen* bird, or vehement

166

substances with strong hot or strong cold [effects], and if it happens that [these effects] are directly opposed to the illness [treated], then their dangerous [nature] becomes evident immediately after they have been taken. Those ordinary substances, on the other hand, that are unable to cure an illness, and that generate but further illnesses, do not cause immediate death.

[There are, of course, illnesses] that are cured if one only waits long enough for the pathogenic influences to recede, and the proper influences to recover by themselves. But there are some that continue for a long time, and it may happen that [during that time the patient will] unnoticeably receive harm from these [drugs] until he dies. Or [the patient, during the long time of his illness], switches from one common physician to the next, tries all types of drugs, with the pathogenic influences penetrating, over long, deeper and deeper until his original influences are exhausted, and he dies.

It may also be that someone received a mistaken treatment in the beginning, that caused the generation of further illnesses, and finally he dies.

Or, it may be that an initial intake [of drugs] shows some small effect and that a prolonged intake results in an overdose that then generates further illnesses, and leads to [the patient's] death.

[The common physicians] observe some small improvement day by day, and they think [the illness] can be cured, while, if it turns a little worse, they think it is difficult to cure. This does not resemble malpractice; in fact, [it] is malpractice! The patients' families think if an [illness] is not cured after a long time, it is just natural that the [patient] fails to rise again, and hence they would never blame the physician. Since [the patient] did not die immediately [after the drugs were administered], they do not accuse the physician. In reality, though, this is genuine homicide, and [the physician] is aware of it!

If vehement drugs that are opposed [to an illness] are administered incorrectly, and if some obvious harm results afterward, everyone will be able to realize who was the killer. But if the patient was mistakenly [asked to] consume rapidly supplementing drugs such as *shen* and *fu*, and dies thereafter, his family will nevertheless accept [this treatment], and will not hold the physician responsible. Even if the physician is himself aware of his error, he need not consider it as a warning and need not alter his practices.

藥石性全用異論

一藥有一藥之性情功效其藥能治某病古方中用之

以治某病此顯而易見者然一藥不止一方用之他方

用之亦效何也蓋藥之功用不止一端在此方則取其

此長在彼方則取其彼長真知其功效之實自能曲中

病情而得其力迨至後世一藥所治之病愈多而亦效

者蓋古人尚未盡知之後人屢試而後知所以歷代本

草所註藥性較之神農本經所註功用增益數倍蓋以

此也但其中有當有不當不若神農本草字字精切耳

又同一熱藥而附子之熱與乾姜之熱逈乎不同同一

寒藥而石膏之寒與黃連之寒逈乎不同一或誤用禍

害立至蓋古人用藥之法並不專取其寒熱溫涼補瀉

之性也或取其氣或取其味或取其色或取其形或取

其所生之方或取嗜好之偏其藥似與病情之寒熱溫

涼補瀉若不相關而投之反有神效古方中如此者不

可枚舉學者必將神農本草字字求其精義之所在而

參以仲景諸方則聖人之精理自能洞曉而已之立方

亦必有奇思妙想深入病機而天下無難治之症矣

168

8. On [Herbal] Drugs and Minerals with Identical Nature and Different Functions

Each single drug has properties and effects that are characteristic of that specific drug. If a drug is able to cure a particular illness, it was used in the prescriptions of antiquity to cure that particular illness. That is obvious and easily discernible. Still, one specific drug finds application not only in one specific prescription. It may well be used, with positive effects, in further prescriptions too. How is that?

Well, the functions of drugs are not one-dimensional. In one particular prescription one takes advantage of one particular ability, in another prescription one takes advantage of another ability [of the same drug]. As long as one is truly familiar with the actual functions of the drugs, one will be able to accommodate their [application] to the characteristics of the illnesses, and thus take advantage of the powers [of the drugs].

In later times, though, each single drug was employed in the treatment of ever more illnesses, and this with positive results, because what the ancient [physicians] had not yet entirely known became known through many trials to those who lived afterwards. Consequently, the properties of drugs described in pharmaceutic literature through the ages have increased many times in comparison with the functions [of drugs] as described in the original classic of Shen-nung. However, among [these properties] are some that one can agree with, and others that one cannot. [Later pharmaceutic works] differ from the *Shen-nung Pen-ts'ao,* in which every single word reflected ingenuity.

Also, drugs may be identical in being hot, but the heat of *fu-tzu* and the heat of *kan-chiang* are quite different. Drugs may be identical in being cold, but the cold of *shih-kao* and the cold of *huang-lien* are [also] quite different. If one [of these drugs] is applied mistakenly [in place of the other], disaster and harm will follow immediately.

When the ancients applied drugs, they did not just rely on [the drugs'] cold, hot, warm, cool, supplementing or draining nature. In some cases they took advantage of [a drug's thermo-]influences, in some cases of its flavor. In some cases, they relied on [a drug's] color, in some cases on its shape. In some cases they took into account the region where the drug grows, and sometimes they just followed one-sided cravings [of a patient]. There are more instances than I could recount here where, in ancient prescriptions, the drugs had no relation whatsoever to the cold, hot, warm, cool, supplementing or draining [nature of the substance seemingly required by] the nature of the illness, and yet [these prescriptions] showed miraculous results.

A student [of medicine] must search each single word of the *Shen-nung Pen-ts'ao* for its subtle meanings, and he must combine [his findings] with all the prescriptions [in the works of Chang] Chung-ching. Then, all the subtle principles of the Sages will be open to him. And, when he sets up his own prescriptions, he must engage in extraordinary thoughts and sophisticated considerations, and he must deeply penetrate the workings of the illnesses, and there will be no pathocondition left under heaven that is difficult to treat.

劫劑論

世有奸醫利人之財取効于一時不顧人之生死者謂

之劫劑劫劑者以重藥奪截邪氣也夫邪之中人不能

使之一時即出必漸消漸托而後盡焉今欲一日見効

勢必用猛厲之藥與邪相爭或用峻補之藥過抑邪氣

藥猛厲則邪氣暫伏而正亦傷藥峻補則正氣驟發而

邪內陷一時似乎有效及至藥力盡而邪復來元氣已

大壞矣如病者身熱甚不散其熱而以沉寒之藥過之

腹痛甚不求其因而以香燥禦之瀉痢甚不去其積而

以收欲之藥塞之之類此峻厲之法也若邪盛而投以

大劑終附一時陽氣大旺病氣必潛藏自然神氣畧定

越一二日元氣與邪氣相併反助邪而肆其毒為禍尤

烈此峻補之法也此等害人之術奸醫以此欺人而騙

財者十之五庸醫不知而効尤以害人者亦十之五為

醫者可不自省病家亦不可不察也

171

9. On Coercive Medication

Wicked physicians exist who are only after the possessions of the people. [The therapies that these wicked physicians apply achieve] preliminary effects, but they do not take the patients' [ultimate] survival or death into account — [they rely on what] are called "coercive medications."

Coercive medications subdue and intercept evil influences by means of heavy [doses of] drugs. However, when evil [influences] strike a person, they cannot be forced to leave all at once. [The evil influences that have invaded the patient] must be diminished gradually, [and the patient's proper influences must be] supported step by step; as a final [result, the evil influences] will be exhausted.

Now, if one wishes to see the effects [of a treatment] within one day, one must either apply drugs with ferocious strength that struggle with the evil [influences], or such drugs that stop the evil influences through their [ability to provide] rapid supplementation.

When drugs with ferocious [strength are applied], the evil influences hide for the time being, but the proper [influences] are harmed too. When drugs with [an ability to provide a] rapid supplementation [are applied], proper influences are developed immediately, but the evil [influences] only penetrate deeper into [the body]. It appears as if [the treatment] was effective for a while, but as soon as the force of the drugs is exhausted, the evil [influences] will recover, and [the patient's] original influences will have been injured significantly in the meantime.

When a patient's body is very hot, and one fails to dissipate this heat, but subdues it with drugs that are very cold, or when someone has severe pain in his abdomen and [the physician] fails to search for the cause [of this pain] and suppresses it by means of aromatic drying [substances], or when someone suffers from extreme diarrhea, and rather than eliminating accumulations [that should be drained], the [physician] applies astringent drugs that block [the passage of the diarrhea], all these [procedures] constitute patterns of ferocious [therapy].

When evil [influences] are present in abundance, and [the physician] gives [the patient] large doses of *shen* and *fu*, with the effect that his yang influences come to flourish greatly for some time, while his pathogenic influences are forced to hide away, then, of course, [the patient's] spirit and his [proper] influences are somewhat stabilized. But after one or two days have passed, the [patient's] original influences and evil influences have merged with each other, and [the former] now assist, contrary [to what one might have expected], the latter to develop their poison, with the result of a particularly violent disaster. This is a pattern of a rapidly supplementing [therapy].

In fifty percent of all cases, such harmful practices are employed by wicked physicians who deceive the people and cheat them out of their belongings. In all other cases, [such practices] are employed by common physicians who just do not know [what they are doing], and who merely imitate [the others]. Those who practice medicine must examine themselves [as to whether they apply such coercive medications], and the patients' families should be on their guard as well.

製藥論

製藥之法古方甚少而眾詳于宋之雷斅今世所傳雷
公炮炙論是也後世製藥之法日多一日内中亦有至
無理者固不可從若其微妙之處實有精義存焉凡物
氣厚力大者無有不偏偏則有利必有害欲取其利而
去其害則用法以製之則藥性之偏者醇矣其製之義
又各不同或以相反為製或以相資為製或以相惡為
製或以相畏為製或以相喜為製而製法又復不同或
製其形或製其性或製其味或製其質此皆巧于用藥
之法也古方製藥無多其立方之法配合氣性如桂枝
湯中用白芍亦即有相製之理故不必每藥製之也若
後世好奇眩異之人必求貴重怪僻之物其製法大費
工本以神其說此乃好奇尚異之人造作以欺誑富貴
人之法不足憑也惟平和而有理者為可從耳

10. On the Modification of Drugs

In ancient prescriptions very few patterns for the modification of drugs were applied. The most detailed [modification instructions were compiled] only during the Sung by Lei Hsiao. They are "Lei-kung's Treatise on the Preparation [of Drugs]," which is [still] transmitted today.[1] In later times, the patterns for the modification of drugs increased each day, but some of them are quite unreasonable and should, of course, not be followed. Those prescriptions, though, that are [based on] rather sophisticated [considerations], they indeed have a subtle rationale.

All substances with strongly developed influences, and with strong powers, must be one-sided [in their effects]. This one-sidedness has its benefits, but may also be harmful. If, therefore, one wishes to take advantage of the beneficial [properties], and to eliminate the harmful [properties], one employs certain patterns to modify [their one-sidedness]. And, as a result, even drugs with a one-sided nature act mildly. There are a number of different rationales available for the modification [of drugs].

In some cases [the one-sided effects of drugs] are modified by [combining drugs] that oppose each other. In other cases this modification is [achieved] by [combining drugs] that depend on each other. Sometimes [drugs] are modified by [compounding substances] that hate each other, or that fear each other, or that enjoy each other.

[Not only the rationales, but] the patterns guiding the modification [of one-sided drug effects follow] different [variables as well]. In some cases, the shapes [of drugs] are modified. In other cases their flavors are modified, and in still other cases, the very substance is modified. All these patterns enable a very skillful application of drugs.

In ancient times, only a few prescriptions [were based on] modified drugs. The pattern [followed by the ancients] when they set up their prescriptions consisted only of combinations of [thermo-]influences and nature. For instance, when they used *pai-shao* in the "Decoction with *kuei-chih*," this was for the sake of mutual modification. Hence they did not need to modify each drug individually.

When in later times men emerged who preferred the strange and who were confused by the extraordinary, and who, therefore, searched for expensive and exotic substances, their modification patterns required large expenditures of work and money to make their doctrines appear miraculous. This way, those who prefer the strange and who appreciate the extraordinary have created patterns in order to cheat and deceive the rich and the noble. They are not worth listening to. Only the moderate and reasonable should be followed.

Note

1.   This is the *Lei-kung P'ao-chiu Lun,* allegedly compiled during the so-called Liu Sung era [420-478] by Lei Hsiao. It is said to have contained descriptions of the pharmaceutic processing of 300 drugs. Since the original was lost long ago, editions available today contain only 180 such descriptions and are based on a reconstruction compiled by Chang Chi in 1932.

人參論

天下之害人者殺其身未必破其家未必殺其

身先破人之家而後殺其身者人參是也夫人參用之而

當實能補養元氣拯救危險然不可謂天下之死人皆

能生之也其為物氣盛而力厚不論風寒暑濕痰火鬱

結皆能補塞故病人如果邪去正良用之固宜或邪微

而正亦憊或邪深而正氣怯弱不能逐之於外則於除

邪藥中投之以為驅邪之助然又必審其輕重而後用

之自然有扶危定傾之功乃不察其有邪無邪是虛是

實又佐以純補溫熱之品將邪氣盡行補住輕者邪氣

永不復出重者即死矣夫醫者之所以遇疾即用而病

家服之死而無悔者何也蓋愚人之心皆以價貴為良

藥價賤為劣藥而常人之情無不好補而惡攻故服參

而死即使明知其誤然以為服人參而死則醫者之力

已竭而人子之心已盡此命數使然可以無恨矣若服

攻削之藥而死即使用藥不惧病實難治而醫者之罪

已不可勝誅矣故人參者乃醫家邀功避罪之聖藥也

病家如此醫家如此而害人無窮矣更有駭者或以用

人參為冠冕或以用人參為有力量又因其貴重深信

以為必能挽回造化故殺然用之敗知人參一用凡病

之有邪者即死其不死者亦終身不得愈乎其破

家之故何也蓋向日之人參不過一二換多者三四換

今則其價十倍其所服又非一錢二錢而止小康之家

服二三兩而家已蕩然矣夫人情于死生之際何求不

得寧恤破家乎醫者全不一念輕將人參立方用而不

遵在父為不慈在子為不孝在夫婦昆弟為惡心害理

并有親戚朋友責罰痛罵即使明知無益姑以此塞責

又有孝子慈父徇其或生竭力以謀之遂使貧窶之家

病或稍愈一家終身凍餒若仍不救棺殮俱無賣妻鬻
子全家覆敗醫者誤治殺人可恕而遲已之意日日害
人破家其惡甚于盜賊可不慎哉吾願天下之人斷不
可以人參為起死回生之藥而必服之醫者必審其病
實係純虛非參不治服必萬全然後用之又必量其家
業尚可以支持不至用參之後死生無靠然後節省用
之一以惜物力一以全人之命一以保人之家如此存
心自然天降之福若如近日之醫殺命破家于人不知
之地恐天之降禍亦在人不知之地也可不慎哉

178

11. On Ginseng

Among all those in the world who destroy man, some kill [an individual's body] but do not necessarily ruin [that individual's] family, and some ruin [an individual's] family but do not necessarily kill [that individual's] body. However, that which first ruins a person's family and subsequently kills [that person's] body is ginseng.

If applied properly, [ginseng] is definitely capable of supplementing and nourishing one's original influences, and of rescuing [a patient] from a dangerous condition. Nobody should assume, though, that the dead in the world can be brought back to life [by means of this drug]!

Since [ginseng] is a substance rich in influences and full of vigor, it is able to supplement [a depletion] and stop [the loss of proper influences], no matter whether [a patient's illness is related to] wind, cold, summer-heat, dampness, phlegm, fire or some binding [of influences within the body]. An application [of ginseng] is always appropriate when the evil [influences that caused a] patient's [illness] leave [his body, but his] proper [influences are still] weak; or when only a few evil [influences remain, but the] proper [influences] are also exhausted. Or, when evil [influences] have penetrated deeply [into the body, and] the proper [influences] are themselves too weak to drive off [the evil influences].

In order to support the elimination of the evil [influences by means of drugs], one must give [the patient ginseng] together with other drugs [that are capable of] driving off [evil influences]. However, before one applies [ginseng], one should examine whether [the case to be treated] is minor or serious, and only [if one takes that variable into account] will the effect of rescue from danger, or of straightening what is already bent, appear as a matter of course. If one fails to investigate, though, whether evil [influences] are present or not, and whether [the person to be treated suffers from a] depletion or from a repletion; and if one adds [to a prescription] warm or hot substances of a purely supplementing [nature], then one will merely supplement the evil influences and help them settle down. In minor cases, the evil influences will [as a result of such mistaken therapy] never leave [the patient's body] again. In serious cases, death is inevitable.

Why is it, then, that physicians prescribe this [drug] against any illness that they are confronted by, and that patient's families do not regret it [when the patient] takes [ginseng] and dies? Well, stupid people believe that expensive drugs must be good drugs, while cheap drugs are supposed to be inferior, and it is common human nature to love supplementation and to dislike attack. If, therefore, someone dies after consuming ginseng, [his son] may have been aware of this mistake, but he will nevertheless believe that when someone dies after having taken ginseng the physician's resources had all already been exhausted, that his filial attitude was fully applied, that everything was a matter of fate, and that no grudge should be harbored against anyone.

However, if [a patient] dies after having taken attacking and diminishing drugs, [peoples' opinion is that] the physician cannot be punished severely enough, even though [it should be clear to any knowledgeable person that] there was no mistake in the application of the drugs, even though the illness was indeed difficult to cure. Ginseng, then, is a sacred drug employed by physicians who practice with an eye to reward, and who wish to avoid accusations. Patients' families act this way, physicians act this way, and the harm done to people is immeasurable.

There are also further appalling [instances of the mistaken use of ginseng], when it is applied, for instance, just because it is fashionable, or when someone believes the application of ginseng is [an appropriate way to demonstrate his financial] resources. Also, there are those who are firmly convinced that [this drug] must be able to turn around [the course of] creation simply because it is so expensive, and hence they are determined to use it. Who knows, though, that an application of ginseng, as long as the patient harbors evil [influences in his body], entails immediate death,[1] while those who do not die [after consuming ginseng erroneously] will remain uncured for the rest of their life?

What, now, is the reason for [my initial statement that ginseng is capable not only of killing a person's body but also of] destroying this [individual's] entire family? Formerly, the price for [one treatment with] ginseng did not exceed one or two strings [of cash]. At most, [the price] was three or four strings. Today, the prices [for ginseng] have increased tenfold, and the dose [people] consume [in the course of one treatment] is no longer restricted to one or two ch'ien. If [patients from] rich families take two or three liang, this is enough to cause their household to go bankrupt. Human nature is such that at the borderline between death and life one wishes to grasp every [possibility for rescue], and who [in such a situation] would feel sorrow [regarding the financial] destruction of his family?

The physicians, though, fail to take such human emotions into account, and they lightly make prescriptions with ginseng. When a father does not obey the use [of ginseng by the physician], that is considered a lack of compassion [toward his sons]. When a son [fails to obey the prescription of ginseng by a physician] that is considered lack of filial piety. When husbands and wives, or elder and younger brothers [resent an application of ginseng], that signals hardening of the heart, and a violation of basic principles. Also, relatives and friends would condemn [such alleged misconduct], and they would strongly abuse [those who insist on not using ginseng]. And, even if they knew that there is no benefit [to be expected from taking this drug], they would nevertheless advocate it to demonstrate performance of their duties!

Then, there are sons marked by filial piety, and also compassionate fathers, who praise themselves fortunate when [their respective parents or children] survive, and who spare no efforts in their search [for help]. As a result, in a household that is poor already, the patient may improve a little, but the entire family must suffer [for want of financial resources] from cold and hunger for the rest of its life. And, if [the patient, in the end], cannot be helped [and dies], no [money is left to buy a] coffin and mourning dresses. Wife and children have to be sold, and the entire family will be destroyed.

Physicians who kill someone through a mistaken therapy may still be excused; but those who harm people at liberty and destroy families day after day, they are worse than thieves and robbers! One must be cautious [about such practitioners]! I wish that no one on earth would regard ginseng as a drug that has to be consumed because it is capable of raising the dead and bringing them back to life.

Physicians [contemplating the use of ginseng] should first of all investigate whether the [patient's] illness is, indeed, a pure depletion that cannot be eliminated except with the help of ginseng. Only [when they are sure that] its intake will result in a complete cure, may they use it. Also, [the physician] must weigh the financial resources of the [patient's] family to find out whether they are sufficient to support life or manage death! If, finally, [ginseng] is applied, this should be done economically; first, in order to spare the [family's financial] resources, second, to guard the patient's life, and third, to protect the patient's family.

If one's intentions focus [on these aims], happiness will descend from heaven by itself. However, since today's physicians kill [their patients'] lives and destroy [their patients'] families to an extent unknown to mankind [before], it is to be feared that disaster will be sent down by heaven to an extent similarly unknown to man. Should we not proceed with utmost caution?

Note

1.　　The two characters *ssu che* are a mistaken addition to the text.

181

用藥如用兵論

聖人之所以全民生也五穀為養五果為助五畜為益
五菜為充而毒藥則以之攻邪故雖甘草人參誤用致
害皆毒藥之類也古人好服食者必生奇疾猶之好戰
勝者必有奇殃是故兵之設也以除暴不得已而後興
藥之設也以攻疾亦不得已而後用其道同也故病之
為患也小則耗精大則傷命隱然一敵國也以草木偏
性攻藏府之偏勝必能知彼知己多方以制之而後無
喪身殞命之憂是故傳經之邪而先奪其未至則所以
斷敵之要道也橫暴之疾而急保其未病則所以守我
之巖疆也挾宿食而病者先除其食則敵之資糧已焚
合舊疾而發者必防其併則敵之內應既絕辨經絡而
無泛用之藥此之謂嚮導之師因寒熱而有反用之方
此之謂行間之術一病而分治之則用寡可以勝眾使

前後不相救而勢自衰數病而合治之則併力搗其中
堅使離散無所統而眾悉潰病方進則不治其太甚固
守元氣所以老其師病方衰則必窮其所之更益精銳
所以搗其穴若夫虛邪之體攻不可過本和平之藥而
以峻藥補之衰敝之日不可窮民力也實邪之傷攻不
可緩用峻厲之藥而以常藥和之富強之國可以振威
武也然而選材必當器械必良剋期不愆布陣有方此
又不可更僕數也孫武子十三篇治病之法盡之矣

12. On Parallels in the Use of Drugs and the Use of Soldiers

In their efforts to protect the lives of people, the Sages [of antiquity] employed the five grains to nourish [the influences of the five viscera], the five fruits for support, [meat of] the five domestic animals to benefit [the five viscera], and the five vegetables for filling [what was depleted], but they made use of toxic drugs to attack the evil.[1] Even *kan-ts'ao* and ginseng may be counted among the toxic drugs, because they cause harm if not applied properly. Those people of antiquity who liked to ingest [toxic substances produced to extend their life span][2] were bound to be affected by extraordinary illnesses, and they may be compared to those who love to fight in wars, and who are therefore bound to receive extraordinary injuries.

Now, the rationale of having soldiers is to eliminate violence, and if there is no other way, military operations must be started.[3] Similarly, the rationale of having drugs is to attack illnesses, and if there is no other way, they must be employed. The principle is the same. To suffer from an illness means, in minor cases, a loss of one's essential [influences], and, in severe cases, harm to one's life. It is as if one were confronted with a hostile country.

One takes advantage of the unilaterally marked nature of herbs and trees to attack unilaterally dominant viscera and bowels. One must know the foreign [territory], and one must know one's own [territory]. And, if one checks the [enemy] at many places, there will be no grief over a destroyed body or over losses of life afterwards. Hence, where illness is transmitted through the conduits, one occupies, first of all, those locations that have not yet been reached [by the evil]. This way, one interrupts the strategic roads of the enemy.

In case of sudden violent illnesses, one must quickly protect what has not yet fallen ill. This corresponds to how we guard our border areas.

If an illness results from food remaining [in the body for too long], this food must be eliminated. This way, the enemy's provisions will be burned up entirely.

If [a new disease] is about to unite with an old disease, one must prevent their union. This way the enemy will be cut off from its internal ally. If one distinguishes between those of the transportation channels [that are affected and others that are not], that is called "[employing a] guide."[4]

If [someone suffers from] cold or heat, and if one [employs, in such a situation] drugs with exactly opposite effects, that is called "the technique of marching right into [the enemy's] lines."

183

If one applies separate therapies to treat one single illness, that is like employing a small number [of troops] to overcome a multitude [of enemies. This way], one succeeds in making [the enemy's] front and rear unable to come to each other's aid, and the forces [of the enemy] weaken as a result.

If [a patient] suffers from a number of illnesses [simultaneously], and one treats all of them with one combined [therapy], this is like running into the main body of an army. [This way,] one succeeds in dispersing [the enemy's troops], not permitting them to unite again, and destroys them entirely.

If an illness has just emerged, one will not treat it as if it had reached full strength. Rather, one strengthens and protects [the patient's] original influences. This way one succeeds in tiring the [enemy's] troops. If an illness is about to become weaker, one must follow it wherever it may turn. Also, one must increase [the victim's] elite soldiers and attack the [enemy's] hiding place.

If the [patient's] body is affected by a depletion evil, one must not lead too strong an attack. One should base one's therapy on peaceful substances, and support them with some swiftly acting drugs. In times when the people are weak and worn out, one cannot make full use of their strength.

[In case a patient] suffers from harm caused by repletion evil, one's attack must not be slow. One must use swift and ferocious drugs, and harmonize [their effects] with regular drugs. Countries that are rich and strong are in a position to deploy awe-inspiring forces. However, the men chosen [to conduct such interventions] must be appropriate, [just as] the instruments and machines [of war] must be of good quality. The periods [of their use] are fixed, and must not be passed.

To set [troops] in battle follows specific schemes. [There are more such parallels] than can be enumerated here. The thirteen books of Master Sun Wu fully cover all patterns applied in the treatment of illness.

Notes

1.   *Su-wen*, treatise 22 ("Ts'ang ch'i fa shih lun"), states: "Toxic drugs attack the evil; the five grains nourish, the five fruits support; the five animals provide benefit; and the five vegetables fill." Hsü Ta-ch'un's rephrasing serves to emphasize the use of strongly active drugs in antiquity as remedies against acute diseases.

2.   The terminology employed here suggests a reference to Taoist alchemical practices.

3.   In this paragraph, Hsü Ta-ch'un employs numerous literal, or almost literal, quotations from a work on military tactics, the *Sun-tzu Ping Fa* by Sun Wu of the 6th century B.C., to elucidate his argument.

4.   In *Sun-tzu Ping Fa*, treatise "Chiu ti p'ien," it is said, "Pu yong hsiang-tao che, pu neng teh ti li," i.e., "without the use of guides one will not be able to benefit from a particular situation."

執方治病論

古人用藥立方先陳列病症然後云某方主之若其症
少有出入則有加減之法附于方後可知方中之藥必
與所現之症纖悉皆合無一味虛設乃用此方毫無通
融也又有一病而云某方亦主之者其方或稍有異同
或竟不同可知一病并不止一方所能治今乃病名稍
似而其中之現症全然不同乃亦以此方施治則其藥
皆不對症矣并有病名雖一病形相反亦用此方則其
中盡屬相反之藥矣總之欲用古方必先審病者所患
之症悉與古方前所陳列之症皆合更檢方中所用之
藥無一不與所現之症相合然後施用否則必須加減
無可加減則另擇一方斷不可道聽塗說聞某方可以
治某病不論其因之異同症之出入而冒昧施治雖所
用恭本于古方而害益大矣

13. On Grasping a [Specific] Prescription to Treat [Specific] Illnesses

In ancient times, when people devised pharmaceutic prescriptions, they first of all listed [a patient's] illnesses and pathoconditions, and then they pointed out which prescription mastered these [pathoconditions]. If the pathoconditions of a specific [patient] differed slightly [from those covered by a particular well-established prescription], patterns were available to add or leave out [certain drugs from this prescription], and [these patterns] were added to the prescriptions [as an appendix]. From this it can be seen that the drugs in a prescription corresponded exactly in even the finest details to the pathoconditions exhibited [by the patient]. Not a single substance was arranged [in a prescription] without specific purpose, and the application of such a prescription left absolutely no room for compromise. But, there were also individual illnesses where [the prescription literature] said that another prescription was also suited to the [patient's pathoconditions], and this [second] prescription may have been quite similar [to the first], or it was totally different indeed.

Obviously, one particular illness can be treated not only with one particular prescription. Today, the name of an illness may still be quite similar to that [of an illness in ancient times], but the pathoconditions that appear in the course of this [illness today] may be very different [from those in ancient times]. If the same prescription is used for treating [this modern illness], the drugs employed will not at all correspond to the [patient's] pathoconditions. Also, even though the names of [an ancient and of a contemporary] illness may be identical, the manifestations of these illnesses may be in complete contrast. If the same prescription is used [today as in ancient times], all of its drugs will be contraindicated.

To summarize, if one wishes to use ancient prescriptions, one must first examine which pathoconditions a patient suffers from, and whether they are identical with those pathoconditions listed in front of the ancient prescription [one is about to use]. Then one should make sure that each drug in the [ancient] prescription corresponds to the pathoconditions exhibited [by the patient one intends to treat. If this is the case], one may apply [the prescription]. Otherwise, one must add or eliminate [substances in accordance with the specific circumstances of the illness to be treated], and if such adding or eliminating is unfeasible, one should select another prescription.

By no means should one follow road-side gossip; that is, if one has heard that a certain prescription is able to cure a certain illness, [one should not] apply it without proper thinking, [i.e.,] without taking the cause of the illness and all the pathoconditions into regard. [The drugs] employed may indeed all be based on an ancient prescription, but the harm resulting [from thoughtless application] will be severe.

湯藥不足盡病論

內經治病之法鍼灸為本而佐之以砭石熨浴導引按
摩酒醴等法病各有宜缺一不可益服藥之功入腸胃
而氣四達未嘗不能行於臟腑經絡若邪在筋骨肌肉
之中則病屬有形藥之氣味不能奏功也故必用鍼灸
等法即從病之所在調其血氣逐其風寒為實而可據
也況即以服藥論止用湯劑亦不能盡病益湯者盪也
其行速其質輕其力易過而不留惟病在榮衛腸胃者
其效更速其餘諸病有宜丸宜散宜膏者必醫者豫備
以待一時急用視其病之所在而委曲施治則病無遁
形故天下無難治之症而投輙有神效扁鵲倉公所
謂禁方者是也若今之醫者祇以一煎方為治惟病後
調理則用滋補丸散盡廢聖人之良法即使用藥不誤
而與病不相入則終難取效故扁鵲云人之所患患病

多醫之所患患道少近日病變愈多而醫家之道愈少
此痼疾之所以日多也

14. On the Inadequacy of Decoctions to Completely Cure Illnesses

The basic therapeutic methods of the *Nei-ching* are needling and cauterization, and these [two methods] are supplemented by pointed stones, hot poultices, baths, gymnastics, massage, and [medicinal] wines. For each illness there exists a suitable [therapeutic method]. Not one [of those listed] must be omitted.

The effects of drugs enter the intestines and the stomach, and their influences penetrate in all directions. Never have they been barred from moving into the viscera and bowels, [major] conduits and network [vessels]. If evil [influences] have entered the sinews, the bones, the muscles or the flesh, then the illness [resulting from this intrusion] is a morphological one, and the [thermo-]influences and flavor [influences] of drugs will show no effect. Hence [in such cases] one must apply [therapeutic] methods such as needling and cauterization.

One regulates blood or influences according to the location of the illness, and drives off wind or cold. These are tangible facts. How much more then, if we focus on the application of drugs now, [should it be clear] that applying nothing but decoctions is quite inadequate to completely cure illnesses.

Decoction (*t'ang*) stands for agitation (*tang*). [Decoctions] move fast. Their substance is light; their strength quickly subsides and does not stay. The effects [of decoctions] are especially fast when it comes to illnesses affecting the constructive or protective [influences], the intestines and the stomach. In case of all other illnesses, either pills or powders or pastes may be appropriate. The physicians must prepare [pills, powders, and pastes] in advance of a situation when [they are confronted with an illness requiring] their urgent application. Once this moment has arrived, the physician must] examine where an illness is located, and apply the treatment with all due consideration. Then the illness will not be able to hide away. Hence, there are no pathoconditions on earth that are difficult to cure, and [the drugs] given [to the patient] will show immediate miraculous results. These, then, are the so-called secret prescriptions of Pien Ch'io and Ts'ang-kung.

Today's physicians, though, treat [their patients] with a single prescription designed as a decoction. Only for the harmonizing that is carried out in the aftermath of an illness episode do they use nourishing and supplementing pills and powders. Thus, they have given up the good [old] methods of the Sages entirely.

The drugs they use may not be wrong, but if they fail to enter [the body] in accordance with the [location of the] illness [they are supposed to eliminate], then positive results are difficult to achieve. Hence Pien Ch'io stated, "What people suffer from is a multitude of illnesses; what physicians suffer from is a paucity of approaches."[1] Today, the illnesses appear in ever more variations, and the physicians have ever fewer approaches at their disposal. Hence chronic illnesses increase day by day.

Note

1.   This is a slightly modified quotation from the biography of Pien Ch'io in the *Shih-chi*, ch. 105. Actually, these are the words of Ssu-ma Ch'ien, the author of the *Shih-chi*, not of the legendary Pien Ch'io.

本草古今論

本草之始仿于神農藥止三百六十品此乃開天之聖人與天地為一體實能探造化之精窮萬物之理字字精確非若後人推測而知之者故對症施治其應若響仲景諸方之藥悉本此書藥品不多而神明變化已無病不治矣迨其後藥味日多至陶弘景倍之而為七百二十品後世日增一日凡華夷之奇草逸品試而有效醫家皆取而用之代有成書至明李時珍增益唐慎微證類本草為綱目考其異同辨其真偽原其生產集諸家之說而本草更大備此藥由少而多之故也至其功用則亦後人試驗而知之故其所治之病益廣然皆不若神農本草之純正真確故宋人有云用神農之品無不效而弘景所增已不甚效若後世所增之藥則尤有不足憑者至其詮釋大半皆視古方用此藥醫某病則增注之或古方治某病其藥不止一品而誤以方中此藥為專治此病者有之更有以已意推測而知者又或偶愈一病實非此藥之功而強著其效者種種難信至張潔古李東垣輩以某藥專派入某經則更穿鑿矣其詳在治病不必分經絡藏府篇故論本草必以神農為本而他說則必審擇而從之更必驗之于病而後信又必考古人方中所曾用者乃可採取餘則止可于單方外治之法用之又有後世所增之奇藥或出于深山窮谷或出于殊方異域前世所未嘗有者後人用之往往有奇效此乃偏方異氣之所鍾造物之機久而愈洩能治古方所不能治之奇病博物君子亦宜識之以廣見聞此又在本草之外者矣

15. On Ancient and Contemporary Materia Medica

In the beginning, the art of materia medica followed Shen-nung. The drugs [he introduced in his book] numbered only 360.[1] This [means] that the Sages [of antiquity] who opened [the secrets of] nature were one with heaven and earth, and they were, indeed, able to uncover the essentials of creation. They fully investigated the principles of all things. Word for word [their writings] were both subtle and accurate. Their knowledge was, therefore, different from that gained by people of later times through deductive reasoning and measurements. Hence, when [the ancients] applied a treatment for a pathocondition, the result came like an echo.

All the drugs in the prescriptions [listed] by [Chang] Chung-ching were based on that book [by Shen-nung]. These drugs were not many but they were modified [for different uses] with great intelligence. There were no illnesses that remained uncured. Later then, the number of drugs increased daily, and T'ao Hung-ching, finally, doubled [the contents of the work written by Shen-nung] by listing 720 substances [in his own book].[2]

During the following generations, [the number of drugs] increased further day by day. All strange herbs and extraordinary items from China and from foreign tribes were accepted for [therapeutic] application by physicians, once they had been tested and shown positive results. Books were compiled through the ages [to impart the knowledge thus gained], until Li Shih-chen, during the Ming dynasty, enlarged T'ang Shen-wei's *Cheng-lei Pen-ts'ao* and compiled the *[Pen-ts'ao] Kang Mu*. [Li Shih-chen] studied differences and similarities [among drugs]. He distinguished between false and correct [identification]. He traced the [geographic] origins [of the drugs]; and he collected the sayings of all [the previous] experts. As a result, he brought the materia medica to an even greater degree of completeness [than had existed before]. This is the reason why the number of pharmaceutical substances increased from a mere few [at the time of Shen-nung] to many [in the book written by Li Sih-chen].

The same applies to [drug] effects. Here, too, the people of later times carried out tests and gained knowledge. Here, too, the number of illnesses they could treat successfully increased [with the number of newly introduced drugs]. And yet, none of these [later additions] reached the purity and authenticity of the [knowledge outlined in] the *Shen-nung Pen-ts'ao*. Hence the people of the Sung era used to say:

Apply Shen-nung's drugs and none will fail to show positive results. Those added by [T'ao] Hung-ching are, already, not overly effective. And those drugs that were added in still later times are even less reliable.

As for explanatory notes [in later drug compendiums], often enough their [authors] had observed that some ancient prescription had used this or that drug to treat a specific illness, and hence they added this [information] as a commentary [to their drug descriptions]. However, sometimes an ancient prescription, in [being designed] for a specific illness, had employed more than one item, and [later commentators] mistakenly assumed that [all] the drugs of that prescription were only capable of curing that specific illness. Also, there was knowledge based on personal speculation. And in other cases the effects of a drug were forcibly pointed out, where in fact, an illness had come to an end rather by coincidence than because of the effects of this drug. All such [commentaries] are hard to believe.

When, finally, [people] like Chang Chieh-ku and Li Tung-yüan held that certain drugs penetrate through specific conduits, then this was particularly artificially construed. A detailed [discussion] of this [erroneous concept may be found] in the paragraph "For the Treatment of Illness it is not Necessary to Distinguish between [Main] Conduits and Network [Vessels], Viscera and Bowels."[3]

If, therefore, one discusses materia medica, one should accept Shen-nung's [contribution] as fundamental. All other statements should be examined critically before one accepts them as guides. They must prove effective against illnesses first before one believes them!

Also, one should investigate whether [a drug] was already used in ancient prescriptions. If so, it may be chosen [without further questions] for use [again]. All other [drugs] should only be used in single-substance prescriptions and in patterns designed for external application.

Then there are those out-of-the-way drugs that were added by later generations. Some originated from deep in the mountains and from distant valleys. Others came from strange regions and foreign lands. Earlier generations did not have these [drugs], and when people of later times applied them [in therapy], they often showed wonderful results. These, then, are [drugs] that require far-away regions with extraordinary influences [to have their special effects grow]. The mechanics of creation become known to man increasingly as time goes by. As [these strange substances] cure strange illnesses that cannot be cured with prescriptions of ancient times, the scholar must be familiar with them to widen his knowledge. They remain, however, outside of [the scope of ordinary] materia medica.

Notes

1.   Shen-nung, a legendary pre-historic god and cultural hero, is the alleged author of the *Shen-nung Pen-ts'ao Ching*, a work probably compiled in the first century A.D. See Paul U. Unschuld, *Medicine in China: A History of Pharmaceutics.* Berkeley, Los Angeles, London: U.C. Press. 1985: 17-27.

2.   T'ao Hung-ching compiled a *Shen-nung Pen-ts'ao Ching* and a *Pen-ts'ao Ching Chi-chu,* both with 730 (not 720) drug descriptions. See Unschuld, *History of Pharmaceutics,* pp. 30-43.

3.   See above essay I.6., p. 72

藥性變遷論

古方所用之藥當時效驗顯著而本草載其功用鑿鑿
者今依方施用竟有不應其故何哉蓋有數端焉
一則地氣之殊也當時初用之始必有所產之地此乃
其本生之土故氣厚而力全以後傳種他方則地氣移
而力薄矣一則種類之異也凡物之種類不一古人所
採必至貴之種後世相傳必擇其易于繁衍者而種之
未必皆種之至貴者物雖非偽而種則殊矣一則天生
與人力之異也當時所採皆生于山谷之中元氣未洩
故得氣獨厚今皆人功種植既非山谷之真氣又加灌
溉之功則性平淡而薄矣一則名實之訛也當時藥
不市賣皆醫者自取而備之追其後有不常用之品後
人欲得而用之尋求採訪或誤以他物充之或以別種
代之又肆中未備以近似者欺人取利此藥遂失其真

矣其變遷之因實非一端藥性既殊即審病極真處方
極當奈其藥非當時之藥則效亦不可矣今之醫者
惟知定方其藥則惟病家取之肆中所以真假莫辨雖
有神醫不能以假藥治真病也

16. On Changes in the Qualities of Drugs

The drugs used in the prescriptions of antiquity showed obvious results in those times, and their functions were recorded by the pharmaceutic literature with all clarity. If, however, one applies [these same drugs] today according to the prescriptions [of old], sometimes [the illnesses] respond, sometimes not. What is the reason?

Well, there are a number of principles [responsible for these differences]. First [one may regard] differences in the regional influences [affecting the qualities of drugs as responsible]. When, in [ancient] times, [the drugs] came into use, there were specific areas where [specific drugs] grew. These, then, were their native places. Hence, [each drug] was rich in influences and full of strength. Later, [the drugs] were transferred to other regions to be planted there too. The regional influences [affecting the drugs] changed, and they weakened in strength.

A further [reason for changes in the qualities of drugs may be sought in] differences in the varieties [of a particular substance used]. In ancient times, people gathered only the most valuable varieties [of a drug]. In later generations, when [the use of drugs] spread widely, it was necessary to select and plant those that could be multiplied most easily. These, however, were by no means always the most valuable varieties. Even [in case a drug remained without effect] if the substance itself was not a false substitute, the variety may have been different.

A further [reason for changes in the qualities of drugs may be sought in] differences between natural growth and [cultivation through] human effort. In those [ancient] times, all [drugs] gathered grew in mountain valleys. There the original influences had not yet leaked away, and therefore, [the drugs] received rich quantities of influences. Today, all [drugs] are cultivated by man, and they do not get the true influences of the mountain valleys any longer. Also, [the fields where the drugs are grown] are irrigated artificially, hence the qualities of the drugs are unpronounced and weak.

A further [reason for changes in the qualities of drugs may be sought in] falsely named substances. In those [ancient] times, drugs were not sold in markets. The physicians gathered and prepared them always by themselves. Later, there were people who wished to acquire some rarely used items and apply them [in therapy]. They searched for them and inquired [where they might get them]. Sometimes they mistakenly substituted them with some other substances. Or, they used another variety [of the same drug] instead. Or, a shop had no supplies [of a requested drug] and cheated people with some similar [item] to gain a profit. As a consequence, this drug lost its genuine character.

There are, indeed, a number of causes contributing to these changes! Given these differences in the qualities of drugs, one may analyze most carefully whether an illness is truly [identical with the one named in an ancient prescription], and one may take great pains to design a most appropriate prescription. If the drugs are not the same as those [used] in [ancient] times, their effects cannot be taken for granted.

Today's physicians know only how to write standardized prescriptions, and the drugs they [prescribe] are always acquired from shops by the patients themselves. Hence genuine and false [substances] are no longer distinguished, and although a physician may be [as capable as] a spirit, he will not be able to cure a genuine illness with false drugs.

藥性專長論

藥之治病有可解者有不可解者如性熱能治寒性燥

能治濕芳香則通氣滋潤則生津此可解者也如同一

發散也而桂枝則散太陽之邪柴胡則散少陽之邪同

一滋陰也而麥冬則滋肺之陰生地則滋腎之陰同一

解毒也而雄黃則解蛇虫之毒甘草則解飲食之毒已

有不可盡解者至如鱉甲之消痞塊史君子之殺蛔虫

赤小豆之消膚腫桃仁生服不眠熟服多睡白鶴花之

不腐肉而腐骨則尤不可解者此乃藥性之專長即所

謂單方秘方也然人止知不可知者之為專長而不能

常用藥之中亦各有專長後人或不知之而不能

用或日用而忽焉皆不能盡收藥之功效者也故醫者

當廣集奇方深明藥理然後奇症當前皆有治法變化

不窮當年神農著本草之時既不能睹形而即識其性

又不可每藥歷試而知竟能深識其功能而所投必效

豈非與造化相為黙契而非後人思慮之所能及者乎

199

17. On Special Strength in the Qualities of Drugs

When drugs cure an illness, in some cases this can be explained, in others not. For instance, [drugs with] a hot quality can cure [illnesses related to] cold, and [drugs with] a dry quality can cure [illnesses related to] dampness. [Drugs that are] fragrant will stimulate [a patient's] influences to penetrate [what would otherwise remain blocked], and [drugs that have a] moistening [quality] produce liquids. All of these [are examples of therapeutic effects that] can be explained.

When, however, [drugs are] identical in their dispersing [quality, but different in their actual effects] — such as *kuei-chih*, which disperses evil [influences from the] great-yang [regions], and *ch'ai-hu*, which disperses evil [influences from the] minor-yang [regions] — or when [drugs are] identical in their [capabilities of] nourishing the yin [but differ in their actual effects] — such as *mai-tung*, which nourishes the yin [influences] of the lung, and *sheng-ti*, which nourishes the yin [influences] of the kidneys — or when [drugs are] identical in their [abilities to] dissolve poison [but differ in their actual effects] — such as *hsiung-huang*, which dissolves the poisons of snakes and insects, and *kan-ts'ao*, which dissolves the poisons of foods and beverages — [then these are] already [some examples of therapeutic drug effects] that cannot be explained entirely.

But when it comes to [the ability of] turtle shells to dissolve blockages, or to [the ability of] *shih-chün-tzu* to kill *hui* worms, or to [the ability of] *ch'ih-hsiao-tou* to eliminate skin swellings, or to [the fact that] *jui-jen* keep one awake if eaten in a fresh state, while they cause one to be very sleepy if eaten after they were processed, or [when it comes to the ability of] *pai-ho-hua* to preserve meat from decay while allowing bones to rot, then [these are examples of drug effects] that are even harder to explain.

Such are the special strengths in the qualities of drugs, and [one makes use of them] in single[-ingredient] prescriptions and in secret formulas. People [today], however, consider only that which cannot be explained as special strengths, and they do not know that each of those drugs that are in frequent use has effects based on special strengths too. [Like all] people of later times, they either do not know of these [drugs,] and are therefore unable to use them, or they use them day after day but disregard their [special effects. As a result,] none of them is able to fully appropriate the effects of the drugs [for therapeutic purposes].

Physicians, therefore, should widely [search for and] collect extraordinary prescriptions, and they should be thoroughly familiar with the principles of drugs. Later then, when they are confronted with extraordinary pathoconditions, they will have therapeutic patterns at their disposal for each of them, and [they will be able to apply prescriptions] in countless modifications.

When Shen-nung wrote [his book on] pharmaceutics, he did not gain his knowledge of the qualities [of the drugs] from inspecting their [physical] appearance, and there was also no way for him to gather his knowledge by testing all drugs one by one. When he was thoroughly acquainted with the effects [of the drugs], and when each application brought forth a success, this was surely because he was familiar with [all the secrets of] creation — something that could never be achieved by the people of later times through all their reasoning!

煎藥法論

煎藥之法最宜深講藥之效不效全在乎此夫烹飪魚羊豕失其調度尚能損人況藥專以之治病而可不講乎其法載于古方之末者種種各殊如麻黃湯先煮麻黃去沫然後加餘藥同煎此主藥當先煎之法也而桂枝湯又不必先煎桂枝服藥後須啜熱粥以助藥力又一法也如茯苓桂枝甘草大棗湯則以甘瀾水先煎茯苓如五苓散則以白飲和服服後又當多飲煖水小建中湯則先煎五味去渣而後納飴糖大柴胡湯則煎減半去渣再煎柴胡加龍骨牡蠣湯則煎藥成而後納大黃其煎之多寡或煎水減半或十分煎去二三分或止煎一二十沸煎藥之法不可勝數皆各有意義大都發散之藥及芳香之藥不宜多煎取其生而疎盪補益滋膩之藥宜多煎取其熟而停蓄此其總訣也故方藥

雖中病而煎法失度其藥必無效蓋病家之常服藥者或尚能依法為之其粗魯貧苦之家安能如法制度所以病難愈也若令之醫者亦不能知之矣況病家乎

18. On the Patterns of Drug Boiling

The patterns of drug boiling need a very thorough discussion, because whether a drug has an effect or not is entirely dependent upon these patterns. Poultry, fish, sheep, and pork, if cooked improperly, may harm man, and it should go without saying that this applies all the more to drugs whose special [virtue] lies in the curing of illness.

Very many different patterns were recorded at the conclusion of the ancient prescriptions. For instance, [to prepare] the "Decoction with *ma-huang*," one boils the *ma-huang* first and removes the foam. Only then are the remaining drugs added and [all the ingredients] boiled together. This is the pattern of boiling the major drug [of a prescription] first.

Or take the case of the "Decoction with *kuei-chih*." Here [the main drug of the prescription] must not be boiled [alone] first. Following an intake of *kuei-chi* for medicinal purposes,[1] one must sip hot congee in order to support its therapeutic forces. That is another pattern.

Or take the case of the "Decoction with *fu-ling, kuei-chih, kan-ts'ao, ta-tsao.*" Here one first of all [should] boil the *fu-ling* together with sweet-softened water.[2]

The "Powder with *wu-ling*," to cite another example, is to be taken together with a thick soup, and after it has been taken one should drink, in addition, large quantities of warm water. [In the case of the] "Small Decoction for Strengthening One's Center," the five ingredients are boiled first, and the dregs are discarded. Then, granulated sugar is added.

[In the case of the] "Large Decoction with *ch'ai-hu*," [the drugs are boiled] until [the water has] diminished by one half. Then one discards the dregs and boils again.

[In the case of the] "Decoction with *ch'ai-hu* amended by *lung-ku* and *mu-li*," *ta-huang* is added only after the [remaining] drugs [of this prescription] have been sufficiently boiled.

As to the extent of the boiling, in some instances the boiling is to reduce the water by one half. Or, two or three tenths [of the water volume] are to be removed [through boiling], or one boils [the water] only until it has bubbled ten or twenty times.

It is impossible to enumerate all the different patterns of boiling [drugs]. Each of these patterns has its specific significance. Generally speaking, dispersing drugs as well as aromatic drugs should not be boiled for long [since one intends] to take advantage of their [abilities] to distribute and stir up — [abilities which they have only as long] as they are raw.

Supplementing and nourishing drugs should be boiled extensively [because one intends] to make use of their [abilities] to hold and to store — [abilities that they acquire only after] they have been processed.

[All the examples listed so far], however, should serve merely as a general outline. Even if the drugs of a prescription [have been selected in such a way that they] hit the illness [they are supposed to treat], if the boiling pattern [applied] is inappropriate, the drugs will remain without effect!

Some of those patients who take drugs frequently may still be able to prepare their [medications] according to a [correct] pattern. How, though, could uneducated and destitute families be able to follow the [appropriate] patterns and rules? Their illnesses are, therefore, difficult to cure. And if even today's physicians are unaware of this [issue], how much more does this apply to the patients?

Notes

1.   *Kuei-chih*, cinnamon, could be used also as a spice.

2.   "Sweet-softened water," *kan lan shui*, is produced by ladling water from a vessel and pouring it back many times. It is supposed to have a beneficial effect on the stomach and intestines.

服藥法論

病之愈不愈不但方必中病方雖中病而服之不得其
法則非特無功而反有害此不可不知也如發散之劑
欲驅風寒出之于外必熱服而煖覆其體令藥氣行于
榮衛熱氣周徧挾風寒而從汗解若半溫而飲之仍當
風坐立或僅寂然安臥則藥留腸胃不能得汗風寒無
暗消之理而榮氣反為風藥所傷矣通利之藥欲其化
積滯而達之于下也必空服頓服使藥性鼓動推其垢
濁從大便解若與飲食雜揉則新舊混雜而藥氣與食
物相亂則氣性不專而食積愈頑矣故傷寒論等書服
藥之法宜熱宜溫宜凉宜冷宜緩宜急宜多宜少宜早
宜晚宜飽宜飢更有宜湯不宜散宜散不宜丸宜膏不
宜圓其輕重大小上下表裏治法各有當此皆一定之
至理深思其義必有得于心也

19. On Patterns of Drug Intake

Whether [the treatment of] an illness results in a cure or not, requires more than [a composition of drugs in a] prescription that hits the illness. Although a prescription may [be well suited to] hit an illness, it will not only fail to exert any effect, but will — on the contrary — even cause harm, if its intake did not correspond to an appropriate pattern. It is absolutely essential to be aware of this.

For instance, if one wishes to expel wind and cold [from the body] by means of dispersing preparations, [the latter] must be taken hot, and [the patient's] body must be warmly covered. This causes the influences of the drugs to move into the constructive and protective [influences]. Hot influences will be distributed everywhere [in the body]. They take hold of the wind or cold [that are to be eliminated], and release them [from the body] together with the [resulting] sweat.

If [someone suffering from wind or cold] drinks only a lukewarm [decoction], sits or stands exposed to wind, or simply lies down quickly [after taking the medication], then the drugs will stay in [his] intestines or stomach. No sweating occurs, and there is no reason why wind or cold should vanish or dissipate. On the contrary, the constructive influences will even be harmed by those drugs [that should have acted against the] wind.

[By treating a patient] with penetrating drugs, one intends to take advantage of their ability to transform accumulations and cause them to move downwards. Such drugs must be taken on an empty stomach, and all at once, so that their qualities can be set in motion. As a result, they will push the filth [out of the body] by releasing it together with the stools. If, however, one brings [such drugs] into [the body] together with beverages or food, new and old will be mixed, and the influences of the drugs will be confused with [those of] the food. As a result, the qualities of the drugs cannot [exert] their special [effects], and the accumulations of food will be increasingly obstinate.

Hence the patterns for taking drugs, as [recommended] in the *Shang-han lun* and other books, [include] requirements [to consume] medications hot or warm, cool or cold, slowly or speedily, in large or small amounts, early or late, on a full stomach or hungry. In addition, some [drugs] should be [taken as] decoctions but not as powders, [others] should be [taken as] powders but not as pills, [and others again] should be [taken as] pastes but not as balls.[1]

206

Whether [an illness is] light or serious, comprehensive or minor, in the upper or lower [sections of the body], in the exterior or interior [sections of the body], for each [of these conditions] suitable therapeutic patterns exist. All of these are firmly established principles; one must carefully consider them, and then one will definitely understand their significance.

Note

1.   "Balls" are large pills with a diameter of up to 3 cm. Usually, they are not consumed in one piece.

醫必備藥論

古之醫者所用之藥皆自備之内經云司氣備物則無遺主矣當時韓康賣藥非賣藥也即治病也韓文公進學解云牛溲馬勃敗鼓之皮俱收並蓄待用無遺醫師之良也今止方人稱醫者為賣藥先生則醫者之自備藥可知自宋以後漸有寫方不備藥之醫其藥皆取之肆中今則藥世皆然夫賣藥者不知醫猶之可也乃行醫者竟不知藥則藥之是非真偽全然不問醫者與藥不相謀方即不誤而藥之誤多矣又古聖人之治病惟感冒之疾則以煎劑為主餘者皆用丸散為多其丸散有非一時所能合者倘有急迫之疾必須丸散候丸散合就而人已死矣又有一病止須一丸而愈合藥不可止合一丸若使病家為一人而合一料則一丸之外皆為無用惟醫家合之留待當用者用之不終棄也又有不常用不易得之藥儲之數年難遇一用藥肆之中因無人問則亦不備惟醫者自蓄之乃可待不時之需耳至于外科所用之煎方不過通散營衛耳若護心托毒全賴各種丸散之力其藥皆貴重難得及鍜煉之物修合非一二日之功而所費又大亦不得為一人止合一二丸若外治之圍藥塗藥昇藥降藥護肌腐肉止血行瘀定痛煞癢提膿呼毒生肌生皮續筋連骨又有薰燕烙灸吊洗黑淵等藥種種各異更復每症不同皆非一時所能備必須平時豫合乃今之醫者既不知其方亦不講其法又無資本以蓄藥料偶遇一大症内科則一煎方之外更無別方外科則膏藥之外更無餘藥即有之亦惟取極賤極易得之一二味以為應酬之具則安能使極危極險極奇極惡之症令起死回生乎故藥者醫家不可不全備者也

20. On the Need for Physicians to Prepare Drugs [by Themselves]

In ancient times, the physicians prepared by themselves all the drugs they applied. The *Nei-ching* states, "If items [to be used as drugs] are prepared [in consideration of the] influences governing [the annual seasons, one will] not fail to master [the illnesses to be treated]."[1] At that time Han K'ang sold drugs, and when he did not sell drugs, he cured illnesses.[2] Han Wen-kung[3] stated in his *Chin-hsüeh Chieh*, "He who collects [rarely used drugs such as] the urine of an ox, [the herb] *ma-po*, as well as the skin of a broken drum, and is not in want of them when they are needed for application, is a good physician."

The people in the north call a physician [even] today "Mr. Drug Seller." From this one may know that the physicians [in former times] prepared their drugs by themselves. Beginning with the Sung, a gradual development took place towards [a situation where] physicians who wrote prescriptions did not prepare the drugs [themselves]. They obtained all [their] drugs in shops, and that is how it is everywhere now.

Those who sell the drugs [in the shops] know nothing about medicine. Be that as it may, when those who practice medicine know nothing about the drugs, they simply do not investigate whether a drug is right or wrong, genuine or falsified. If a physician does not care about drugs, the prescriptions [he writes] may be correct, but the drugs themselves may be marred by many mistakes. Also, when the Sages of ancient times treated illnesses, they considered decoctions as most appropriate only in cases of affections by adverse [weather conditions]. Against all other [illnesses] they applied mostly pills and powders.

However, among the pills and powders are some that cannot be prepared instantaneously. In case of an urgent illness that requires pills or a powder, the patient would be long dead by the time his medication was prepared. Also, it may well be that a particular illness needs only one single pill and is cured. However, when preparing drugs, it is impossible to prepare only one single pill. If the patient's family were to prepare one single medication for one single person, all the pills except one are of no use. Only when a physician prepares them, may he keep them until [another patient] needs them, and then he can make use of them. In the long run, he does not throw any of them away.

Furthermore, there are drugs that are only rarely used, and that cannot be easily obtained. Even if one stores them over several years, they hardly come to use but once. In drug shops [such drugs] are not kept in stock because no one ever asks for them. Only when the physicians themselves gather such [items, can they be sure to have them at their disposal] when they are confronted, after all, with an unexpected case [requiring just one of these substances].

Prescriptions for boiled [drugs] to be applied in external medicine are only suitable for penetrating and dispersing the constructive and protective [influences]. But when it comes to [illnesses] where one has to protect one's heart and chase away a poison, and where one has to fully rely on the strengths of all types of pills or powders, then the drugs [required] for these [medications] are all expensive and difficult to obtain. And, then, those items that have to be prepared through processes of forging and melting,[4] they cannot be completed by just one or two days' work, and they require even higher expenditures. Here, too, one cannot prepare one or two pills for just one person.

For external treatments, there are drugs to encircle [a swelling or pain], drugs to be smeared [on a particular location], drugs that rise, and drugs that descend. They protect the muscles or remove spoiled flesh; they stop bleeding and cause blocked blood to move again. They settle pain, and they eliminate itching. They draw pus, and they extract poison. They generate flesh, and they generate skin. They elongate sinews, and they connect bones. Also, there are drugs for smoking and steaming, those for burning and cauterization, those for drawing pus and washing, those for etching, and those for moistening. All of these [drugs and their applications] are different, and all pathoconditions are unlike each other. None of them can be prepared on the spot. They ought to be kept prepared all the time.

Today's physicians do not know the prescriptions [to prepare] these [drugs], and they fail to consider the respective [therapeutic] patterns. In addition, they lack the necessary capital to collect the drug materials. When they happen to encounter a serious pathocondition, in internal medicine, they have only one prescription with boiled [drugs], and in external medicine, they have only paste-drugs. Where they have [additional medications], they pick only one or two of the cheapest and most easily obtainable substances as means to cope [with an emergency] as well as they can. How, then, could they be able to raise the dead and bring back life to those who suffer from the most dangerous, from the most critical, from the most extraordinary, and from the most vicious pathoconditions?

Therefore, physicians must have all [medications] prepared by themselves.

Notes

1.   See *Su-wen,* treatise 74, "Chih-chen yao ta-lun." The meaning of this quotation has been interpreted by Chinese commentators of the *Su-wen* in reference to the doctrine of Five [Calendrical] Movements and Six [Climatic] Influences (*wu yün liu ch'i*) governing the course of a year. Accordingly, one should prepare, for example, bitter drugs only at that time of the year when minor-yin or minor-yang influences dominate, or one should, as another example, collect cooling drugs, such as *ta-huang,* only at a time of the domination of great-yang influences, in order to harvest them at the time of their highest potency.

2.   Han K'ang's brief biography in chapter 83 of the dynastic history of the Later Han period refers to him only as selling drugs in Ch'ang-an for more than thirty years without ever reducing his prices in bargaining. He discontinued his appearance at the market when a young woman was angered by his unwillingness to lower a price and addressed him by his name, thereby revealing his identity.

3.   Posthumous title "Lord of Literature" of Han Yü (768-824), the famous poet and one-time President of the Board of Rites of the T'ang era.

4.   This is a reference to alchemy.

亂方論

世有書符請仙而求方者其所書之方固有極淺極陋

極不典而不能治病且誤人者亦有極高極古極奇極

穩以之治病而神效者其仙或託名呂純陽或託名張

仲景其方亦宛然純陽仲景之遺法此其事甚奇然亦

有理焉夫亂方者機也人心之感召無所不通即誠心于

求治則必有能治病之鬼神應之雖非真純陽仲景必

先世之明于醫理不遇于時而死者其精靈一時不散

遊行于天地之間因感而至以顯其能而其人病適當

愈則獲遇之此亦有其理也其方未必盡效然皆必有

意義反不若世之時醫用相反之藥以害人惟決死生

之處不肯鑿鑿言之此則天機不輕洩之故也至于不

通不典之方則必持亂之術不工或病家之心不誠非

真亂方也

21. On Prescriptions Revealed through Divinatory Practices

There are [people] who write charms to have the Immortals come, and to ask them for prescriptions. Among the prescriptions obtained through such writings there are some that are very superficial, very vulgar, and very heterodox. They are unsuited to cure any illness, and they may cause harm to the people [using them] instead. But, then there are also those that are very sophisticated, very old, very extraordinary, and very safe. If [these latter prescriptions] are applied to treat an illness, miraculous results can be achieved. The immortals [revealing such prescriptions] may assume the names of Lü Ch'un-yang[1] or of Chang Chung-ching, and the prescriptions they [write] may correspond indeed to the patterns left behind by [Lü] Ch'un-yang and [Chang] Chung-ching.

This is very strange, but there is also a reason behind it. "To divine" (chi) stands for "[mental] powers" (chi). The desires of the human mind penetrate everywhere. If someone with a sincere mind searches for a treatment, there must be a response from some demon or spirit able to cure illnesses. Although [this demon or spirit] may not really be that of [Lü] Ch'un-yang or [Chang] Chung-ching, it must represent someone who, in his earlier life, was knowledgeable in the principles of medicine, and who has died without being able to unfold his expertise during his time. His essential spirit does not disperse for some time, and travels between heaven and earth. He follows, now, the desire [of the patient] and approaches him to prove his skills. That person's illness was about to be cured anyway, and therefore, he meets [such spirits]. Such [occurrences] then, have their rational explanation too.

Such prescriptions need not be effective in all instances, but they always have a meaning. This is very different from [the practices of] those physicians of [recent] generations [who follow only the trends of their own] times, and who employ drugs that are contraindicated [in the case of the illnesses against which they are used] and serve only to harm man.

However, when it comes to determining [a patient's] point of death or survival, [the Immortals] are not willing to provide any clear details. The reason is that the secret workings of heaven are not to be disclosed so easily. As for those illogical and heterodox prescriptions [mentioned above], they must come from the hands of people unskilled in the techniques of divination, or [they result from the fact that] the patient's mind was insincere. They are not truly divinatory prescriptions.

Note

1.   Lü Tung-pin, who adopted the name Ch'un-yang, was born in A.D. 798 and is one of three historic personages among the Eight Immortals of China. He is said to have been instructed by another Immortal in the secrets of alchemy and the preparation of the elixir of life.

熱藥誤人最烈論

凡藥之誤人雖不中病非與病相反者不能殺人即與

病相反藥性平和者亦不能殺人與病相反性又不平和

而用藥甚輕不能殺人性既相反藥劑又重其方中有

幾味中病者或有幾味能解此藥性者亦不能殺人焉

此數害或其人病甚輕或其人精力壯盛亦不能殺人

蓋誤藥殺人如此之難也所以世之醫者大半皆誤亦

不見其日殺數人也即使殺之乃輾轉因循以至于死

死者不覺也其有幸而不死或漸自愈者反指所誤用

之藥以為此方之功效又轉以之誤治他人矣所以終

身誤人而不自知其咎也惟大熱大燥之藥則殺人為

最烈蓋熱性之藥往往有毒又陽性急暴一入藏府則

血湧氣升若其人之陰氣本虛或當天時酷暑或其人

傷暑傷熱一投熱劑兩火相爭目赤便閉舌燥齒乾口

渴心煩肌裂神躁種種惡候一時俱發醫者及病家俱

不察或云更宜引火歸元或云此是陰症當加重其熱

藥而佐以大補之品其人七竅皆血呼號宛轉狀如服

毒而死病家全不以為咎醫者亦洋洋自得以為病勢

當然總之愚人喜服補熱雖死不悔我目中所見不一

垂涕泣而道之而醫者與病家無一能聽從者豈非所

謂命哉夫大寒之藥亦能殺人其勢必緩猶為可救不

若大熱之藥斷斷不可救也至于極輕淡之藥誤用亦

能殺人此乃其人之本領甚薄或勢已危殆故小誤即

能生變此又不可全歸咎于醫殺之也

215

22. On [the Fact that] the Most Violent [Harm Caused] to Man by a Mistaken [Pharmaceutical Treatment Originates from] Drugs with Hot [Nature]

Whenever someone [is treated with] the wrong drugs, [these drugs], even though they may not [be suitable to] hit his illness, will not be able to kill this person as long as they are not contraindicated in the case of the illness [to be treated]. Even if they are contraindicated in the case of the illness [to be treated], they will not be able to kill a person as long as their nature is balanced. Even if they are contraindicated in the case of the illness [to be treated], and even if their nature is not balanced, they will still not be able to kill a person as long as they are applied in very light doses. Even if the nature of the drugs is contraindicated and if the dose is heavy, they will still not be able to kill a person as long as there are some substances in the prescription that hit the illness [to be treated] or as long as [the prescription] contains a few substances that are able to dissolve [adverse] drug qualities. Even if all [these potentially] harmful [conditions] appear together, [the drugs] will nevertheless not be able to kill a person as long as his illness is but very light or as long as that person is full of essence and strength. It is that difficult to kill a person through [a treatment with] the wrong drugs.

Hence, even though these days the majority of the physicians commit mistaken [treatments], one still does not see them kill numerous patients each day. But when they kill someone, then this is rather indirect, and it takes quite a while until [the patients] die. Those who die do not realize [why they are dying]. In case [a patient is] lucky and survives, or when he recovers slowly by himself, the [physicians] point out — contrary [to the facts] — the mistakenly applied drugs as being responsible for the good results of the prescription, and they use them, consequently, for further erroneous treatments of other people. Hence for their entire life, they [provide] erroneous [treatments] to the people without ever noticing that it is their own fault.

Only drugs with a very hot or very dry [nature] kill people in a most violent way. The reason is that hot natured drugs are often toxic. Also, their yang nature is urgent and fierce. As soon as they enter the body's viscera and bowels, the blood bubbles up and the influences rise. If a person's yin influences were depleted beforehand, or if it is a hot day, or if the patient had been harmed by summer-heat or [other] heat already, as soon as he takes hot [drugs] the two fires clash, and all types of terrible symptoms will appear at the same time. [The patient's] eyes turn red and his stools are blocked, his tongue loses its moisture and his teeth dry out.

216

His mouth is thirsty and his heart is troubled, his flesh shows cracks and his spirit is disturbed.

The physicians, as well as the patients, fail to notice [the real cause of this condition]. They may say it is good to draw even more fire [into the patient's body] in order to have his original [influences] return, or they may say that this is a yin pathocondition, and that even more drugs with a hot [nature] should be added [to the situation]. And, they will support [such drugs] with strongly supplementing substances. As a result, the person [undergoing such a treatment loses] blood through all his seven orifices. He screams and turns around as if he had taken some poison, and dies. The patients' families never blame [the physician]; and the physicians are self-satisfied too, believing that it had to be this way given the condition of the illness.

In general, then, ignorant people love to take supplementing [drugs that provide the body with] heat. Even death cannot cause them to repent. I have seen this with my own eyes more than once. But even if I were to tell this with tears [in my eyes], neither physicians nor patients would be able to listen and follow [my advice]. Is this not what is called fate? Drugs with a strongly cold [nature] can also kill people, but their force is necessarily milder, and [the patients] can be saved. This is in contrast to drugs with a strongly hot [nature], where no rescue is possible at all. If someone is killed through the application of very light and neutral drugs, then this is either a result of a very weak constitution [on the part of the patient], or the condition [of his illness] had reached a dangerous state already. Hence, even a small mistake may cause [unwanted] changes, and in such cases responsibility for the patient's death cannot be entirely placed on the physician.

薄貼論

今所用之膏藥古人謂之薄貼其用大端有二一以治表一以治裏治表者如呼膿去腐止痛生肌并攄風護肉之類其膏宜輕薄而日換此理人所易知治裏者或驅風寒或和氣血或消痰癖或壯筋骨其方甚多藥亦隨病加減其膏宜重厚而久貼此理人所難知何也蓋人之疾病由外以入內其流行于經絡藏府者必服藥乃能驅之若其病既有定所在于皮膚筋骨之間可按而得者用膏貼之閉塞其氣使藥性從毛空而入其腠理通經貫絡或提而出之或攻而敗之較之服藥尤有力此至妙之法也故凡病之氣聚血結而有形者薄貼之法為良但製膏之法取藥必真心志必誠火候必到方能有效否則不能奏功至于敷熨吊温種種雜法義亦相同在善醫者通變之而已

218

23. On Thin Ointments

The paste drugs applied today were called "thin ointments" by the people in ancient times. Basically, the intention of using them is two-fold. First, [they are applied] for treating exterior [ailments]. And second, [they are applied] for treating interior [ailments].

Treatments of exterior [ailments] include, for instance, the drawing of pus, the elimination of rotting [flesh], the ending of pain, and the generation of muscles, as well as the expulsion of wind, and the protection of flesh. Pastes [employed for] such [ends] should be applied thinly, and they should be changed daily. The reason behind this [therapy] is easily understandable.

Treatment of interior [ailments by means of pastes] includes, for instance, the elimination of wind-cold, the harmonization of influences and blood, the dissolving of blockages caused by mucus, and the strengthening of sinews and bones. Many prescriptions for such [therapeutic purposes] exist, and drugs have to be added to or are to be taken away from [such prescriptions] in accordance with the illness [to be treated. If used] for this purpose [of treating interior ailments], a paste must be applied in thick layers, and it should be left on [the skin] for an extended period of time.

The reason behind this [therapy] is difficult to comprehend. Why? Well, man's illnesses proceed from the outside [of the body] to its internal regions. As long as they flow through the [main] conduits and the network [vessels], as well as through the viscera and bowels, there is no other way to eliminate them except through an intake of drugs. However, once an illness has settled down at a specific location, and when it can be felt in the region between skin, sinews, and bones, one applies a paste there to seal up the [illness's] influences, and to let the qualities of the drugs proceed through the pores of the hair into the ts'ou-li [area between skin and flesh], penetrate the conduits and their network [vessels], pick up [the illness] there and move it out [of the body], or attack and disperse it.

The strength of the drugs [applied this way] is far superior to [that of drugs that are] taken internally. This is a very subtle [therapeutic] pattern. Hence, whenever someone suffers from accumulations of influences, or from clottings of blood, with [his illness] assuming a physical shape, the [therapeutic] pattern of "thin ointments" is excellent.

However, [one should keep in mind] that the patterns of paste preparation require the use of nothing but genuine drugs, a sincere mind, and appropriate strength of the fire [used to boil the drugs]. Only if these [conditions are met] will a prescription show good results. Otherwise, it will not be able to produce any effects.

As for the [further] patterns [of external drug application, such as] smearing [ointments], attaching hot [poultices], spooning,[1] and soaking, their meanings are identical [with those of the application of pastes]. An expert physician knows all this, and modifies [his treatment in accordance with the specific therapeutic problem confronting him].

Note

1.   The term *tiao* has two meanings. It may indicate here the moving of a spoon filled with warm water on the skin above an aching or otherwise ailing area. In paragraph IV.20 the term was rendered with its second meaning as "drawing pus."

貌似古方欺人論

古聖人之立方不過四五味而止其審藥性至精至當
其察病情至真至確方中所用之藥必軰對其病而無
毫髮之差無一味泛用之藥且能以一藥兼治數症故
其藥味雖少而無症不該後世之人果能審其人之病
與古方所治之病無少異則全用古方治之無不立效
其如天下之風氣各殊人之氣稟各異則不得不依古
人所製主病之方畧為增減則藥味增矣或病同而
症甚雜未免欲蕳顧則隨症增一二味而藥又增矣故
後世之方藥味增多非其好為雜亂也乃學不如古人
不能以一藥該數症故變簡而為繁耳此猶不失周詳
之意且古方之設原有加減之法病症雜出亦有多品
之劑藥味至十餘種自唐以後之方用藥漸多皆此義
也乃近世之醫動云效法漢方藥止四五味其四五味

之藥有用浮泛輕淡之品者雖不中病猶無大害若趨
時之輩竟以人參附子乾姜蒼朮鹿茸熟地等峻補辛
熱之品不論傷寒暑濕惟此數種輪流轉換以成一方
種種與病相反每試必殺人毫不自悔既不辨病又不
審藥性更不記方書以為此乃漢人之法嗚呼今之所
學漢人之方何其害人如此之毒也其端起于近日之
時醫好為高論以欺人又人情樂于溫補而富貴之家
洗甚深如堤則道不行所以人爭效尤以致貽害不息
安有讀書考古深思體驗之君子出而挽回之亦世道
生民之大幸也

24. On [Attempts to] Imitate Ancient Prescriptions and to Cheat People

When the Sages of antiquity established a prescription, [they based it on] no more than four or five substances. They identified the qualities of the drugs in a most skillful and most reliable way, and they diagnosed the character of the illnesses in a most accurate and most exact manner. Hence, the drugs employed in their prescriptions corresponded perfectly to the illnesses [they were meant to cure], and not even the slightest discrepancy occurred [between therapeutic means and goals]. Not a single substance was used without careful consideration. Also, the [Sages of antiquity] were able to treat different pathoconditions with one and the same drug, so that, although the number of substances [employed by them] was small, each pathocondition was covered.

Those people of later times who were able to realize that someone's illness was completely identical with an illness treated by a prescription from antiquity, and who relied on nothing but such ancient prescriptions [to treat such illnesses], they too achieved immediate good results. Since the winds and the influences are different everywhere on Earth, and since the people are, therefore, affected by different influences too, it is a necessity that the prescriptions that were designed to master illnesses by the ancients were slightly [modified in later times in that drugs were] added to or taken away from them. Naturally, this has led to an increase in pharmaceutic substances. Also, while illnesses may be identical, the pathoconditions associated with them are extremely complex [and may differ from illness to illness]. All [pathoconditions] have to be taken into consideration, and one or two substances were added [to an originally small prescription] for each pathocondition [by people in later times]. Hence, the number of drugs increased even further.

When, therefore, in later times the number of pharmaceutic substances [employed] increased significantly, this was not because [the people] loved to create confusion and chaos. It is just that the learning [of the people in later times] was inferior to that of the ancients, [and that the physicians] were unable to treat several pathoconditions with one single drug. Hence they changed to complexity what was simple before.

And still, [their behavior] was not entirely void of an attempt at a comprehensive and exact [approach]. However, the design of ancient prescriptions had included, from its very beginning, the pattern of adding or subtracting [drugs] already. If, in the case of an illness, various pathoconditions appeared [in antiquity], preparations with larger numbers of substances were [used], comprising more than ten drugs. These [circumstances, as outlined above,] are the reason for the steady increase in drugs employed in prescriptions ever since the T'ang.

Today, the physicians claim at every occasion to repeat the prescriptions of the Han, and they restrict their drugs to four or five substances [again]. But, as these four or five substances they use but unspecific and neutral items that, while not hitting the illnesses [they are supposed to cure], do not cause any great harm either.

Those, however, who prefer to be fashionable, they use only rapidly supplementing, acrid, and hot substances, namely *jen-shen, fu-tzu, kan-chiang, ts'ang-shu, lu-jung,* and *shou-ti.* And no matter whether [a patient] was harmed by cold, heat, or dampness, [these physicians] oscillate between these few [drugs] to compose their prescriptions. Often enough, these [drugs] are contraindicated in the case of the illness [to be treated], and every trial is bound to kill someone. Still, there is not the slightest self-reproach.

[These physicians of today] do not recognize the different illnesses, they fail to examine the qualities of drugs, and they certainly do not consult any of the prescription works. And yet, they believe that [what they prescribe] is identical with the patterns of the people of the Han. Alas! How can it be that today's study of the prescriptions of the people of the Han causes harm to mankind as poisonous as this?

Well, this has its origin in the physicians of today who prefer to make lofty speeches, to betray the people. Also, people are pleased [if one uses] warm and supplementing [drugs], and this applies, in particular, to the rich and noble. Those who do not follow these preferences will not be able to continue their profession for long. Hence, people [today] strive to achieve the best effects [with their treatments], but they cause only unending calamity.

If there were to appear a noble person who has read the literature and who has studied antiquity, who has given himself to profound thoughts and who has conducted substantial investigations, if [such a person] were to reform [this situation], this would be very fortunate for all the people.

V. Therapeutic Patterns

司天運氣論

邪說之外有欺人之學有耳食之學何謂欺人之學好
為高談奇論以駭人聽聞或勦襲前人之語以示淵博
彼亦自知其為全然不解但量他人亦莫之能深考也
此為欺人之學何謂耳食之學或竊聽他人之說或偶
閱先古之書略記數語自信為已得其秘大言不慚以
此動輒所謂道聽塗說是也如近人所談司天運氣之
類是矣彼所謂司天運氣者以為何氣司天則是年民
當何病假如厥陰司天風氣主之則是年之病皆當作
風治此等議論所謂耳食也蓋司天運氣之說黃帝不
過言天人相應之理如此其應驗先候於脉凡遇少陰
司天則兩手寸口不應厥陰司天則右寸不應太陰司
天則左寸不應若在泉則尺脉不應亦如之若脉不當
其位則病相反者死此診脉之一法也至於病則必觀

是年歲氣勝與不勝如厥陰司天風淫所勝民病心痛
脇滿等症倘是年風淫雖勝而民另生他病則不得亦
指為風淫之病也若是年風淫不勝則又不當從風治
矣經又云相火之下水氣乘之水位之下火氣乘之五
氣之勝皆然此乃亢則害承乃制之理即使果勝亦有
相尅者乘之更與司天之氣相反矣又云初氣終三氣
天氣主之勝之常也四氣盡終氣地氣主之復之常也
有勝則復無勝則否則歲半以前屬司天歲半以後又
屬在泉其中又有勝不勝之殊其病更異定矣又云厥
陰司天左少陰右太陽謂之左間右間六氣皆有左右
間每間主六十日是一歲之中復有六氣循環作主矣
其外又有南政北政之反其位天符歲會三合之不齊
太過不及之異氣欲辨明分斷終年不能盡其蘊當時
聖人不過言天地之氣運行旋轉如此耳至於人之得

病則豈能一一與之盡合一歲之中不許有一人生他
病乎故內經治歲氣勝復亦不分所以得病之因總之
見病治病如風淫于內則治以辛涼六氣皆有簡便易
守之法又云治諸勝復寒者熱之熱者寒之溫者清之
清者溫之無問其數以平為期何等劃一凡運氣之道
言其深者聖人有所不能知及施之實用則平正通達
人人易曉但不若今之醫者所云何氣司天則生何病
正與內經圓機活法相背耳

1. On the [Calendrical] Movement and [Changing] Influences Governing the Heavens

Apart from those teachings that are just heterodox, [other] types of scholarship exist that [were designed to] cheat people. Also, there are types of scholarship that [people] eat with their ears.

What do [I] mean by "scholarship [designed to] cheat people"? If someone loves high-flown talk to startle his listeners, or if someone plagiarizes the sayings of people of former times to demonstrate depth and broadness, and if [that person] is himself perfectly aware that he does not understand a single word of these [ancient sayings], but assumes that neither will others be able to investigate [these sayings] deeply, then this is scholarship [designed to] cheat people.

And what do [I] mean by "scholarship that [people] eat with their ears"? If someone plagiarizes the sayings he has heard from others, or if someone just casually reads through the literature written by the ancients, memorizes a few statements, believes that he has grasped all their subtle secrets, does not feel ashamed to [present his limited understanding] in great speeches to excite his audiences, then this is what is called "'to tell on the road what one has heard by the way." The rhetoric in recent times concerning the [calendrical] movements and [changing] influences governing the heavens is but one example of this.

Those who speak of the [calendrical] movements and [changing] influences governing the heavens, they hold that if specific influences govern the heavens [in a specific year], then the people must get the specific illnesses [corresponding to these influences] in that year. When, for example, "ceasing-yin [influences] govern the heavens, then that year is dominated by wind influences,"[1] and all the illnesses in that year should be treated as [caused by] wind. This kind of reasoning is meant by "[scholarship that the people] eat with their ears."

The fact [is] that of the doctrines of [calendrical] movements and [changing] influences governing the heavens, the Yellow Emperor has referred only to the principle of mutual correspondence between heaven and man, and the manifestations of this [correspondence that] appear, first of all, in the [movement in the] vessels. This same [principle appears in the *Nei-ching*] in all such [statements as:] "When minor-yin [influences] govern the heavens, [the movement in the vessels is so weak that it] cannot be felt at either of the inch-openings of the two hands. When ceasing-yin [influences] govern the heavens, no [movement] can be felt at the inch-section of one's right [hand]. When great-yin [influences] govern the heavens, no [movement in the vessels] can be felt at the inch-section of one's left [hand]. If [these influences appear] at the fountain, then no [movement in the] vessels can be felt in the foot-section [of one's hand]."[2] "If the [movement in the] vessels does not appear at the appropriate locations, one suffers from a [condition] opposite [to the prevailing influences], and such [a condition implies] death."[3]

This is one pattern of examining the [movement in the] vessels [in addition to many other patterns]. If [one diagnoses] an illness [with this method], one must observe which influences dominate in that given year, and [which influences] do not. "When," for instance, "the ceasing-yin [influences] govern the heavens, wind-excess dominates, and the people suffer from pathoconditions such as heart-ache and fullness in the flanks."[4] If in such a year people develop illnesses other [than those just mentioned], even though wind-excess dominates, these [other] cannot also be identified as related to wind-excess. If in a given year wind-excess does not dominate, [then, of course,] neither [can the illnesses of that year] be treated as if [caused] by wind.

The Classic states further, "[In a season that is] under the [domination of the] minister-fire, the influences of water [emerge to] check [the fire. In a season that is] under the [domination of the phase of] water, . . . [the influences of] fire [emerge to] check [the metal]."[5] The same applies to the domination of any of the five influences. The principle at work here is, "excessive strength results in harm; checked strength results in order."[6] That is, as soon as [certain influences] happen to gain excessive strength, they will be checked by those [influences] that are capable, according to the order of mutual control among the five phases, to do so — they are antagonistic with those [influences] governing the heavens.

The [Classic] states further, "From the first influence [period] through the third influence [period, a year] is mastered by the influences of heaven. This is the time of strength. From the fourth influence [period] through the final influence [period, a year] is mastered by the influences of earth. This is the time of recovery [by the opponents of strength]. Where there is strength, there will be a recovery [of opponents]; where there is no [strength], there will be no [recovery of opposing influences]."[7] That is, the first half of a year belongs to [influences] governing the heavens, while the latter half of the year belongs to [influences] at the fountain. And within [these two halves of a year], there are [influences of] strength, and [there are influences of] no strength. The illnesses appearing during these [different periods], though, are even less predetermined.

The [Classic] also states, "When ceasing-yin [influences] govern the heavens, minor-yin [influences] are to the left, and great-yang [influences] are to the right."[8] These are the so-called "lateral [influences][9] to the left and to the right." Each of the six influences has lateral [influences] to the left and to the right. Each lateral [influence] rules for sixty days. That is, within one year, each of the six influences rules once in turn. In addition, [each year is assigned one of two] opposite positions of "south[-facing] government" and "north[-facing] government."[10] There are different degrees of correspondences [between the calendrical nature of a year and its actual quality in terms of changing influences, with these different degrees of correspondences being called] "celestial correspondence," "annual coincidence," and "triple union."

And [finally], there are differences as to whether the [respective] influences are present in too great an abundance, or in insufficient quantities. If one were interested in a perfect understanding of all these [details of the doctrine of the calendrical movement and changing influences governing the heavens], one would not be able to gather all [the information] needed within one year. The Sages of those times [when the *Nei-ching* was written] discussed only the cyclical movement of the influences of heaven and earth in exactly those [terms I have just outlined]. How could it ever be possible that each single illness a human being can contact could coincide with all these [cyclical movements]? And, should not one single person be allowed to develop, in the course of an entire year, illnesses other [than those predetermined by the particular calendrical nature of that year]?

When the *Nei-ching* treats annual influences associated with a "strength" or with a "recovery,"[11] it does not distinguish among these [influences] as causes of one's having fallen ill. Generally speaking, when it sees an illness, it treats that illness. For example, an internal excess of wind is treated with acrid and cooling [remedies]. For each of the six influences simple patterns are [outlined in the *Nei-ching*] to change [an adverse condition] or to guard [against a specific situation. The *Nei-ching*] furthermore states: "[Conditions of] cold are to be heated; [conditions of] heat are to be chilled. [Conditions of] warmth are to be cooled; [conditions of] coolness are to be warmed." No [calendrical] numbers are demanded here. [Treatments are] "finished when a balanced condition is reached again."[12] It is that clearly defined!

Some of the more profound aspects of the doctrines of [calendrical] movement and [changing] influences are inaccessible to Sages; how to apply these [ideas] in practical use, though, represents no problem at all — this is easy knowledge for everyone. This, however, is different from the statements of today's physicians pointing out that those influences that govern the heavens cause the emergence of corresponding illnesses [in man]. Such [ideas] are in contrast to the essential, flexible patterns of the *Nei-ching*.

Notes

1. See *Huang-ti Nei-ching, Su-wen,* treatise "T'ien yüan chi ta lun."

2. See *Su-wen,* "Chih chen yao ta lun." *Ssu t'ien,* "governing the heavens," is a designation for the first six months of the year when the influences of heaven are supposed to rule. The term *tsai ch'üan,* "at the fountain," designates the latter six months of the year when the influences of the earth are supposed to rule.

3. See *Su-wen,* "Wu yün hsing ta lun"; also "Liu wei chih ta lun."

4. See *Su-wen,* "Chih chen yao ta lun."

5. See *Su-wen,* "Liu wei chih ta lun."

6. Ibid.

7. See *Su-wen,* "Chih chen yao ta lun."

8. See *Su-wen,* "Wu yün hsing ta lun." "Left" and "right" refer to the position of the influence periods adjoining a given season to the left and to the right in a circular graphic depiction of the six influence periods.

9. See "Chih chen yao ta lun" for a discussion of "lateral influences."

10. This is a reference to categorizations of the calendrical natures of a year into two groups. Years associated with the cyclical phases of wood, fire, metal, and water are termed subordinates that face the government; they therefore "face north" when they receive their orders. A year associated with the cyclical phase of soil is termed a ruler, and therefore "faces south" when issuing orders. See *Su-wen,* "Chih chen yao ta lun."

11. See *Su-wen,* "Wu yün hsing ta lun" and "Liu wei chih ta lun."

12. See *Su-wen,* "Chih chen yao ta lun."

醫道通治道論

治身猶治天下也。天下之亂。有由乎天者。有由乎人者。由乎天者。如夏商水旱之災是也。由乎人者。如歷代季世之變是也。而人之病。有由乎先天者。有由乎後天者。其人生而虛弱柔脆是也。由乎後天者。六淫之害。七情之感是也。先天之病。非其人之善養。與服大藥不能免於夭折。後天之病猶之天生之亂。非大聖大賢。不能平也。天之病。乃風寒暑溼燥火之疾。所謂外患也。喜怒憂思悲驚恐之害。所謂內憂也。治外患者。以攻勝。四郊不靖。而選將出師。速驅除之可也。臨辟雍而講禮樂。則敵在門矣。故邪氣未盡。而輕用補者。使邪氣內入而亡。治內傷者。以養勝。綱紀不正。而崇儒講道。徐化導之可也。若任刑罰而嚴誅戮。則

禍益深矣。故正氣不足。而輕用攻者。使其正氣消盡而亡。然而大盛之世。不無玩民。故刑罰不廢。則補中之攻也。然使以小寇而遽起戎兵。是擾民矣。故補中之攻。不可過也。征誅之年。亦修內政。故攻中之補也。然以戎首而稍存姑息。則養寇矣。故攻中之補。不可誤也。天下大事。以天下全力為之。則事不墮。天下小事以一人從容處之。則事不擾。患大病以大藥制之。則病氣無餘。患小病以小方處之。則正氣不傷。然而施治有時。先後有序。大小有方。輕重有度。疏密有數。純而不雜。整而不亂。所用之藥。各得其性。則器使之道。所處之方。各得其理。則調度之法。能即小以喻大。誰謂良醫之法。不可通於良相也。

2. On Similarities between the Ways of Medicine and the Ways of Government

To order the body is like ordering the empire. Disorder in the empire may have its origin in heaven, and it may originate from man. Examples [of disorders] originating from heaven are the flood and drought disasters at the time of the Hsia and Shang. Examples [of disorders] originating from man are the changes accompanying the closing years of all dynasties. Similarly, illnesses affecting man may have their origin in [both] the earlier and the later dependencies[1] [of one's life]. Examples [of illnesses] originating from the earlier dependencies are weak and tender constitutions from one's birth onward. Examples of [illnesses] originating from one's later dependencies are the harms resulting from the six excesses, and the affections resulting from the seven emotions.

Illnesses originating from one's earlier dependencies need careful nourishment and the intake of major drugs; otherwise, early death is inevitable. This may be compared to disorder [in the empire] originating from heaven. If it were not [for the activities of] major Sages and major exemplary men, peace could not be restored.

Illnesses [originating] from one's later dependencies include ailments resulting from wind, cold, heat, dampness, dryness, and fire, the so-called sufferings [from] outside; and harm resulting from joy, anger, grief, pondering, rage, fright, and fear, the so-called grief [from] inside. Sufferings [from] outside are to be overcome by attack. When rebellions occur at any of the four frontiers, an appropriate [defense] is to choose a general and to dispatch troops to quickly drive away [all rebels]. If, however, one were to go into the Hall of Learning, to discuss ceremonies and music, then the enemy would [advance quickly] to the gates [of the city]. If therefore [for an illness caused by evil influences that have entered the body from outside] one carelessly employs supplementing [drugs] before the evil influences have been eliminated completely, this will cause these evil influences to proceed deeper into [the patient's body, causing him to] die.

Harm [originating] inside is to be overcome by nourishment. If public morality is out of order, an appropriate [approach is to] emphasize reverence for [the teachings of] Confucius, and to explicate the [demands of the] Way, to cause changes slowly and offer guidance. If [the government] were to resort to punishment, and severely reprimand [the people] by means of executions, the trouble would only become more serious. If, therefore, in case of an insufficiency of proper influences, one carelessly employs attacking [drugs], this will cause the [remaining] proper influences to completely disperse, and [the patient will] die.

Now, even in years of great abundance, there will be a few troublemakers. Hence one does not abandon punishment entirely, and this is [to be understood as pursuing] an attack within [a time of] supplementation. If, however, one were to quickly raise armed troops because of [isolated disorders caused by] some petty thieves, this would annoy the people. That is, in [a time of] supplementation, one must not exaggerate an attack.

In a year when rebels have to be eliminated, one must nevertheless [pay attention to] an improvement of internal policies. If therefore [even in serious crisis] one does not relax one's effort to instruct and support [the people], then this is [to be understood as continued] supplementation even within a [time of] attack. If, however, [the official] leading a military operation showed lenience, this would only strengthen the rebels. That is, if [one applies] supplementation within a [time of] attack, one must not make any mistakes.

The major affairs of the empire are to be handled with all the powers of the empire. This way, these [major] affairs will not fail. The minor affairs of the empire can be handled through the knowledge of individuals. This way, these [minor] affairs will not cause any disturbances. If [a patient] suffers from a major illness, this illness must be checked with major [drugs] until nothing is left of its [evil] influences. If [a patient] suffers from a minor illness, this is to be handled by means of a minor prescription lest [the patient's] proper influences be harmed.

That is to say, whenever one carries out such ordering [interventions, in the body and in the empire], there are priorities for what comes first and what comes later. There are prescriptions designed for major and minor [issues]; there are rules for mild and heavy [attacks]; and there are figures for scattered and narrow [spacings of intervention. One should prefer] purity over confusion, order over chaos.

If one uses all the drugs [in a medical treatment] in accordance with their qualities, this is [comparable to] the [governmental] principle of examining a person's capabilities and employing him accordingly. If one applies [in medicine] all prescriptions in accordance with their [original] meaning, this is [comparable, in the government of the empire, to] the method of considering appropriate tactics and strategies.

Since it seems to be possible to refer to the petty [teachings of medicine][2] in order to illustrate the major [affairs of the empire], how could anyone deny that the methods [employed by a good physician] are similar to [those employed by] a good minister?[3,4]

Notes

1.   A modern translation of the concept of illnesses originating "in [one's] earlier dependencies" would be "congenital."

2.   The term "petty teachings" appears in the *Analects* of Confusius and was defined by Chu Hsi (1130-1200), the famous Confucian philosopher and writer of the Sung era, as referring to agriculture, horticulture, medicine, etc. Ever since, medical writers in China have written treatises to demonstrate the significance of the "petty teachings" of medicine. See Paul U. Unschuld, *Medical Ethics in Imperial China,* Berkeley, Los Angeles, London: University of California Press, 1979, p. 39.

3.   This is a reference to a Chinese saying, "Whoever cannot act as a good minister, may act as a good physician." This saying dates to the Sung statesman Fan Wen-cheng 范文正 (989-1052). According to Wu Tseng 吳曾 (fl. 1150), Fan had prayed to become chief minister. When the answer of the oracle was negative, he asked to become a good doctor instead. See Robert P. Hymes, "Not Quite Gentlemen? Doctors in Sung and Yüan," *Chinese Science,* 1987, 8: 43-44.

4.   This paragraph was not included in the 1778 *Ssu K'u Ch'üan-shu* version of the text. It is reproduced here in its original length from the Wu chou Publishing Co. edition, Taipei, 1969.

五方異治論

人稟天地之氣以生故其氣體隨地不同西北之人氣
深而厚凡受風寒難於透出宜用疎通重劑東南之人
氣浮而薄凡遇風寒易於疎洩宜用疎通輕劑又西北
地寒當用溫熱之藥然或有邪縕於中而內反甚熱則
用辛寒為宜東南地溫當用清涼之品然或有氣隨邪
散則易於亡陽又當用辛溫為宜至交廣之地則汗出
無度亡陽尤易附桂為常用之品若中州之卑濕山陝
之高燥皆當隨地制宜故以入其境必問水土風俗而細
調之不但各府各別即一縣之中風氣亦有迥殊者并
有所産之物所出之泉皆能致病土人皆有極效之方
皆宜詳審訪察若恃已之能執已之見治竟無功反為
土人所笑矣

湖州長興縣有合溪小兒飲此水則腹中生痞土人

治法用線掛頸以兩頭按乳頭上剪斷即將此線掛
轉將兩頭向背脊上一併拽齊線頭盡處將墨點記
脊上用艾灸之或三壯或七壯即消永不再發服藥
無效

3. On [the Need for] Different Therapies in the Five Cardinal Regions

Man's life depends on the influences of heaven and earth. Hence, [the condition of] his own influences and his body differ according to the geographic region [where he resides].

In the Northwest, the influences of [heaven and earth enter the human body] deeply, and they do so in rich quantities. When [people in the Northwest] are affected by wind-cold, it is difficult to drive [the evil influences] out again, and heavy preparations of dredging [drugs] are indicated.

In the Southeast, the influences [of heaven and earth remain at the body's] surface, and they do so only in small quantities. When [these people] are affected by wind-cold, it is easy to drain [the evil influences], and light preparations of dredging [drugs] are indicated.

Also, the Northwest is a cold region, and one should employ drugs with warm or hot [thermo-influences]. However, sometimes [people there are affected by] accumulations of evil [influences] in the center [of their body], and contrary [to their normal condition], they become very hot internally. In such cases one should use [drugs with an] acrid [taste and a] cold [thermo-influence].

The Southeast is a warm region, and one should employ cooling substances [for treatment]. However, it happens that both [proper] influences and evil [influences] disperse together, and [in such situations] one may easily lose one's yang [influences]. In this case, then, it is advisable to use [drugs with an] acrid [taste and with a] warm [thermo-influence]. In the regions of Vietnam and Canton, sweat flows without end, and one is especially at risk of losing one's yang [influences]. Here *fu*[-*tzu*] and *kuei* are often-used substances.

Also, the low-lying and damp [territories] of the central districts, or the dry [territories] in the high altitudes of Shanhsi, these all require regimens in accordance with [the specific conditions] of these geographic regions. Hence, one must ask about climate, and customs, and closely adjust to them, as soon as one enters such territories. Differences exist not only between each prefecture; varying winds and influences exist even within one county.

In addition, any item produced and any spring that emerges may cause illness, and the local people have very effective prescriptions that should be studied with utmost attention. If one were to rely on only one's personal abilities, and if one were to cling to only one's personal views, a successful therapy would be impossible, and one would merely make the locals laugh.

In Ch'ang-hsing county of Hu-chou, children drink water from the Ho creek, which results in blockages in their abdomens. The therapeutic pattern applied by the local people is such that they place a thread around [the patient's] neck and, then, press both its ends against the nipples of the breast. There [the thread] is cut off. Next, the thread is tied [around the patient's neck] the other way round, with the two ends pointing to the back. They pull both of them to the same length, and mark the points where they end with black dots. At these [dots] the [patient] is cauterized, perhaps three times or seven times, and [the blockages in his abdomen] vanish and never occur again. An intake of drugs would remain without effect.

病隨國運論

天地之氣運。數百年一更易。而國家之氣運亦應之

。上古無論。即以近代言。如宋之末造。中原失陷

。主弱臣弛。張潔古李東垣輩立方。皆以補中宮。

健脾胃。用剛燥扶陽之藥爲主。局方亦然。至于明

季。主暗臣專。膏澤不下於民。故丹溪以下諸醫。

皆以補陰益下爲主。至我本朝。運當極隆之會。聖

聖相承。大權獨攬。朝綱整肅。惠澤旁流。此陽盛

于上之明徵也。又冠飾朱纓。口燼煙草。五行惟火

獨旺。故其爲病。皆屬盛陽上越之症。數十年前。

雲間老醫知此義者。往往專以芩連知柏。挽回誤投

溫補之人。應手奇效。此實與運氣相符。近人不知

此理。非惟不能隨症施治。並執寧過溫熱。毋過寒

冷之説。偏於溫熱。又多矯枉過正之論。如中暑一

症。或有伏陰在內者。當用大順散。理中湯。此乃

千中之一。今則不論何人。凡屬中暑。皆用理中等

湯。我目覩七竅皆裂面死者。不可勝數。至于託言

祖述東垣。用蒼朮等燥藥者。舉國皆然。此等惡習

。皆由不知天時國運之理。誤引舊説以害人也。故

古人云。不知天地人者。不可以爲醫。

4. On Parallels between [the Emergence of] Illnesses and the Changing [Condition] of States

The influences sent out by heaven and earth undergo change every few hundred years, and the condition of states [changes] accordingly. Let us not discuss this with reference to ancient times. [I will] refer to recent periods to explain [what I mean]. For example, when in the final years of the Sung [dynasty] the Chinese territory fell into the hands of the enemy, the head [of state] was weak, and his ministers failed to show any strength. [At the same time] Chang Chieh-ku, Li Tung-yüan, and others, in establishing their prescriptions, emphasized supplementation of the central palace, i.e., a nourishment of spleen and stomach. They considered tough and dry drugs [with an ability to] support the yang as most important. The prescriptions [published] by the [Imperial Medical] Office were of the same type.

During the time of the Ming [dynasty], then, the head [of state] was hidden [from the population], and his ministers assumed responsibility. No benefits were passed downward to the people. Hence all physicians, beginning with [Chu] Tan-hsi, considered supplementation of the yin [regions of the body], as well as an increase of downward passage, as most important [therapies].

The era of our current dynasty is a time of extreme prosperity. Sage after Sage follow each other. A strong central authority exists. The morality of the imperial court is upright and deserves respect, and favor flows everywhere. This is clear evidence that the upper echelons are full of yang. Also, one wears red tassels to decorate one's cap, and in their mouths [people] smoke tobacco. Of all the five phases, only fire prospers. Hence all illnesses [people develop] are accompanied by pathoconditions resulting from the ascent of exuberant yang.

Many decades ago, an old physician from Yün[-nan] who knew of the meaning [of this phenomenon] often resorted to [huang-]ch'in, [huang-]lien, chih[-mu], and [huang-]po to restore [the health of] persons who had been mistakenly treated with warm and supplementing [drugs]. He always achieved miraculous results immediately, and it is certain that there is a close correspondence [between the illnesses of the people and their successful therapy on the one hand], and on the other hand the [general] movement of influences.

The people of today no longer know this principle. They are not only unable to apply a treatment in accordance with the [patient's] pathoconditions, but they also accept the doctrine that it is better to apply too warm or hot [a treatment] than too cold or cool [a treatment]. They stick onesidedly to [drugs with a] warm or hot [thermo-influence]. Also, there are many doctrines that [may be called] too rigid. For instance, in the case of the pathocondition "struck by summerheat," yin [influences] may lie hidden in the inner [regions of the body], and one should apply the "Powder to Achieve Great Smoothening," or the "Decoction Regulating the Center." This is one [possibility] out of a thousand. Today, though, regardless of the individual case, whenever [someone displays a] "struck by summerheat" [condition, physicians] always use the "[Decoction] Regulating the Center" and similar decoctions. I have seen many [patients] with my own eyes who died with their seven orifices bursting open.[1] As for those who insist on [using] the doctrines of [Li] Tung-yüan as their guidelines, and who rely on desiccating drugs such as *ts'ang-shu*, they can be found all over the country. Their bad practices result from their unawareness of the changing phases of times and states, and from their erroneous reliance on outmoded doctrines, whereby they only harm the people.

Hence the people of antiquity had a saying: Those cannot act as physicians who do not know heaven, earth, and man.[2]

Notes

1.   The character 面 *mien*, "face," is a mistake for 而 *erh*, "and."

2.   This paragraph was not included in the 1778 *Ssu K'u Ch'üan-shu* version of the text. It is reproduced here in its original length from the Wu chou Publishing Co. edition, Taipei, 1969.

針灸失傳論

靈素兩經其詳論臟腑經穴疾病等說為針法言者十
之七八為方藥言者十之二三上古之重針法如此然
針道難而方藥易病者亦樂於脈藥而苦於針所以後
世方藥盛行而針法不講今之為針者其顯然之失有
十而精微尚不與焉兩經所言十二經之出入起止淺
深左右交錯不齊其穴隨經上下亦參差無定今人祇
執同身寸依左右一直豎量並不依經曲折則經非經
而穴非穴此一失也兩經治病云某病取某穴者固多
其餘則指經而不指穴如靈樞終始篇云人迎一盛瀉足
少陽補足太陰厥病篇云厥頭痛或取足陽明太陰或
取手少陽足少陰耳聾取手陽明嗌乾取足少陰皆不
言其穴其中又有瀉子補母等義今則每病指定幾穴
此二失也兩經論治并營輸經合最重冬刺井春刺營

夏刺輸長夏刺經秋刺合凡只言其經而不言其穴者
大都皆指井營輸五者為言今則皆不講矣此三失也補
瀉之法內經云吸則內針無令氣忤靜以久留無令邪
布吸則轉針以得氣為故候呼引針呼盡乃去大氣皆
出為瀉呼盡內針靜以久留以氣至為故候吸引針氣
不得出各在其處推闔其門令神氣存大氣留止為補
又必迎其經氣疾內而徐出不按其痏為補隨其經氣
徐內而疾出即按其痏為瀉揣而循之切而散之推
以大指推出為瀉撮入為補此四失也納針之後必候
其氣刺實者陰氣隆至乃去針刺虛者陽氣隆至乃出
針氣不至無問其數氣至即去之勿復針難經云先以
左手壓按所針之處彈而努之爪而下之其氣之來如動
脈之狀順而刺之得氣因而推內之是謂補動而伸之
是謂瀉今則時時轉動候針下寬轉而後出針不問氣

242

之至與不至此五失也凡針之深淺隨時不同春氣在
毛夏氣在皮膚秋氣在肌肉冬氣在筋骨故春夏刺淺
秋冬刺深反此有害今則不論四時分寸各有定數此
六失也古之用針凡瘧疾傷寒寒熱咳嗽一切臟腑七
竅等症無所不治今則止治經脈形體痿痺屈伸等病
而已此七失也古人刺法取血甚多靈樞血絡論言之
最詳而頭痛腰痛尤必大瀉其血凡血絡有邪者必盡
去之若血射出而黑必令變色見赤血而止否則病不
除而反有害今人則偶爾見血病者巳惶恐失據
病何由除此八失也內經刺法有九變十二節九變者
輸刺遠道刺經刺絡刺分刺大瀉刺毛刺巨刺焠刺十二
節者偶刺報刺恢刺齊刺揚刺直針刺輸刺短刺浮刺
陰刺傍刺贊刺以上二十一法視病所宜不可更易一
法不備則一病不愈今則祇直刺一法此九失也古之

針制有九鑱針員針鍉針鋒針鈹針員利針毫針長針
大針亦隨病所宜而用一失其制則病不應今則大者
如員針小者如毫針而已豈能治癰疾暴氣此十失也
其大端之失巳如此而其尤要者更在神志專一手法
精嚴經云神在秋毫屬意病者審視血脈刺之無殆又
云經氣巳至慎守勿失深淺在志遠近若一如臨深淵
手如握虎神無營於眾物又云伏如橫弩起如發機其
專精敏妙如此今之醫者隨手下針漫不經意即使針
法如古志不凝而機不達猶恐無效況乎全與古法相
背乎其外更有先後之序迎隨之異貴賤之殊勞逸之
分肥瘦之度多少之數更僕難窮果能潛心體察以合
聖度必有神功其如人之畏難就易盡達古法所以世
之視針甚輕而其術亦不甚行也若灸之一法則較之
針所治之病不過十之一二知針之理則灸又易易耳

5. On the Loss of the Tradition in Needling and Cauterization

In their detailed discussion of the viscera and of the bowels, of the conduits and their insertion points, and of illnesses, the *Ling*[-*shu*] and the *Su*[-*wen*] refer to the method of needling seven or eight times out of ten, while they refer to prescriptions and drugs only two or three times out of ten. That shows how much [the people] in high antiquity valued the method of needling. However, learning the doctrine of needling is difficult, while it is easy [to use] prescriptions and drugs. Also, patients enjoy taking drugs, but they suffer from the needles. Hence, in later times the [use of] prescriptions and drugs flourished widely while no one spoke of the method of needling anymore. Today, the application of the needles is marked by ten obvious losses, and that does not even include all the subtleties [that have been forgotten since antiquity].

The two classics outline the origins and the ends of the twelve conduits, where they appear and where they stop; [they state whether the conduits] lie near the surface or in the depth, to the left or to the right, and how they are intertwined and have no uniform [pathways]. Similarly, the insertion points are located irregularly without any fixed order, following the upward and downward [paths] of the conduits. Today, people grasp only the [individually] standardized body inch,[1] and apply their measurements in straight [lines from] left or right. Never do they follow the curves and bends [in the courses] of the conduits. Hence the conduits [they identify] are not the conduits [specified in the classics], and the insertion points [they identify] are not the insertion points [specified in the classics]. That is the first loss.

When the two classics refer to the treatment of illnesses, they do, of course, quite often state: "In case of such-and-such an illness, select such-and-such an insertion point." In all other cases, though, they refer to the conduits and not to the insertion point. As it is stated, for instance, in the chapter "Chüeh ping" of the *Ling*[-*shu*]: "In case of deafness, select the hand yang-brilliance [conduit for treatment]"; "in case of a dry throat, select the foot minor-yin [conduit for treatment]." In all these [and many other] instances, [the classics] do not say "such-and-such an insertion point." Today, for each illness, a number of holes are specified. That is the second loss.

The two classics discuss the well, brook, rapids, stream, and the confluence [insertion points[2] located on the lower segment of the four extremities] with greatest emphasis. Whenever they speak of just a particular conduit, and do not mention a particular point, they refer, for the most part, to one of the five [generic insertion points] such as well, brook

244

[etc.]. Today, these [insertion points] are no longer mentioned. That is the third loss.

On the methods of supplementing and draining, the *Nei-ching* states: "When [the patient] inhales, insert the needle. Do not allow the influences to be irritated [by confronting them during an exhalation]. Let [the needle] remain quietly in its position for a while. Do not allow evil influences to spread. [When the patient] inhales [again], twirl the needle because this way it collects influences [around itself]. Wait until [the patient] exhales and remove the needle. By the end of that exhalation, the needle should be removed. Large [quantities of] influences will leave [with the needle through the insertion point]. This is drainage. [To supplement,] one inserts the needle at the moment an exhalation ends. Let [the needle] remain in position quietly for a while because the influences [need time] to arrive. Wait until an inhalation and pull the needle [because during an inhalation] the influences cannot leave and stay where they are. [Once the needle is removed, one uses one's fingers] to close the gate [that was opened by the needle] with some pressure, and causes the spirit influences to stay [inside]. Large [quantities of] influences [that were inserted together with the needle] will remain [inside too]. That is supplementation."[3] [In the classics it is stated] further that if [one angles the needle on its insertion], contrary to the [movement of the] influences in the vessels, inserts quickly, and withdraws slowly, without closing the wound [afterwards], that is draining. If [one inserts the needle] following the [direction of the movement of the] influences in the conduits, inserts slowly, and withdraws quickly, and then presses the wound [to close it], that is supplementation. The methods [of draining and supplementation] may be applied in many ways, but today, [people] twirl the needle and use their thumbs to push [influences] out [of the vessels], and that is their draining; or they rub [the influences while twirling the needle] into [the insertion point], and that is their supplementation. That is the fourth loss.

After the needle has been inserted, one must wait until the influences [have arrived]. If one pricks a repletion, yin influences must arrive in large quantities, and only then is the needle to be removed. If one pricks a depletion, yang influences must arrive in large amounts before one may withdraw the needle. If no influences arrive [immediately, the needle is inserted] many times, again and again, and it is withdrawn only when the influences have [finally] arrived — and not inserted again. Today, [people] constantly twirl and move [the needle and do not let it remain quietly for a while]. As soon as the needle is lowered into [the flesh], it is twirled extensively, and then it is withdrawn again. No one checks whether the influences have arrived or not. That is the fifth loss.

Whether [one inserts] a needle deeply or not depends on the different [requirements of the four] seasons. In spring the influences are in the hair; in summer the influences are in the skin; in autumn the influences are in the flesh; in winter the influences are in the sinews and bones. Hence needling is shallow in spring and summer, while one needles into the depth in autumn and winter. If one acts contrary to these [laws], harm will result. Today, [people] do not consider the four seasons. The number of tenths and inches [by which the needles are inserted] is always fixed. That is the sixth loss.

In ancient times the needles were used to treat all cases of *yao* illness,[4] harm caused by cold, [fits of] cold and heat, coughing, as well as all illnesses affecting the viscera, bowels, and the seven orifices. Today, [the needles are used] only to treat the conduit-vessels and the physical body, [and only] if they are affected by illnesses such as paralysis and obturation, [that is, those conditions affecting one's ability] to bend and stretch [one's limbs]. That is the seventh loss.

One of the pricking methods [employed] by people in ancient times was to take blood in large amounts. This is outlined in great detail by the *Ling-shu* in its discussion of the blood[-vessel] network. In particular, in cases of headache and pain in one's waist, one must drain the [patient's] blood in large quantities. Whenever some evil [influences] are located in the blood[-vessel] network, they must be eliminated completely. When black-colored blood flows, it must be left to flow until the color changes and red blood appears. Then one must stop [the flow]. If the [blood] is not [let out in these quantities], the illness will not be removed, and, on the contrary, more harm will result. Today, if the people happen to see some blood, both patients and physicians are frightened and lose all direction. How, then, can an illness be removed [in this circumstance]? That is the eighth loss.

According to the *Nei-ching*, the methods of needling may undergo nine variations and may be divided into twelve sections. The nine variations include the needling of transport [points alone],[5] needling from a distance,[6] needling conduits,[7] needling network [vessels],[8] needling [the space] between [the skin and flesh], needling to induce drainage of large [amounts of pus or blood], needling [of the skin as cautiously as with a] hair, square needling,[9] and cauterization needling.[10] The twelve sections include paired needling,[11] retaliation needling,[12] broad needling,[13] combination needling,[14] scattered needling,[15] direct needling,[16] transport needling,[17] short needling,[18] surface needling,[19] yin needling,[20] sideways needling,[21] and supportive needling.[22] These twenty-one methods mentioned above [should be used] in accordance with the requirements of the illnesses [treated]. One cannot exchange [one method] for another. If one fails to master all these methods no illness will be cured. Today, [people] cling to the one method of direct needling. That is the ninth loss.

In ancient times the needles were shaped in nine [different ways, including] the chisel needle, the round needle, the arrow-head needle, the lance-point needle, the sword needle, the round-sharp needle, the hair needle, the long needle, and the large needle. These, too, were employed in accordance with the requirements of the illnesses [to be] treated. Every time one misses the [correct] shape [of the needle to be used in a specific therapy], the illness will fail to respond [to the treatment]. Today, [people use] only large [needles], resembling the round needle, and small ones resembling the hair needle. How could they treat chronic illnesses or violent influences [successfully]? That is the tenth loss.

These, then, are the major losses [marking the tradition of needling today]. Even more important, though, [is that the ancients were able] to concentrate their minds [on the problems confronting them] and to act with their hands in a most skillful and dignified manner. The Classic states: "If one's spirit focuses on the minutest details, and if one pays close attention to the patient's blood vessels, an insertion [of needles] will cause no harm."[23] And it further states: "Once the influences in the conduits have arrived [at the needle], be careful not to lose them. Concentrate on whether they are in the depth or near the surface, and it should be all the same whether they are distant or near.[24] [Be as careful] as if you approached a deep abyss, and your hand [should be as firm] as if you were holding a tiger. Do not let your thoughts be distracted by anything."[25] [The Classic] also states, "[Until the influences have arrived, be as attentive as if] lying in ambush with your crossbow in hand. [Once they have arrived, insert your needle as fast as a hunter] rises and releases the trigger."[26] This is how extremely thoughtful [the ancients were].

Today's physicians insert their needles at liberty and do not care about any schema. And even if they were to employ needling methods like the ancients, they would be unable to concentrate their thoughts, and they would not even reach the trigger. Most likely, they would not achieve any good result. How much more is this true, though, for those who turn their backs on the ancient methods!

In addition, [there are issues that must be considered, such as] the order of [which pathoconditions to treat] first and which later, or the difference between [angling the needles] against or in the direction [of flow in the conduits], or the differences [in treatment] of rich and poor [patients], or the need to distinguish between [patients suffering from] fatigue, and others who live in idleness, or the degree of obesity or emaciation, and finally the number [of needles to be inserted]. I could hardly list them all!

247

If one is able to conduct thoughtful inquiries and thorough investigations, and to conform with the measures taken by the Sages [of antiquity], he will achieve miraculous results. But because people shy away from the difficult, and prefer what is easy, they never follow the ancient methods. Hence, acupuncture has fallen into disrepute today, and the technique [of needling] is no longer widely practiced. As for the method of cauterization, in comparison to needling, it is suited only for one or two out of ten illnesses. If one knows the principles of needling, cauterization will be very easy.

Notes

1.   Since people may be tall or short, corpulent or thin, methods were devised in ancient China to locate the insertion points relative to the size of the individual. It was assumed that the length of the middle joint of the index finger varied in direct proportion to the length of the body. Thus, this distance was called an "individually standardized body inch." Today, the body inch is also measured via standard horizontal and vertical units located on the head, chest and abdomen, back, sides of the chest and abdomen, arm and leg. These units are based on the distance between two anatomical points divided into a set number of body inches. Each relative measure is used in the area of the relative standard to establish distances between insertion points and anatomical features.

2.   For a detailed discussion of these five acupoints, see *Ling-shu*, treatise 1, 'Chin ching shih-erh yüan," and Paul U. Unschuld, *Nan-ching. The Classic of Difficult Issues*, Berkeley, Los Angeles, London: University of California Press, 1986, "Difficult Issues" 62 ff.

3.   See *Su-wen*, treatise 27, "Li ho chen hsieh lun."

4.   *Yao* illnesses appear to have included malaria.

5.   "Needling of transport [points]" is needling of the five insertion points "well" through "confluence" on the distal extremities.

6.   "Needling from a distance" is needling of a point far away from the affected area.

7.   "Needling of conduits" is needling of the conduit primarily affected by an illness.

8.   "Needling of network [vessels]" is needling of small vessels in the region directly below the skin to drain blood.

9.   "Square needling," today also called "contralateral insertion," is needling of a site on the right side of the patient if the illness is located on the left, and vice versa.

10.   "Cauterization needling" is needling with a heated needle.

11.   "Paired needling" is a needling of two sides of pain on the back and front of the patient.

12.   "Retaliation needling" is a method to treat pain changing its location. A needle is inserted at the site of the pain. The physician locates with his hand a second site of pain, withdraws the needle from the first and inserts it at the the second site.

13.   "Broad needling" is a needling next to a cramped or painful sinew. The needle is moved back and forth to widen the opening at the insertion point.

14.   "Combination needling" is the insertion of one needle each to the left and right of a needle inserted directly into an affected area.

15.   "Scattered needling" is the insertion of four needles around a first needle.

16.   "Direct needling" is a needling into a lifted skin fold without damaging the flesh.

17.   "Transport needling" is a fast and deep insertion and withdrawal of a needle.

18.   "Short needling" is a deep insertion of a needle until it comes close to a bone.

19.   "Surface needling" is a slanted superfical insertion.

20.   "Yin needling" is a needling of the foot minor-yin conduit both on its right and left course.

21.   "Sideways needling," is needling to the side of a needle already inserted.

22.   "Supportive needling" is shallow needling to drain blood and support the dispersion of pain and swellings.

23.   See *Ling-shu*, treatise 1, "Chiu chen shih-erh yüan."

24.   "Distant or near" may refer to influences in the depth or near the surface, or to needling of the extremities or of the body respectively.

25.   See *Su-wen*, treatise 25, "Pao ming ch'üan hsing lun."

26.   Ibid.

水病針法論

凡刺之法不過補瀉經絡袪邪納氣而已其取穴甚少

惟水病風疿膚脹必刺五十七穴又云皮膚之血盡取

之何也蓋水旺必尅脾土脾土衰則徧身皮肉皆腫不

特一經之中有水氣矣若僅刺一經則一經所過之地

水自漸消而他經之水不消則四面會聚并一經已瀉

之水亦復滿矣故必周身腫滿之處皆刺而瀉之然後

其水不復聚其此五十七穴者皆藏之陰絡水之所客

也此與大禹治洪水之法同蓋洪水泛濫必有江淮河

濟各引其所近之衆流以入海必不能使天下之水祇

歸一河以入海也又出水之後更必調其飲食經云方

飲與食方食無飲使飲食異居則水不從食無食也

食百三十五日此症之難愈如此余往時治此病輕者

多愈重者必復腫蓋由五十七穴未能全刺而病人亦

愈理可不慎哉

不能守戒一百三十五日也此等大症少違法度即無

6. On the Needling Pattern in Case of Water Illnesses

[The therapeutic technique of] needling includes only the [two] patterns of supplementing and draining the [major] conduits and network [vessels, that is,] of eliminating evil [influences] and of adding [proper] influences. Only very few insertion points are selected [to pursue] these [therapeutic goals].

However, when it comes to water illnesses [such as] wind[-caused] edema with skin swellings, a total of 57 insertion points must be needled![1] [In addition, the *Ling-shu*] states, "The blood of the skin has to be removed entirely."[2] What does that mean?

Well, when water dominates, it must subdue the soil of the spleen.[3] When the soil of the spleen is weak, the skin and flesh are swollen all over the body, and water influences are present in not only one conduit. If one were to needle merely one conduit, only the water from the territory passed by this particular conduit would slowly vanish. However, the water in the other conduits would not vanish at all. It would accumulate everywhere, and even the one conduit from which the water was drained would [soon] be filled again as before. It is for that reason that all the places [on the body] that are swollen must be needled and are to be drained. Only then will the water no longer be able to accumulate again. The 57 insertion points [mentioned above] are located on the conduits and network [vessels] of the viscera, and they store the water.[4]

The pattern employed here is identical with that of Yü the Great[5] when he regulated the flood. When a great flooding occurs, [large streams such as the Ch'ang]-chiang, the Wei, the [Huang-]ho, and the Han[6] will drain [the water from the smaller] rivers nearby into the ocean. It would be absolutely impossible to cause all the water covering the land to find a course to the ocean through only one river.

Also, once the water has flowed away, one must regulate the [patient's] beverages and food. The Classic states: "At the moment [the patient] drinks, he should not eat; at the moment he eats, he should not drink."[7] The intention here is to have beverages and food settle at different locations so that the water does not follow the food to the place where the soil of the spleen accumulates its dampness. "He should not eat any food [other than that prescribed by the physician] for 135 days."[8] It is that difficult to heal this pathocondition.

In former years, when I treated this illness, I achieved many successes in mild cases. More serious cases were bound to display recurrent swellings because it was either impossible to needle all the 57 insertion points, or the patients were unable to fast for 135 days. Whenever one is confronted with such serious pathoconditions, the slightest aberration from the [correct treatment] pattern will make a cure impossible. One has to be careful!

Notes

1.   See *Su-wen*, treatise 61, "Shui je hsüeh lun," for details on the 57 insertion points.

2.   See *Ling-shu*, treatise 19, "Ssu shih ch'i." The preceding sentence "wind[-caused] edema . . . must be needled" is quoted from the same paragraph.

3.   According to the five phases doctrine, the lung is associated with the phase of metal, the heart with fire, the spleen with soil, the liver with wood, the kidneys with water. Under normal conditions, soil controls water just as a dike controls a river. Here, a flood has overcome the dikes.

4.   The character *yin* 陰 must be a mistake here. All other editions have *ching* 經 instead. The character *k'e* 客 may be a mistake for *jung* 容.

5.   A legendary culture hero. Together with Yao and Shun, he is called one of the Three Great Sovereigns of ancient times.

6.   The character *chi* 濟 is a mistake here; other versions of the text have a *han* 漢 instead.

7.   See *Ling-shu*, treatise 19, "Ssu shih ch'i."

8.   Ibid. My interpretation here is based on Yang Wei-chieh 楊維傑, *Huang-ti Nei-ching Ling-shu Chieh*, Taipei, Lo-ch'ün Publishing Co., 1976, p. 204.

出奇制病論

病有經有緯有常有變有純有雜有正有反有整有亂

并有從古醫書所無之病歷來無治法者而其病又經

可愈既無陳法可守是必熟尋內經難經等書審其經

絡臟腑受病之處及七情六氣相感之因與夫內外分

合氣血聚散之形必有鑿鑿可徵者而後立為治法或

先或後或併或分或上或下或前或後取藥極當立方

極正而寓以巧思奇法深入病機不使扞格如庖丁之

解牛雖筋骨關節之間亦游刃有餘然後天下之病千

緒萬端而我之設法亦千變萬化全在平時於極難極

險之處參悟通徹而後能臨事不眩否則一遇疑難即

束手無措冒昧施治動輒得咎誤人不少矣

253

7. On the Need to Produce Extraordinary [Therapies] To Master [Unusual] Illnesses

There are illnesses that pass lengthwise [through the organism], and others that spread cross-wise. There are those that are constant [in their appearance], and others that are marked by changes. Some are purely [one illness]; others are complex [combinations of several illnesses]. Some run a proper [course], others develop contrary [to the course expected]. Some are associated with a complete set [of symptoms], and others display atypical [signs]. Also, there are those illnesses that have not been described in the medical literature since antiquity, and for which no therapeutic methods exist that have come down through the ages. Even such illnesses can be cured, however [if one pursues the following approach.]

When no time-honored [treatment] patterns that should be observed are available, one must [first] carefully search books like the *Nei-ching* and the *Nan-ching*. One [must] investigate at what places the conduits and their network [vessels], the viscera and the bowels, harbor an illness. [One must examine] the reasons for mutual effects of the seven emotions and six influences upon each other; and [one must take into consideration] the different manifestations [of illnesses] that occur only in the interior or in the exterior [sections of the body], or in both [simultaneously], and also of those that represent accumulations or dispersions of influences or blood. [Such examinations] must be [continued until one acquires] indisputable evidence [of a specific illness]. Then, one designs [an appropriate] treatment pattern, [taking into consideration that] some [drugs are to be taken] prior to and others after [meals; that] some [drugs are to be consumed] together and others separately; [that] some [should] rise [in the body], and others descend; [and that] some [are to be applied] before [an illness is transmitted] and others after [transmission has occurred]. If the drugs one chooses are most appropriate, and if the prescription designed is most accurate, and if one has established an extraordinary [therapeutic] pattern on the basis of ingenious thoughts, deeply penetrating the workings of the illness, without creating any barrier; this is comparable, then, to the [expert] cook who, when he dissected a cow, had sufficient room for his blade even when he moved it through the interstices of sinews, bones, and joints.[1]

[After such preparations,] I may be confronted with thousands of ends and tens of thousands of beginnings of the illnesses under heaven, and yet I will be able to design [therapeutic] patterns in thousands of adaptations. If, in normal times, one examines, and becomes most familiar with, situations that are most difficult and most dangerous, one will not be confused in times of crisis. Otherwise, whenever one meets a doubtful or difficult [situation], one's hands are tied and one is at a loss as to what to do. One designs a therapy in blindness, and is guilty [of mistakes] again and again. Many people [will be harmed by such] erroneous [therapies].

Note

1.   The story of Pao-ting, the expert cook, is told in *Chuang-tzu*, book III, "*Yang sheng chu.*"

治病緩急論

病有當急治者有不當急治者外感之邪猛悍剽疾以

犯臟腑則元氣受傷無以托疾於外必乘其方起之時

邪入尚淺與氣血不相亂急驅而出之於外則易而且

速若俟邪氣已深與氣血相亂然後施治則元氣大傷

此當急治者也若夫病機未定無所歸著急用峻攻則

邪氣益橫如人之傷食方在胃中則必先用化食之藥

愈若即以硝黃峻藥下之則食尚在上焦即使隨藥而

使其食漸消由中焦而達下焦變成渣穢而出自然漸

下乃皆未化之物腸胃中脂膜與之同下而人已大疲

病必生變此不當急治者也以此類推餘病可知至於

虛人與老少之疾尤宜分別調護使其元氣漸轉則正

復而邪退醫者不明此理而求速效則補其所不當補

攻其所不當攻所服之藥不驗又轉求他法無非誅伐

無過至當愈之時其人已為藥所傷而不能與天地之

生氣相應矣故雖有良藥用之非時反能致害緩急之

理可不講哉

8. On Slow and Quick Treatments of Illnesses

Some illnesses must be treated quickly. Some must not be treated quickly. For example, if a patient has been affected by external evil [influences] to the extent that a violent illness has internally invaded the patient's viscera and bowels, then, the patient's original influences are already harmed and it will be virtually impossible to expel the illness to the exterior again. Thus, it is imperative to seize the moment when [this violent illness] is just about to emerge. That is, as long as the evil [influences] have only superficially penetrated [the body] and are not yet mixed with [the body's] proper influences and blood, [they are readily expelled]. If one quickly pushes [the evil influences] out [of the body early], this will be both easy and fast. If one were to wait, though, until the evil influences [penetrate] deep [into the body], and if one were to design a treatment only after they have mixed with [the body's proper] influences and blood, then the original influences will have already received great harm. This, then, is [an example of an illness] that must be treated quickly.

As long, however, as the workings of an illness are not yet perfectly understood, and as long as [this illness] has not settled at a specific location, the quick application of a [therapy of] fierce attack would only cause the evil influences to become more aggressive. For example, if someone has been harmed by the food he has eaten, and if [this harmful food] is right in his stomach, one must first apply drugs that transform this food and cause it to disappear slowly by moving it from the central burner into the lower burner, where it becomes refuse and leaves [the body. The illness] then heals gradually by itself. If one were to use fierce drugs such as *hsiao-huang* to bring [the food] down, even the food that is still in the upper burner would be forced to follow the drugs and move downward. All items that are not transformed, as well as fat and membranes from the intestines and from the stomach, would descend together. The person affected would suffer from severe exhaustion, and his illness would develop [secondary ailments as a result]. This, then, is [an example of an illness] that must not be treated quickly.

By analogy one would know [how to proceed with] all other illnesses. As for the illnesses of persons [suffering from a] depletion, as well as of the old and of children, here one must be particularly careful. One must ensure that their original influences gradually recover so that the proper [influences] return and the evil [influences] disappear.

If a physician does not know these principles, and seeks but quick results, he will supplement what should not be supplemented, and he will attack what should not be attacked. The drugs [he requires the patient to] consume will remain without effect, and he will turn to other [therapeutic] methods.

Each [treatment will be comparable to] capital punishment of someone innocent. When the moment has come when a cure should occur, the person affected has already been harmed by drugs to such an extent that he will be unable to respond to the vital influences of heaven and earth. Hence, even excellent drugs, contrary [to what is expected], can cause harm if used at the wrong time. The principle of slow and quick [treatments in medicine] must always be taken into consideration.

治病分合論

一病而當分治者如痢疾腹痛脹滿則或先治脹滿或

先治腹痛即脹滿之中亦不同或因食或因氣或先治

食或先治氣腹痛之中亦不同或因積或因寒或先去

積或先去寒種種不同皆當視其輕重而審察之以此

類推則分治之法可知矣有當合治者如寒熱腹痛頭

疼泄瀉厥胃胸滿內外上下無一不病則當求其因何

而起先於諸症中擇最甚者為主而其餘症每症加專

治之藥一二味以成方則一劑而諸症皆備以此類推

則合治之法可知矣藥亦有分合焉有一病而合數藥

以治之者閱古聖人製方之法自知有數病而一藥治

之者閱本草之主治自知為醫者無一病不窮究其因

無一方不洞悉其理無一藥不精通其性庶幾可以自

信而不枉殺人矣

9. On Combined and Separate Treatments of Illnesses

The treatment of one single illness may have to be carried out in separate stages. For instance, when dysentery [is associated with] abdominal pain, in addition to distention and fullness, some cases [require] that the distention and fullness be treated first, other cases [require first treating] the abdominal pain. Even within distention and fullness differences exist because sometimes [these conditions] are caused by food, sometimes by [evil] influences. [This means that] sometimes one should first focus a treatment on the food and sometimes first [focus] on the [evil] influences. Similarly, within abdominal pain differences exist because sometimes [this condition] is caused by accumulations, and sometimes by cold. [This means that] sometimes one should first eliminate an accumulation and sometimes one should first disperse a cold. There are many such differences, and in each case one must investigate which problem is minor or serious, and conduct a careful examination.

By analogy with the [example just given], one may know the [general] pattern of separate treatments. But there are also cases where one should treat [several pathoconditions] together. For instance, if someone suffers from fits of heat and cold, from abdominal pain, headache, diarrhea, and [influences] moving upward from the stomach causing fullness in the chest, with his inner and outer, upper and lower [sections of the body] all being equally ill, in such a situation one must search for the cause and origin [of all these conditions]. The most serious of all these pathoconditions must be selected as the main [focus of the treatment]; the prescription is completed by adding one or two drugs to treat each of the additional pathoconditions. As a result, one preparation alone serves to cover all pathoconditions together. By analogy with this [example] one may know the [general] pattern of combined treatments.

Drugs may also be [used] separately or in combination. For instance, there are cases where one individual illness must be treated through a combined intake of several drugs. This becomes self-evident, if one simply examines the patterns by which the ancient Sages designed their prescriptions. Also, there are several illnesses that can be treated with one and the same drug. This becomes self evident if one but examines the main indications [of drugs] listed in the materia medica literature.

Everyone who practices medicine must carefully examine the cause of each illness, must perfectly understand the principle underlying each prescription, and must be completely familiar with the nature of each drug. Only then may he come close to a point of self-confidence, and only then will he not kill others by mistake.

發汗不用燥藥論

驅邪之法惟發表攻裏二端而已發表所以開其毛孔
令邪從汗出也當用至輕至淡芳香清洌之品使邪氣
緩緩從皮毛透出無犯中焦無傷津液仲景麻黃桂枝
等湯是也然猶恐其營中陰氣為風火所煽而消耗於
內不能滋潤和澤以托邪於外於是又啜薄粥以助胃
氣以益津液此服桂枝湯之良法凡發汗之方皆可類
推汗之必資於津液如此後世不知凡用發汗之方每
專用厚朴葛根羌活白芷蒼朮豆蔻等溫燥之藥即使
其人津液不虧內既為風火所熬又復為燥藥所爍則
汗從何生汗不能生則邪無所附而出不但不出邪氣
反為燥藥鼓動益復橫肆與正氣相亂邪火四布津液
益傷而舌焦唇乾便閉目赤種種火象自生則身愈熱
神漸昏惡症百出若再發汗則陽火盛極動其真陰腎

水來救元陽從之大汗上洩亡陽之危症生矣輕者亦
戌痙症遂屬壞病難治故用燥藥發汗而殺人者不知
凡幾也此其端開於李東垣其所著書立方皆治濕邪
之法與傷寒雜感無涉而後人宗其說以治一切外感
之症其害至今益甚況治濕邪之法亦以淡滲為主如
猪苓五苓之類亦無以燥勝之者蓋濕亦外感之邪總
宜驅之外出而兼以燥濕之品斷不可專用勝濕之藥
使之內攻致邪與正爭而傷元氣也至於中寒之症亦
先以發表為主無竟用熱藥以勝寒之理必其寒氣乘
虛陷入而無出路然後以薑附回其陽此仲景用理中
之法也今乃以燥藥發雜感之汗不但非古聖之法并
誤用東垣之法醫道失傳只此淺近之理尚不知何況
深微者乎

10. On the [Need to] Avoid Parching Drugs When Inducing Perspiration

The patterns for expelling evil [influences from the body] are based on none other than the two principles of effusing them to the outside or of attacking them internally.

To effuse [evil influences] to the outside means that the [patient's] hair pores are opened to let the evil leave [the body] together with sweat. [To achieve this goal] it is advisable to use very light, and [in their flavor] very neutral, as well as aromatic, and cool substances that cause the evil influences to slowly leave [the body] through the hair of the skin, that do not offend the central burner, so that the central burner remains unaffected, and no harm is caused to the [body's] liquids.

[Examples of such drugs may be seen in prescriptions] such as [Chang] Chung-ching's *ma-huang* and *kuei-chih* decoctions. And yet, there is still the risk that the yin influences among the [patient's] constructive [influences] will be burned by the fire of the wind and waste away internally, so that they are no longer able [to fulfill their function] of providing [the body] with the moisture [that is needed] to escort the evil to the outside. Hence [the patient] should sip a thin broth to support the influences of his stomach and to enrich his [body's] liquids. This is a good pattern for consuming *kuei-chi* decoction, and all other prescriptions for [expelling evil by] inducing perspiration can be inferred [from this example] by analogy.

Later generations were no longer aware of the necessity to support any [induced] sweating, by means of [enriching the patient's] liquids. Whenever [today's physicians] apply prescriptions to induce perspiration, they use warm and parching drugs such as *hou-p'o, ke-ken, chiang-huo, pai-chih, ts'ang-shu,* and *tou-k'ou.* If the patient's internal liquids had not yet wasted away, but are heated by the fire of the wind, and if they are then, in addition, parched by the parching drugs [listed above], from whence could perspiration develop?

And, if no perspiration develops, there is nothing to which the evil influences can attach to leave [the body]. But, the evil influences will not only fail to leave [the body]; on the contrary, they will be excited by the parching drugs. They will become even more violent, and they will mix with the [body's] proper influences. The evil fire spreads into all sections [of the body], and the [body's] liquids will be increasingly damaged. The tongue is desiccated, and the lips dry. The stools are blocked, and the eyes turn red. Many signs related to fire emerge. Consequently, the temperature of the body rises, the spirit becomes confused, and many unfavorable pathoconditions appear.

If one causes [the patient] to perspire even further, the yang fire reaches [its] utmost strength and the [patient's] true yin [influences] are set in motion. The water of the kidneys comes to offer assistance, and it is followed by the original yang [influences. The patient] perspires profusely in the upper [parts of his body], and pathoconditions indicating the danger of complete loss of yang [influences] emerge. Even mild cases produce spastic conditions and belong, therefore, to the kind of destructive illnesses that are difficult to cure.

I do not know how many people have already been killed because [their physicians] employed parching drugs to induce perspiration. The beginnings of this [practice] date from Li Tung-yüan.[1] All the prescriptions he established in his books represent patterns to treat [illnesses caused by] dampness evil, and they have nothing to do with the various affections associated with harm caused by cold. But later, people relied on his doctrines in their treatments for all types of pathoconditions resulting from affections from the outside, and the damage [caused] by this [approach] has increased ever since until this very day.

Also, [proper] patterns for treating dampness evil rely on [substances that are] weak in flavor, and that induce drainage of liquids, as major [components of therapy]. Examples are *chu-ling* and *wu-ling*. Similar [to the patterns of induced perspiration discussed above, the correct patterns of treating dampness evil] do not employ parching [drugs alone] to overcome [dampness]. Dampness is an evil affecting [the body] from the outside, and there is no [therapy] other than expelling it by using parching and humid substances simultaneously. It is definitely impossible to employ drugs that merely overcome dampness and have them launch an interior attack. This would lead only to a struggle between evil and proper [influences], resulting in damage to [the patient's] original influences.

As for the pathocondition of harm caused by cold, here too the main [emphasis of a treatment] should be to effuse [the evil influences] to the outside first. There is no such principle as to use nothing but drugs with a hot [thermo-influence] to overcome the cold. This would cause the cold influences to seize [regions of] depletion and to sink into [the body]. There would be no way for them to leave [the body]. After [the evil influences have been effused to the outside], yang [influences] are brought back into the [patient's body] by means of drugs such as [*kan-*]*chiang* and *fu*[*-tzu*]. This is the pattern of "regulating the center" applied by [Chang] Chung-ching.

When today's [physicians] employ parching drugs to cause perspiration [for the treatment] of various [external] affections, then this [approach] not only fails [to reflect any therapeutic] pattern of the Sages of antiquity, but even represents a mistaken application of the pattern [initiated by Li] Tung-yüan. The tradition of the [true] teachings of medicine has been lost. If even such shallow principles [as the one discussed above] are no longer known, how much more does this apply to subtle [doctrines]!

Note

1.   Li Tung-yüan (1180-1251), with the personal name Li Kao, is a major representative of the Sung-Chin-Yüan era in Chinese medical history. See VII.3 p. 364, and *Medicine in China: A History of Ideas,* pp. 177-179.

病不可輕汗論

治病之法不外汗下二端而已下之害人其危立見故

醫者病者皆不敢輕投至於汗多亡陽而死者十有二

三雖死而人不覺也何則凡人患風寒之疾必相戒以

為寧暖無涼病者亦重加覆護醫者亦云服藥必須汗

出而解故病人之求得汗人人以為當然也秋冬之時

過暖尚無大害至於盛夏初秋天時暑燥衛氣開而易

洩更加閉戶重衾復投發散之劑必至大汗不止而陽

亡矣又外感之疾汗未出之時必煩悶惡熱及汗大出

之後衛氣盡洩必陽衰而畏寒始之暖覆猶屬勉強至

此時雖欲不覆而不能愈覆汗愈寒直至汗出

如油手足厥冷而病不可為矣其死也神氣甚清亦無

痛苦病者醫者及旁觀之人皆不解其何故而忽死惟

有相顧駭然而已我見甚多不可不察也總之有病之

人不可過涼亦不宜太暖無事不可令汗出惟服藥之

後止令小汗仲景服桂枝湯法云服湯已溫覆令微似

汗不可如水淋漓此其法也至於亡陽未劇尤可挽回

傷寒論中真武理中四逆等法可考若已脫盡無可補

救矣又盛暑之時病者或居樓上或卧近竈之所無病

之人一立其處汗出如雨患病者必至時出汗即不

亡陽亦必陰竭而死雖無移徙之處必擇一席稍涼

地而處之否則神丹不救也

11. On [Reasons] Not to Carelessly Induce Perspiration

The treatment of illnesses is based exclusively on the two methods of [inducing] perspiration and downward [purging]. The danger that a person is harmed through downward [purging] is apparent [to any observer] as soon as [it emerges]. Hence, neither physicians nor patients apply [this treatment] carelessly. [On the other hand], two or three out of ten [patients who are treated with induced] perspiration lose large quantities of yang [influences] and die. And despite these deaths, no one realizes [that induced perspiration is dangerous]. How is this?

All people who suffer from wind-cold remind each other to keep themselves too warm rather than too cold. The patients themselves resort to thick covers, and the physicians state that they should take drugs forcing [the evil influences] to leave [the body] and dissolve through perspiration. Hence everyone considers it normal when patients ask for [drugs inducing] perspiration.

If too much heat is generated in the autumn or winter, this does not result in any great damage. However, if at the height of summer or in early autumn, when the climate is hot and dry, and when the protective influences are opened up and easily flow away, when [at this time] in addition [to the natural heat affecting the body] the doors are closed and heavy blankets [heaped over the patient], and if he is given preparations of effusing and dispersing [drugs], then he will greatly perspire without end and lose his yang [influences].

Also, anyone who has been affected [by evil influences] from the outside will feel rather distressed and will have an aversion to heat as long as no sweat has left his body. However, once he has greatly perspired, and once his protective influences have entirely leaked away, his yang will be weakened, and he will have an aversion to cold. If one had to force oneself in the beginning [to accept] such warm covers, there is a moment [when one's yang is weakened to such an extent] that one may wish not to be covered, but is unable [to remove the covers]. The more [the patient] is covered, the more he will perspire, and the more he perspires, the more he will feel cold. Finally, the sweat leaves [the body] like oil. Hands and feet [show signs of] ceasing [influences, and turn] cold. Nothing can be done against the illness any longer. When the patient dies, his spirit is quite clear, and he does not suffer from any pain. Patients, physicians, and observers have no explanation why he suddenly dies. They have no choice but to exchange startled glances.

I have seen very many [such cases], and one should be aware [of this issue]. In conclusion, sick people must neither be too cool nor too warm. Without any [serious] reason one should not cause [a patient] to perspire. Only at the time [a patient] takes medication is it advisable to have him perspire a little. [Chang] Chung-ching's pattern of consuming the "Decoction with *kuei-chih*" says, after the decoction has been taken, [the patient] is to be warmed by blankets until he perspires mildly. [The sweat] must not flow like water. That is the [appropriate] method in this case.

A loss of yang [influences] can be reversed as long as it has not become too critical. [To treat such cases] the "true warrior," the "regulation of the center," and the "four adverse movement" patterns of the *Shang-han Lun* may be consulted.[1] Once [the yang influences] have been entirely lost, nothing can be done to supplement [them] or to rescue [the patient]. Also, if the patient, at a time of great heat, lives on a top floor, or lies near the stove — that is, at a place where even a healthy person who came to stand there would experience immediate perspiration like rain — a patient will perspire all the time, and even if he does not lose his yang [influences], he will lose all his yin [influences] and must die. If he has no other home where he can move, he must select a somewhat cool location and stay there. Otherwise not even the pills of the spirits will save him.

Note

1.   This is a reference to the *chen wu* 眞武 decoction, the *li chung* 理中 decoction, and the *ssu ni* 四逆 powder advocated in the *Shang-han Lun*.

傷風難治論

凡人偶感風寒頭痛發熱咳嗽涕出俗語謂之傷風非
傷寒論中所云之傷風乃時行之雜感也人皆忽之不
知此乃至難治之疾生死之所關也蓋傷風之疾由皮
毛以入於肺肺為嬌臟寒熱皆所不宜太寒則邪氣凝
而不出太熱則火爍金而動血太潤則生痰飲太燥則
耗精液太洩則汗出而陽虛太澀則氣開而邪結并有
視為微疾不避風寒不慎飲食經年累月病機日深或
成血症或成肺痿或成哮喘或成怯弱比比皆然誤治之
害不可勝數諺云傷風不醒變成勞至言也然則治之
何如一驅風蘇葉荊芥之類二消痰半夏象貝之類三
降氣蘇子前胡之類四和營衛桂枝白芍之類五潤津
液妻仁元參之類六養血當歸阿膠之類七清火黃芩
山支之類八理肺桑皮大力子之類八者隨其病之輕

重而加減之更加以避風寒戒辛酸則庶幾漸愈否則
必成大病醫者又加以升提辛燥之品如桔梗乾姜之
類不效即加以酸收如五味子之類則必見血既見血
隨用熟地麥冬以實其肺即成勞而死四十年以來我
見以千計矣傷哉

12. On the Difficulties in Treating Harm Caused by Wind

Whenever someone has been incidentally affected by wind-cold, [resulting in] headache, fever, cough, and running nose, this is called, in everyday language, "harm caused by wind." This, however, is not the "harm caused by wind" that was mentioned in the *Shang-han Lun*. [The vernacular term "harm caused by wind" refers to] various affections that may be prevalent at specific times. No one takes these illnesses seriously, because no one knows that they are most difficult to treat, and that they may decide a person's survival or death.

The fact is that the illnesses of harm caused by wind start from the skin and its hair to enter the lung. The lung is a delicate viscus; it is compatible with neither hot nor cold. [A treatment adding] too much cold causes evil influences [that have entered the lung] to congeal and to not find their way out. [If one adds] too much heat, fire will fuse the metal[1] and excite the blood. [A treatment adding] too much moisture results in the generation of phlegm-fluid. [A treatment causing the lungs to become] too dry also causes the essential fluids to vanish. Too strong a drainage [from the lung] causes perspiration and a depletion of yang [influences]. Too strong a blocking [treatment in the lung] causes the influences to remain shut in, and evil [influences] to lump together.

And yet, all these [conditions] are considered minor illnesses, and [the people affected by such problems] neither avoid wind and cold, nor do they care about what they eat and drink. Over the years, and with every month, the workings of the illness [penetrate the body deeper and] deeper every day. In some cases pathoconditions appear indicating the blood [has been affected]. Or the lung may cease to function, or panting may develop, or disquietude coupled with weakness. It is always the same, and the damage caused by erroneous treatments cannot be measured. As the proverb goes, "If one does not pay attention to harm caused by wind, [the illness] will change to fatigue." Well said! But how to conduct a treatment?

First, the wind is to be expelled [with drugs] like *su-yeh* and *ching-chieh*.

Second, the phlegm is to be dissolved [with drugs] like *pan-hsia* and *hsiang-pei*.

Third, the [breath] influences are to be brought down [with drugs] like *su-tzu* and *ch'ien-hu*.

Fourth, constructive and protective [influences] are to be harmonized [with drugs] like *kuei-chih* and *pai-shao-[yao]*.

Fifth, the [body's] liquids are to be enriched [with drugs] like *lou-jen* and *yüan-shen*.

Sixth, the blood is to be nourished [with drugs] like *tang-kuei* and *a-chiao*.

Seventh, the fire is to be cooled [with drugs] like *huang-ch'in* and *shan-chih*.

Eighth, the lungs are to be regulated [with drugs] like *sang-p'i* and *ta-li-tzu*.

In the course of these eight [steps, the amount of drugs employed] has to be increased or decreased in accordance with the severity of the patho-conditions. Also, in addition, [the patient] should avoid wind and cold, and he should refrain from acrid and sour [food]. As a result [of such treatment], there is a good chance that [the patient] will gradually recover. Otherwise, [an initially minor problem] will develop into a very serious illness.

The physicians [of today] add [to the treatment] acrid and parching substances, suitable to make [the patient's influences] rise, as for instance *chieh-keng* and *kan-chiang*. If these drugs show no effect, they further add sour and astringent [drugs], like *wu-wei-tzu*. This, however, must lead to the appearance of blood [in the patient's sputum]. And when the blood appears, they apply *shou-ti* and *mai-tung* in order to replenish the patient's lung. Fatigue and death are the consequences. Over the past forty years, I have seen this a thousandfold; how distressing!

Note

1.   This is a metaphor to explain why excessive heat harms the lung; the lung is associated with the metal phase.

攻補寒熱同用論

虛症宜補實症宜瀉盡人而知之者然或人虛而症實
如弱體之人冒風傷食之類或人實而症虛如強壯之
人勞倦亡陽之類或有人本不虛而邪深難出又有人
已極虛而外邪尚伏種種不同若純用補則邪氣益固
純用攻則正氣隨脫此病未愈彼病益深古方所以有
攻補同用之法蓋之者曰兩藥異性一水同煎使其相
制則攻者不攻補者不補不如勿服若或兩藥不相制
分途而往則或反補其所當攻攻其所當補則不惟無
益而反有害是不可不慮也此正不然蓋藥之性各盡
其能攻者必攻強補者必補弱猶抵坎於地水從高處
流下必先盈坎而後進必不反向高處流也如大黃與
人參同用大黃自能逐去堅積決不反傷正氣人參自
能充益正氣決不反補邪氣蓋古人製方之法分經別

臟有神明之道焉如瘧疾之小柴胡湯瘧之寒熱往來
乃邪在少陽木邪侮土中宮無主故寒熱無定於是用
柴胡以驅少陽之邪柴胡必不犯脾胃用人參以健中
宮之氣人參必不入肝胆則少陽之邪自去而中土之
氣自旺二藥各歸本經也如桂枝湯桂枝走衛以祛風
白芍走營以止汗亦各歸本經也以是而推無不盡然
試以神農本草諸藥主治說細求之自無不得矣凡寒
熱兼用之法亦同此義故天下無難治之症後世醫者
不明此理藥惟一途若遇病情稍異非顧此失彼即游
移浮泛無往而非棘手之病矣但此必本於古人製方
成法而神明之若竟私心自用攻補寒熱雜亂不倫是
又殺人之術也

13. On the Simultaneous Application of Attacking and Supplementing, and of Cold and Hot [Drugs]

Everyone knows that one must supplement a pathocondition of depletion, and that one must drain a pathocondition of repletion. However, it happens that a person [will suffer from] depletion while his pathocondition [indicates] repletion. An example would be a person of weak constitution who was attacked by wind or harmed by some food. Or, it may be that a person's [influences are] replete while his pathocondition [signals] depletion. An example would be a person of strong constitution who has worked to fatigue and who has lost his yang [influences]. Or, even though someone did not [suffer from] depletion originally, evil [influences have penetrated] deep [into his body] and do not leave [that person] easily. Or, someone has already reached a state of extreme depletion and some external evil still lies hidden [in his body].

All these are examples of different [conditions of depletion], and if one were to apply only a supplementing [therapy], the evil influences would settle ever more firmly. If, however, one were to apply only an attacking therapy, [the patient] would lose his proper influences, and before one illness was cured, a second illness would have penetrated [the body] even deeper. Hence in ancient times some prescriptions followed the pattern of simultaneous [application of] attacking and supplementing [drugs].

Someone might question [the value of] this pattern and say: These two types of drugs differ in their nature. If they are boiled together in water, this results in their restraining each other. Those [drugs whose nature it is to] attack will no longer attack, and those [drugs whose nature it is to] supplement will no longer supplement. [To take such drugs would be] worse than not to take any drugs at all. Even if these two types of drugs did not restrain each other, and proceeded [through the body] on different paths, it might well happen that they supplemented what should be attacked, and that they attacked what should be supplemented. This, then, would result not only in no benefit; on the contrary, it would even cause damage. One should be most reluctant to apply this approach.

In reality it is exactly the other way around. The fact is that drugs will always make full use of the potential associated with their nature. [Drugs with an] attacking [nature] must attack what is strong, [and drugs with a] supplementing [nature] must supplement what is weak. Imagine, for comparison, a pit dug into the earth. Water flows down from some place of higher elevation; it will first fill that pit, and then proceed [elsewhere]. It will never flow upward to a higher elevation. If for example, *ta-huang* and *jen-shen* are applied at the same time, *ta-huang* is itself only able to remove hardened accumulations. It will never turn around and harm the proper influences. *Jen-shen* is itself only able to fill proper influences. It will never turn around and supplement evil influences. Hence, the patterns for designing prescriptions, [established] by the people of antiquity, distinguished between the [various] conduits and discriminated between the [various] viscera in a most enlighted way.

Take, for instance, the "Minor decoction with *ch'ai-hu*" [that is applied in case of the] *yao* illness.[1] When the fits of cold and heat associated with *yao* illness arrive in mutual succession, the evil resides in the minor-yang [region]. The evil of the [region associated with the phase of] wood insults [the region associated with the phase of] soil.[2] The central palace has no ruler, and as a result, cold and heat lack any fixed [location].[3] If one applies, at this moment, *ch'ai-hu* to expel the evil from the minor-yang [region],[4] *ch'ai-hu* will never attack the spleen and the stomach. And, if one applies *jen-shen* to strengthen the influences of the central palace, this *jen-shen* will never enter the liver or the gallbladder. As a result, the evil [influences] will leave the minor-yang region by themselves, and the influences of the central [region associated with the phase of] soil will come to flourish. Both drugs find their way to their respective conduits.

Take, as [another] example, the "Decoction with *kuei-chih*."[5] *Kuei-chih* proceeds to the [paths of the] protective [influences], where it eliminates wind. *Pai-shao* proceeds to the [paths of the] constructive [influences], where it stops perspiration. Here, too, each [drug] finds its way to its respective conduit. This [principle] applies to all other [such cases] in the same manner, and one may check the statements of the *Shen-nung Pen-ts'ao* on the main [drug] indications for proof. If one examines them in detail, one will find every [detail that one may search for].

All patterns of a simultaneous application of [drugs with] cold and hot [qualities] have the same rationale. Hence there are no pathoconditions that are difficult to treat — it is just that physicians of later generations do not understand the principles [outlined above]. They [use] drugs only on one path, and when they are confronted with an illness whose nature is slightly different [from the rule], they either focus on one [aspect] and fail to take into account another, or they oscillate [between different approaches]; wherever they turn, they will find illness exceeding their abilities.

One must base [one's approach] on the fixed patterns [developed] by the ancients for the designing of prescriptions, and one must fully understand these [patterns to be able to adapt them to a given situation]. If one sticks to one's personal ideas, and attacks or supplements, or [applies] cold or hot [drugs] indiscriminately, this, then, is merely a technique for homicide.

Notes

1.   This term appears to have referred to illnesses that included malaria.

2.   The phase of wood [associated with the liver] is able to control or overcome the phase of soil [associated with the spleen].

3.   The term "central palace" refers to the phase of soil, and hence to the spleen and stomach.

4.   The minor yang region includes the gallbladder and triple burner, as well as the foot and hand minor-yang conduits.

5.   The "Decoction with *kuei-chih*" consists of several drugs, including *kuei-chih* and *pai-shao-yao*.

臨病人問所便論

病者之愛惡苦樂即病情虛實寒熱之徵醫者望色切
脈而知之不如其自言之為尤真也惟病者不能言之
處即言而不知其所以然之故則賴醫者推求其理耳
今乃病者所自知之病明明為醫者言之則醫者正可
因其言而知其病之所在以治之乃不以病人自知之
真對症施治反執已之偏見強制病人未有不誤人者
如傷寒論中云能食者為中風不能食者為中寒則傷
寒內中風之症未嘗禁其食也乃醫者見為傷寒之症
斷不許食凡屬感症皆不許其食甚有病已半愈胃虛
求食而亦禁之以至困餓而死者又傷寒論云欲飲水
者稍稍與之蓋實火煩渴得水則解未嘗禁冷水也乃
醫家凡遇欲冷飲之人一概禁止并有伏暑之病得西
瓜而即愈者病人哀求欲食亦斷絕不與至煩渴而死

如此之類不可枚舉蓋病者之性情氣體有能受溫熱
者有能受寒涼者有不受補者有不禁攻者各有不同
乃必強而從我意見況醫者之意見亦各人不同於是
治病之法無一中肯者矣內經云臨病人問所便蓋病
人之所便即病情真實之所在如身大熱而反欲熱飲
則假熱而真寒也身寒戰而反欲寒飲是假寒而真熱
也以此類推百不失一而世之醫者偏欲與病人相背
何也惟病人有所嗜好而與病相害者則醫者宜開導
之如其人本喜酸或得欬症則酸宜忌如病人本喜酒
得濕病則酒宜忌之類此則不可縱欲以益其疾若與
病症無碍而病人之所喜則從病人之便即所以治其
病也此內經辨症之精義也

275

14. On [the Meaning of the Statement] "When You Approach a Patient, Ask For His Preferences."

A patient's preferences and aversions, what gives him misery, and what provides him with joy — these are indications whether he suffers from a depletion or from a repletion, [from an intrusion of] cold or of heat. A physician may recognize the nature of the [patient's] illness by observing his complexion or by feeling the [movement in his] vessels. But this is not as truthful as the words spoken by the [patient] himself.

Only when a patient is unable to express himself [clearly], or if he [attempts to] express himself but does not know the reasons for his condition, [only then] is it up to the physician to search for the principle [behind the patient's illness]. Now, if a patient knows his illness, and tells it to the physician quite clearly, then the physician, following the statement by the patient, should know the location of the illness, and treat it accordingly. But, if the physician does not accept the truth [reported by] the patient [as his guideline] for designing a therapy that focuses on specific pathoconditions, and if he, on the contrary, clings to his own biased views and forces them onto his patient, then harm will be unavoidable.

For instance, in the *Shang-han Lun* it is stated: "Those [patients] who can eat have been struck by wind. Those who cannot eat have been struck by cold." Hence the intake of food has never been forbidden to those who displayed a pathocondition of being struck by wind within [a period when they were also] harmed by cold. But when the physicians see a pathocondition of harm caused by cold, they do not allow [the patient] to consume any food at all. Whenever [they diagnose] a pathocondition associated with an affection [from outside], they do not allow [the patient] to consume any food. They go so far as to forbid it even when [the patient] longs for food because the illness is half cured and the stomach is empty. The result is that [the patient] dies of starvation.

The *Shang-han Lun* states further, "Give a little to those who wish to drink water." When, in the case of a repletion, fire causes thirst, this can be dissipated by giving [the patient] water. [A dose of] cold water has never been forbidden [in such a situation]. However, whenever [today's] physicians meet someone who longs for a cold drink, they prohibit this categorically. Also, some cases of hidden summerheat can [easily] be cured by allowing [the patient to eat] watermelons. But even if the patients were to beg on their knees [to be allowed] to eat [melons, the physicians of today] will not give them anything, with the result that the [patients] die of thirst.

There are many more such examples; I cannot list them all here one by one. The fact is that the disposition of patients, their influences and their physical body, may be such that they can bear warmth or heat, while others may be able to bear cold or coolness. Some cannot stand anything supplementing; others cannot stand to [eat food or take drugs whose nature is] attacking. Each [patient's disposition] is different.

The [physicians, though,] are very determined to follow their own personal opinion — also, the opinions offered by physicians [today] differ from one to the next — so there is no single pattern [that could be termed] appropriate for treating illnesses.

The *Nei-ching* states, "When you approach a patient, ask for his preferences."[1] The fact is that the true nature of an illness lies in a patient's preferences. If, for example, his body is very hot and, contrary [to what one might expect, the patient] longs for hot beverages, then he suffers from a pseudo-heat which is, in reality, a cold. Or, if his body trembles from cold, and nevertheless, [the patient] wishes to drink something cold, then he suffers from a pseudo-cold, which is in fact a heat. If one orients oneself on these [examples], one will not lose one patient in a hundred. And yet, the physicians of today purposely set themselves in opposition to their patients.

What is the reason for this? Only when a patient longs for something that is incompatible with his illness should a physician offer guidance. If, for instance, a person likes [to eat] sour [food] and then gets a cough, sour [food] must be forbidden to him. If a person loves to drink wine and gets a dampness illness, he must abstain from wine. In these cases to cure their illnesses one cannot follow the desires [of the patients]. If, however, the desire of a patient is no obstacle to [the healing of] his illness, then it will lead to a cure of his illness, if one orients oneself on the patient's preferences. This is the essential meaning of the differentiation of pathoconditions [as advocated] in the *Nei-ching*.

Note

1.   See *Ling-shu,* treatise 29, "Shih ch'uan."

治病不必顧忌論

凡病人或體虛而患實邪或舊有他病與新病相反或一人兼患二病其因又相反或内外上下各有所病醫者踟躕束手不敢下藥此乃不知古人制方之道者也

古人用藥惟病是求藥所以制病有一病則有一藥以制之其人有是病則其藥當至於病所而驅其邪決不反至無病之處以為禍也若留其病不使去雖強壯之

人遷延日久亦必精神耗竭而死此理甚易明也如怯弱之人本無攻伐之理若或傷寒而邪入陽明則仍用硝黄下藥邪去而精氣自復如或懷妊之婦忽患癥瘕必用桃仁大黄以下其癥瘀去而胎自安或老年及火

病之人或宜發散或宜攻伐皆不可因其血氣之衰而兼用補益如傷寒之後食復女勞復仲景皆治其食清其火並不因病後而用溫補惟視病之所在而攻之中

病即止不復有所顧慮故天下無棘手之病惟不能中病或偏或誤或太過則不病之處亦傷而入危矣俗所謂有病病當之此歷古相傳之法也故醫者當疑難之際多所顧忌不敢對症用藥者皆視病不明辨症不的審方不眞不知古聖之精義者也

15. On [Situations Where There Is] No [Need to] Worry [about the]Patient's Condition] When Treating an Illness

Whenever a patient's body is marked by depletion, and [the patient] suffers from a repletion evil; or when he already has [had] one illness for some time and is now affected by a new illness that is opposite to the old one; or when someone suffers at the same time from two illnesses with mutually contradictory causes; or when someone is ill everywhere in his [body's] interior and exterior, upper and lower regions; [in all these cases] the physicians are ambivalent [about what to do]. They sit there waiting with their hands tied, and do not dare to [ask the patient to] take any drugs. The reason is that they are unfamiliar with the principles of the ancients as to how to design a prescription.

When the ancients applied drugs, they focussed on nothing but the illnesses. They employed drugs in order to check an illness. For each single illness, there was one specific drug to check it. When a person had a particular illness, a specific drug proceeded nowhere else but to the location of that illness, and expelled the evil [influences] from there. By no means did it turn around and proceed to some location without illness, and cause problems there. If [one] left the illness [in its place], and did not cause it to leave, after some time even a strong person's essential spirit would vanish, with death being the result.

This principle is easily understandable. Basically, there is no reason to conduct a [treatment with drugs of an] attacking nature in people who are anxious and weak. If [such a person] is harmed by cold, with evil [influences] entering the yang-brilliance [region], one must use drugs causing a downward movement, [such as] *hsiao-huang*. [This way] the evil influences [are made to] leave, and the essential influences recover.

Or, if a pregnant woman suddenly [develops] blockages and concentrations, one must apply *t'ao-jen* and *ta-huang* to cause these concentrations to move down. [Her blood] will no longer be blocked in its flow, and the fetus will remain secure [in its place].

Or [consider] people of old age or those already suffering from an illness for a long time. In some cases [their illnesses] must be dissipated; in others they must be attacked. But, just because of the weakened condition of these [patients'] blood and influences, it is not [necessarily] correct to use supplementing and supporting [drugs] simultaneously.

Another example: after one was harmed by cold one [falls ill] again because of [inappropriate] eating, or because of [excessive intercourse with] women. [In such cases, Chang] Chung-ching always directed his treatments at [the patient's] eating [habits], and cooled his fire, but he never applied warming or supplementing [remedies] simply because the [patient] had just recovered from an illness. He would see only where an illness was located, and attack there. When the illness was hit, he would stop [his treatment], and waste no more thought on it.

That is to say, there are no illnesses on earth against which we cannot do anything. Only if one is unable to hit an illness, or if a treatment is unbalanced, or just wrong, or too strong, does this leads to damage at locations where no illness exists, and is dangerous for the person [treated].

The widely used phrase: "When there is an illness, [a treatment should be initiated that is] appropriate for that illness!" is a pattern that has been transmitted from antiquity. When, therefore, physicians, because they are confronted with a doubtful and difficult situation, worry too much [about the patient's condition], and do not dare to direct any drugs against his pathoconditions, that means that they are not clear about his illness, that they do not [know how to] distinguish his pathoconditions correctly, that they are unable to examine [all available] prescriptions accurately, and that they are unfamiliar with the essential meaning [underlying the treatments applied] by the Sages of antiquity.

病深非淺藥能治論

天下有治法不誤而始終無效者此乃病氣深痼非泛然之方藥所能愈也凡病在皮毛營衛之間即使病勢極重而所感之位甚淺邪氣易出至於臟腑筋骨之痼疾如勞怯痞隔風痹痿厥之類其感非一日其邪在臟腑筋骨如油之入麵與正氣相併病家不知屢易醫家醫者見其不效雜藥亂投病日深而元氣日敗遂至不救不知此病非一二尋常之方所能愈也今之集方書者如風痹大症之類前錄古方數首後附以通治之方數首如此而已此等治法豈有愈期必當徧考此病之種類與夫致病之根源及變遷之情狀并詢其歷來服藥之誤否然後廣求古今以來治此症之方選擇其內外種種治法次第施之又時時消息其效否而神明變通之則痼疾或有可愈之理若徒執數首通治之方屢

試不効其計遂窮未有不誤者也故治大症必學問深博心思精敏又專心久治乃能奏效世又有極重極久之病諸藥罔效忽服極輕淡之方而愈此乃其病本有專治之方從前皆係誤治忽遇對症之藥自然應手而痊也

16. On the Impossibility of Curing Deep-Seated Illnesses with Superficial Drugs

It happens that a pattern [selected for a] treatment is correct but shows no positive effect whatsoever. In such cases the influences of the illness have entered [a patient] deeply and [have become an] obstinate problem that can not be cured with just ordinary prescriptions and drugs.

Whenever an illness is located between the skin and its hair and the region of the constructive and protective [influences], its evil influences can easily be eliminated, even if the strength of the illness is extreme, as long as the seat of the affection remains superficial. Obstinate illnesses, though, [that have lodged] in the viscera and bowels, in the sinews and bones, [namely such problems] as fatigue, anxiety, blockages, and stoppages, as well as wind, or obturation, atony, and ceasing [yin influences; or cases] where the affection has already lasted for more than one [or two] days and has entered the viscera and bowels, sinews and bones, and where [the evil influences] have become tied to the proper influences just like oil entering flour, [in such cases] the patients do not know what to do, and they frequently change physicians.

When the physicians see [that their treatments remain] without effect, they randomly toss a number of different drugs [into the patient, with the result] that the illness only penetrates deeper, day after day, while the damage to the original influences increases, until finally a point is reached where no rescue is possible at all. [Physicians] do not know that such illnesses cannot be cured with one or two ordinary prescriptions. In today's prescription literature, when it comes to such serious pathoconditions as wind or obturation, first a number of ancient prescriptions, and then a number of cure-all prescriptions, are listed. And, that is it. How could anyone expect to cure [a serious illness] with such treatment patterns?

What is necessary is that one examines all the different variations of the illness at hand, as well as the origin of the illness, and the circumstances of any change it may have undergone. Also, one must investigate whether there have been any mistakes in the [patient's] previous treatment with drugs. Once this [has all been clarified], one must search widely for prescriptions that have served to treat this illness in former times, and select various therapeutic patterns for treating the [patient's] interior and exterior [body sections], and apply them gradually one by one. One must periodically check whether [the treatment] shows an effect, and skillfully adapt [it to any new developments]. Then there may be a rationale for a cure of even obstinate ailments.

If, though, one clings to but a few cure-all prescriptions, whose repeated applications show no effect, one's strategies will soon be exhausted, and one is bound to have committed mistakes. For the treatment of severe pathoconditions one must, therefore, possess a profound and extensive knowledge, as well as a sophisticated and intelligent mind. Also, one must treat them with full concentration and over long periods of time, and only then will one be able to achieve results.

Some illnesses are very severe and last very long, and no drugs show any effects. Suddenly [the patient] takes a prescription of very light [drugs that are] weak in flavor and is cured. In this case, a prescription existed that could cure the illness, but all previous treatments had been wrong. Suddenly, one comes across a drug that fits the respective pathocondition exactly, and a cure results immediately as a matter of course.

愈病有日期論

治病之法自當欲其速愈世之論者皆以為治早而藥
中病則愈速治緩而藥不中病則愈遲此常理也然亦
有不論治之遲早而愈期有一定者內經藏氣法時論
云夫邪氣之客於身也以勝相加至其所生而愈至其
所不勝而甚至其所生而持自得其位而起其他言病
愈之期不一傷寒論云發於陽者七日愈發於陰者六
日愈又云風家表解而不了了者十二日愈此皆宜靜
養調攝以待之不可亂投藥石若以其不愈或多方以
取效或更用重劑以希功即使不誤藥力勝而元氣反
傷更或有不對症之藥不惟無益反有大害此所宜知
也況本原之病必待其精神漸復精神豈有驟長之理
至於外科則起發成膿生肌收口亦如痘症有一定之
日期治之而誤固有遷延生變者若欲強之有速效則

如揠苗助長其害有不可勝言者乃病家醫家皆不知
之醫者投藥不效自疑為未當又以別方試之不知前
方實無所害特未至耳乃反誤試諸藥愈換而病愈
重病家以醫者久而不效更換他醫徧閱前方知
其不效亦復更換他藥愈治愈遠由是斷斷不死之病
亦不救矣此皆由不知病愈有日期之故也夫病家不
足責為醫者豈可不知而輕以人嘗試乎若醫者審知
之而病家必責我以近效則當明告之故決定所愈之
期倘或不信必欲醫者另立良方則以和平輕淡之藥
姑以應病者之求待其自愈如更不信則力辭之斷不
可徇人情而至於誤人如此則病家一時或反怨謗以
後其言果驗則亦知我識高而品崇矣

284

17. On Specific Time Periods Required for Illness to Heal

It is, of course, the goal of all therapeutic methods to effect the cure of an illness as fast as possible. In all contemporary discourses on this [issue], it is stated that if a treatment commences at an early [stage], and if the drugs hit the illness, [the ailment] heals quickly. If, however, the treatment is conducted in no hurry, and if the drugs fail to hit the illness, then [the ailment] heals slowly. That is, indeed, the usual principle.

But, there are cases where [an illness] heals after a fixed period of time no matter whether the treatment is started early or late. In the treatise "Tsang ch'i fa shih lun" of the *Nei-ching* it is stated, "When evil influences lodge in a [human] body, they have attached themselves [to the body during those times of the year] when they dominate. When [the season] comes [that is associated with the phase that is] produced [by the phase associated with the viscus where the illness is located, the illness] heals. When [a season] comes [that is associated with a phase that] cannot be overcome [by the phase associated with the viscus where the illness is located, then the illness will become] severe. And [the illness] emerges [during the season] when [the phase associated with the affected viscus] assumes the dominant position."[2] [The *Nei-ching*] has several further statements on [the fixed] periods of time [required] for the healing of an illness.

In the *Shang-han Lun* it is stated, "Those [illnesses] that develop in the yang [sections of the body] heal within seven days; those that develop in the yin [sections of the body] heal within six days." And it is further stated, "When a patient suffering from wind has his exterior [affection] cleared but is not yet in good health, [his illness] will be cured within twelve days." In all such cases, though, one must rest and take care of oneself while one waits for one's [recovery], and it is entirely inappropriate to wildly toss [herbal] drugs and minerals [into a patient]. If [one loses one's patience] because [the illness appears] not to heal, and if [one gives the patient] many prescriptions to bring about a [quick] effect, or if one hopes for an [early] result by applying voluminous preparations, the strength of the drugs — even though they may not be wrong — becomes too dominant and, contrary [to one's intentions, the preparation] harms [the patient's] original influences. If, however, the drugs are not exactly matched against the [patient's] pathoconditions, he will not only have no benefit from them; on the contrary, he will receive great damage. One should know this!

Also, in the case of illnesses affecting the source and origin [of one's existence], one must wait for the gradual recovery of the [patient's] essential spirit. There is no principle whatsoever allowing for a quick growth of one's essential spirit!

Turning to external medicine, the rise [of boils] and the generation of pus, the creation of flesh and the closing of wounds, and also the [development of the] pathoconditions [associated with] small pox, all these [processes require] fixed periods of time. Any erroneous treatment will, for sure, cause [the illness] to linger and undergo [undesirable] changes. If one attempts to achieve quick results by force, this is like pulling sprouts to increase their growth. The resulting harm could not be told in words. However, neither the patients nor the physicians know of this.

When the physicians toss their drugs [into the patients] and achieve no [immediate] positive effects, they doubt their own [actions] and consider them inappropriate. Next, they try another prescription without realizing that the prescription first applied was not causing any harm at all. [It had no positive effects] simply because the time [for the illness to heal] had not yet come. Consequently, physicians try many erroneous drugs; the more they change [their prescriptions], the more serious the illness becomes.

The patient [on the other hand] notices that a physician achieves no positive effects for quite some time, and resorts to another physician. This other physician examines all previously [applied] prescriptions, and is told that they had no effects. So he, too, turns to still other drugs, and the more he treats [the patient], the further away [is his treatment from a correct principle]. Hence, even illnesses that should never have resulted in death will develop into hopeless cases. All this results from an unawareness of the fact that the healing of an illness is tied to certain periods of time.

Now, patients cannot really be held responsible for this. But why are the physicians so ignorant, and [why do they] carelessly try [their medications] on people? Given that physicians know of all this and that the patients, as is unavoidable, demand that we speed up the effects [of a treatment], then we should clearly tell them the reason [for their slow recovery], and identify in advance the time [when] they will be healed. If they do not believe, and if they demand that the physician design another good prescription, then one employs drugs that are balanced and light in their qualities, and neutral in flavor — simply to respond to the demands of the patient — and waits until [the illness] heals by itself. If the [patient] still does not believe [that enough has been done], one must firmly decline [to meet the patient's demands]. It is definitely impossible to give in to do him a favor and thus cause harm to that person through an inappropriate treatment. If one acts like this, the patient may well develop hatred [for a physician] and malign him for a while. But later, when the [physician's] words have come true, the [patient] will realize that our knowledge is great and our rank high.

Note

1.   See *Su-wen,* treatise 22.

治人必考其驗否論

天下之事惟以口舌爭而無從考其信否者則是非難
定若夫醫則有效驗之可徵知之最易而為醫者自審
其工拙亦最易然而世之擇醫者與為醫者皆憒憒而
莫之辨何也古人用藥苟非宿病痼疾其效甚速內經
云一劑知二劑已又云覆杯而卧傷寒論云一服愈者
不必盡劑可見古人審病精而用藥當未有不一二劑
而效者故治病之法必宜先立醫案指為何病所本何
方方中用某藥專治某症其論說本之何書服此藥後
於何時減去所患之何症倘或不驗必求所以不驗之
故而更思必效之法或所期之效不應反有他效必求
其所以致他效之故又或反增他症或病反重則必求
所以致害之故而自痛懲焉更復博考醫書期於必愈
而止若其病本不能速效或其病止可小效或竟不可

治亦必豫立醫案明著其說然後立方不得冒昧施治
如此自考自然有過必知加以潛心好學其道日進矣
今之醫者事事反此惟記方數首擇時尚之藥數種不
論何病何症總以此塞責偶爾得效自以為功其效或無
效或至於死亦諉於病勢之常病家亦相循為固然全
不一怪間有病家於未服藥之前問醫者服此藥之後
效驗若何醫者答云且看脉後何如豈有預期之理病
家亦唯自以為失言何其愚也若醫者能以此法自
考必成良醫病家以此法考醫者必不為庸醫之所誤
兩有所益也

18. On the Need to Examine One's Success When Treating a [Sick] Person

Where an event is discussed solely with oral arguments, and where no solid evidence exists that could be checked for proof, right or wrong are difficult to decide. In medicine, though, [therapeutic] successes exist as evidence and can be recognized quite easily. Hence, it is also quite easy for those who practice medicine to check for themselves whether they conduct skillful or inadequate [treatments]. In recent times, however, those who select a physician, and those who practice medicine, they are all equally ignorant and have no way to distinguish [good and bad]. How is that?

When the people of antiquity applied drugs, they always achieved very fast results, except for illnesses that had already lasted for a long time, or for obstinate ailments. The *Nei-ching* states: "One dose, and one knows [the effect]; a second dose and [the illness] is healed."[1] It states further, "Turn a cup and sleep."[2] The *Shang-han Lun* says, "Recovery comes with one dose [of drugs], and does not even require the entire dose." From these [quotations] one can see that the ancients were skilled in examining the illnesses and made proper use of drugs. It simply never happened that one or two doses showed no effects.

To treat illnesses requires, therefore, the following pattern: First, a medical case record has to be established, indicating what [the nature of the] illness [to be treated] is, on which prescription [the treatment] is to be based, and which drugs in that prescription are employed to specifically treat which pathoconditions. It is also to be stated on which literature one's [therapeutic] discourse is based. Once the drugs have been consumed, [it is to be noted] which pathoconditions [the patient] suffers from vanish at what time. If no success can be obtained, one must search for the reason why no success could be obtained, and one must think of a [therapeutic] pattern that is bound to show an effect.

It may be that one does not get the intended effect, and that a different effect occurs instead. In this case, one must search for the reason why this other effect occurred. Furthermore, it happens that new pathoconditions appear in addition [to those one intended to treat], or that — contrary [to one's expectations] — the illness takes a turn for the worse. Then one must search for the reason why such damage could occur, and one should regard [such mishaps] as painful warnings. Again, one must start an extensive search through medical literature, and [only] at the moment when [the illness] has definitely been healed must one end [one's] efforts.

In case the illness, by its nature, cannot be cured within a short time, or in case only minor successes can be achieved, or if [the illness] is just incurable, one must still go ahead and establish a medical case record and document clearly what [the situation] is like, before one writes a prescription. One simply should never carry out a therapy without having given it detailed thought.

If one examines one's own [activities] like this, one will inevitably come to realize one's errors; and if one adds careful studies and a diligent mind, one will make progress every day. Today's physicians, though, act contrary to this [principle] in every instance. They merely memorize a few prescriptions, and select just a few fashionable drugs. Regardless of what type of an illness [they are confronted with], and which pathoconditions [their treatments should focus on], it is always the same how they acquit themselves of their responsibilities.

If, by accident, [their treatments] show an effect, they consider this a personal success. If, however, [their treatments] show no effects, or if [the patient] dies, they put the blame on [what they call] the normal [outcome of such a] forceful illness. The patients comply with these [activities of their physicians] and consider them a matter of course. They never develop any doubts.

There are some patients who ask their physicians prior to the intake of drugs what effects can be expected once they have taken their drugs. The physicians answer, "Let us wait and see what happens after you have taken the drugs." How could one know this in advance? And the patients responds with a "yes, yes," assuming they have said something inappropriate. How stupid!

If the physicians could examine their own [activities] alongside the pattern outlined above, they would inevitably become good physicians. And the patients, if they were to examine the physicians on the basis of this pattern, would never be harmed through the mistakes committed by common physicians. Both [patients and physicians] would benefit.

Notes

1.   See *Su-wen*, treatise 40, "Fu chung lun."

2.   See *Ling-shu*, treatise 71, "Hsieh k'o." "Turn a cup and sleep" means that one should drink all one's drugs until the cup holding the medication is empty, and then go to sleep immediately. This way, drugs are supposed to act rapidly.

防微論

病之始生淺則易治及而深入則難治內經云聖人不

治已病治未病夫病已成而藥之譬猶渴而穿井鬪而

鑄兵不亦晚乎傷寒論序云時氣不和便當早言尋其

邪由及在腠理以時治之罕有不愈患人忍之數日乃

說邪氣入臟則難可制昔扁鵲見齊桓公云病在腠理

三見之後則已入臟不可治療而逃矣歷聖相傳如同

一轍蓋病之始入風寒既淺氣血臟腑未傷自然治之

甚易至於邪氣深入則邪氣與正氣相亂欲攻邪則礙

正欲扶正則助邪即使邪漸去而正氣已不支矣若夫

得病之後更或勞動感風傷食謂之病後加病尤

極危殆所以人之患病在客館道途得者往往難治非

所得之病獨重也乃既病之後不能如在家之安適而

及早治之又復勞動感冒致病深入而難治也故凡人

少有不適必當即時調治斷不可忽為小病以致漸深

更不可勉強支持使病更增以貽無窮之害此則凡人

所當深省而醫者亦必詢明其得病之故更加意體察

也

19. On Protective Measures Against [Illnesses That Are] Still Insignificant

An illness that has just begun to grow and is [located at the body's] surface is easy to cure. [An illness that has already lasted] for a long time and has penetrated [the body] deeply is difficult to cure.

The *Nei-ching* states, "The Sages do not treat those who already have an illness; they treat those who are not yet ill. To appy drugs against an illness that has already formed is like digging a well when one is thirsty, and it is like casting weapons after war has begun. Would this not be too late, too?"[1]

In the preface to the *Shang-han Lun* it is said, "When the seasonal influences are out of balance, this must be stated early. The origin of the evil [entering the body] is to be examined, and also whether it is still in the pores. Then it can be treated in time, and it will be rare that no cure is achieved. If the patient bears [his illness silently], and speaks of it only after a few days, then the evil influences have already entered his viscera and can be brought under control only with great difficulty."

When, in the old days, Pien Ch'io saw Marquis Huan of Ch'i, he said, "[Your illness] is in the pores." After three further audiences, [the Marquis' illness] had entered his body's viscera and was incurable. Hence, [Pien Ch'io] fled away.[2]

The Sages handed down [the principle of early treatment] through the ages as straight as a single-cart track. That is, when an illness is just beginning to enter [the body], the wind or the cold are still at the [body's] surface; neither [the proper] influences nor the blood, nor the viscera nor the bowels, have yet been harmed; and it is of course most easy to successfully treat [the emerging ailment] at this [stage]. Once the evil influences have deeply penetrated [the body], the evil influences and the proper influences become mixed, and if one [now] wished to attack the evil, one would also injure the proper; just as one would strengthen the evil, if one were to support the proper. Even if the evil influences would gradually leave [the body], the proper influences would no longer be in a position to survive by themselves.

If one has one illness already, and then, in addition, moves around and is affected by wind, or is harmed by some influence, or by food, this is called "adding an illness to a pre-existing illness." Such a [condition] is extremely dangerous. When, therefore, someone suffers from an illness that he got in some guesthouse or on the road, this is often enough quite difficult to cure. Not that the illnesses [people] get [on the road] are singularly serious, [but that] after someone has acquired an illness this way, he is unable to rest comfortably in his home, and initiate an early treatment. If, instead, he moves around and is affected by some adverse [influences], his illness penetrates deep [into his body] and is difficult to cure.

Whenever, therefore, someone feels a little uncomfortable, a balancing treatment must be initiated immediately. One must never neglect such a condition as a "minor illness," so that [the evil influences] will penetrate [the body] ever deeper. And it would be even more inappropriate to endure [the illness] as long as possible, because the only effect would be that the illness worsens, and excessive harm results. Everyone should be thoroughly familiar with these [facts]. The physicians, however, must ascertain, through inquiries, the reasons why someone has acquired an illness, and they must pay special attention to thorough examinations.

Notes

1.   See *Su-wen,* treatise 2, "Ssu ch'i tiao shen ta lun."

2.   See *Shih-chi,* ch. 109, "Pien Ch'io Ts'ang-kung lieh chuan."

知病必先知症論

凡一病必有數症有病同症異者有病異者有症同病異者有症
與病相因者有症與病不相因者蓋合之則曰病分之
則曰症古方以一藥治一症合數症而成病即合數藥
而成方其中亦有以一藥治幾症者有合幾藥而治一
症者又有同此一症因不同用藥亦異變化無窮其淺
近易知者如吐逆用黃連半夏不寐用棗仁茯神之類
人皆知之至於零雜之症如內經所載喘咳慌噫語吞欠
嚏嘔笑泣目瞑嗌乾心懸善恐涎下涕出齧唇齧舌善
怒善喜握多夢嘔酸魄汗等症不可勝計或由司天
運氣或由臟腑生尅或由邪氣傳變內經言之最詳後
之醫者病之總名亦不能知安能於一病之中辨明眼
症之源流即使病者身受其苦備細言之而彼實茫然
不知古人以何藥為治仍以泛常不切之品應命并有

用相反之藥以益其疾者此病之所以無門可告也
學醫者當熟讀內經每症究其緣由詳其情狀辨其異
同審其真偽然後徧考方書本草詳求古人治法一遇
其症應手輒愈不知者以為神奇其實古聖皆有成法
也

20. On the Need to Know [a Patient's] Pathoconditions before Treating His Illness

Each individual illness must be accompanied by several pathoconditions. Sometimes identical illnesses are accompanied by different pathoconditions. And, it may also be that [different patients experience] identical pathoconditions, while their illnesses are different. It may be that pathoconditions and illness coincide with each other, and it happens that pathoconditions and illness do not coincide with each other. Now, seen together, they are called illness. Seen separately, they are called pathoconditions.

In ancient prescriptions, one drug served to cure one pathocondition. If several pathoconditions came together to form one illness, then several drugs were brought together to form one prescription. Also, there were instances where one single drug was employed to treat several pathoconditions, or where several drugs were combined to treat one single pathocondition. Also, there were identical pathoconditions whose causes were different, hence the drugs employed had to be different too. Countless variations are possible.

The more superficial [relationships between specific drugs and specific pathoconditions] are widely known. For instance, everyone knows that one uses *huang-lien* and *pan-hsia* for vomiting and [other cases of food or influences] moving contrary to their proper direction, and that one employs *tsao-jen* and *fu-shen* if one cannot sleep. But then there are those countless sundry pathoconditions recorded in the *Nei-ching* as: panting and dry retching, belching and talkativeness, [repeated] swallowing and yawning, sneezing and vomiting, laughing and weeping, obscured vision and dry throat, "hanging heart"[1] and tendency to fear, saliva running down [from one's mouth], snivel flowing out, lip biting and tongue biting, tendency to forget, and tendency to become angry, anxiety, frequent dreaming, sour vomiting, and sweating [from the viscus that stores] the *p'o*.[2]

Some of these [pathoconditions] result from the periodic influences governing the heavens. Others result from [relationships of] mutual production and overcoming of the [body's] viscera, and still others result from a transfer and metamorphosis of evil influences [inside the body]. The *Nei-ching* elucidates all this in great detail.

The physicians of later times do not even know the general names of the illnesses. How could they be able to distinguish the origins of the various pathoconditions within one specific illness? Even though the patient, who suffers with his own body, may explain his illness in great detail, the [physicians] remain rather vague. They do not know what drugs the ancients would have used for treatment, hence they respond to the [patient's] call [for therapy] with unusual and impractical substances. Or they apply drugs that stand in direct contradiction to [those required], and that therefore even support the [patient's] illness. The patient has nowhere he could turn [for complaints].

Any student of medicine should read the *Nei-ching* thoroughly and for each pathocondition he should investigate its origin, carefully examine its circumstances, distinguish between [pathoconditions that are] similar and [those that are] different, and analyze whether [a pathocondition] is genuine or false. Then he must consult prescription books and herbals everywhere, and he must look for therapeutic patterns established by the ancients. This way, as soon as he is confronted with a specific pathocondition, he will effect a cure with but a turn of his hand. Those who are ignorant think this is miraculous, when, in fact, the ready-to-use patterns of the Sages of antiquity [are available even today].

Notes

1.   The term *hsin hsien* appears in the *Su-wen*, treatise 19, "Yü chi chen tsang lun." It was equated by Chang Ching-yo with the term *hsien hsin* 縣心 in the *Ling-shu*, treatise 29, "Shih ch'uan," where it appears to refer to an empty stomach. Chang interpreted this term as "anxieties accompanying hunger."

2.   That is, sweat originating from the lung. The *p'o*, one of two souls in man, is said, in the *Nei-ching*, to be stored in the lung.

補藥可通融論

古人病愈之後即令食五穀以養之則元氣自復無所
謂補藥也黃農仲景之書豈有補益之方哉間有別載
他書者皆托名也自唐千金翼等方出始以養性補益
等各立一門遂開後世補養服食之法以後醫家凡屬
體虛病後之人必立補方以為調理善後之計若富貴
之人則必常服補藥以供勞心縱欲之資而醫家必百
計取媚以順其意其藥專取貴重辛熱為主無非參朮
地黃桂附鹿茸之類托名祕方異傳其氣體合宜者一
時取效久之必得風痹陰涸等疾隱受其害雖死不悔
此等害人之說固不足論至體虛病後補藥之方自當
因人而施視臟腑之所偏而損益之其藥亦不外陰陽
氣血擇和平之藥數十種相為出入不必如治病之法
一味不可移易也故立方只問其陰陽臟腑何者專重

而已沈膏丸合就必經月經時而後服完若必每日視
脈察色而後服藥則必須一日換一丸方矣故凡服補
藥皆可通融者也其有神其說過為艱難慎重取貴僻
之藥以為可以卻病長生者非其人本愚昧即欲以之
欺人耳

21. On the Possibility of Special Arrangements [in the Application] of Supplementing Drugs

When the ancients had successfully cured a patient, they ordered him to eat from the five grains for nourishment. His original influences returned by themselves and there existed no so-called supplementing drugs. How, then, could there have been any prescriptions for a therapy of supplementation in the books compiled by Huang[-ti, Shen-]nung, and [Chang] Chung-ching? All other books [allegedly] written during that time besides [those just mentioned] were published [by later writers] falsely assuming the names [of earlier authors]. Beginning with the appearance of the prescriptions of the *Ch'ien Chin I[-fang]* and other such works during the T'ang dynasty, those [prescriptions] meant to nourish [a person's] nature and to provide supplementation were separately classified as a special category for the first time. This way, the dietetic pattern of supplementation and nourishment was initiated.

Ever since, physicians have designed supplementing prescriptions for people suffering from depletion following an illness. They consider [such treatments as suitable] strategies for [the patients'] full restoration. And when [these patients] are rich and noble people, [the physicians] inevitably have them regularly consume supplementing drugs to supply them with resources to [recover from] the kind of mental fatigue and passionate desires [these persons] give rein to. The physicians must develop numerous schemes to flatter [the rich], in order to comply with the sentiments [of these people].

Falsely claiming secret prescriptions or strange traditions, physicians mainly [prescribe] expensive drugs with acrid [flavor] and hot [thermo-influence], namely: [jen-]shen, [pai-]chu, ti-huang, [jou-]kuei, fu[-tzu], and lu-jung. When the patient's influences and [the condition of his physical] body fully correspond [with these drugs, such prescriptions may] result in short-term success. However, if [the patients] take [these drugs] for long, they will be harmed without noticing it by illnesses such as wind or obturation that [hide in the body's] inner [regions and become] chronic. Even when they [are bound to] die they will not regret [what they took]. The harmful doctrines [on which such activities are based] are not even worth mentioning.

Prescriptions with drugs supplementing a depleted body following an illness should be applied only after [careful consideration of] each individual patient. One must examine whether any of the viscera are unbalanced [in their influences], and delete or add [what is too much or too little] accordingly. The drugs used for this purpose should [regulate] nothing but yin or yang [imbalances], influences or blood. One selects tens of balanced drugs and exchanges them in the course [of the treatment]. Here, one must not act as in the treatment of illnesses where it is not possible to substitute [one drug] for another. Hence, when [a physician] designs a prescription [of supplementing drugs], he must ask only where there is any preponderance of yin and yang [influences] in the patient's viscera and bowels. Also, pastes or pills must be prepared [in such quantities] that a long [time] passes before [the patient] has consumed them entirely. Where [in case of an illness] it is imperative to check the [movement in the] vessels and examine the [patient's] complexion every day, and only then have him consume his drugs, it is essential to change the prescription for [the patient's] pills each day, as well. Hence, whenever someone takes supplementing drugs, it is possible to make special arrangements [for that person].

Those who make their advice sound mysterious, who go through too much trouble and apply too much care, and who resort to expensive one-sided drugs allegedly able to eliminate illnesses and provide long life — such persons are not stupid, they just intend to cheat people.

輕藥愈病論

古諺有不服藥為中醫之說自宋以前已有之蓋因醫
道失傳治人多誤病者又不能辨醫之高下故不服藥
雖不能愈病亦不至為藥所殺況病苟非死症外感漸
退內傷漸復亦能自愈故云中醫此過於小心之法也
而我以為病之在人有不治自愈者有不治難愈者有
不治竟不愈而死者其疾之在人自愈之疾誠不必服藥若難愈
及不愈之疾固當服藥乃不能知醫之高下藥之當否
不敢以身嘗試則莫若擇平易輕淺之方以
備酌用小誤亦無害對病有奇功此則不止於中醫矣
如偶感風寒則用蔥白蘇葉湯取微汗偶傷飲食則用
山查麥芽等湯消食偶感暑氣則用六一散廣藿湯清
暑偶傷風熱則用燈心竹葉湯清火偶患腹瀉則用陳
茶佛手湯和腸胃如此之類不一而足即使少誤必無

大害又有其藥似平常而竟有大誤者不可不知如腹
痛嘔逆之症寒亦有之熱亦有之暑氣觸穢亦有之或
見此症而飲以生姜湯如果屬寒不散寒而用生姜熱
性之藥與寒氣相關已非正治然猶有得效之理其餘
三症飲之必危曾見有人中暑而服濃姜湯一碗覆杯
即死若服紫蘇湯寒即立散暑熱亦無害益紫蘇性發散
不拘何症皆能散也故雖極淺之藥而亦有深義存焉
此又所宜慎也凡人偶有小疾能擇藥性之最輕淡者
隨症飲之則服藥而無服藥之誤不服藥而有服藥之
功亦養生者所當深考也

22. On Curing Illnesses with Light Drugs

An ancient proverb that was already in use during the Sung and earlier says, "Not to take drugs is as good as being treated by a common physician." The fact is that because the tradition of the correct principles of medicine was lost, many people are harmed through mistaken therapies, and the patients are unable to distinguish between physicians of higher or lower [quality]. As a result, when they refuse to take drugs, they may be unable to cure their illnesses, but they avoid being killed by drugs. Also, if an illness is not accompanied by fatal pathoconditions, any external affection will slowly retreat, and any internal damage will gradually recover. [That is, the illness] will heal by itself. That is why [the effects of no treatment at all are compared to those achieved by] "common physicians." These are excessively cautious therapeutic patterns.

In my own view, if an illness is present in a person, there are some cases that heal without treatment; there are others that may — in the absence of treatment — not heal easily; and there are those that — without treatment — will not heal at all, with death as the final result.

If one suffers from an illness that heals by itself, it is definitely unnecessary to take drugs. In case of illnesses that do not heal easily or that will not heal [by themselves] at all, one must of course take drugs. Now, if one does not know how to tell a physician of higher from one of lower [quality], if one is unable to judge whether a drug is appropriate or not, and if one does not dare to offer one's body for experiments, then it is best to resort to, and apply after careful consideration, prescriptions with light and superficial [drugs] that are helpful and do not cause any harm.

[With such an approach] even minor mistakes will not result in any damage. The effects achieved for this illness, though, may be extraordinary and go beyond the skills of a common physician.

For instance, if one was harmed by wind-cold, one applies a "Decoction with *ts'ung-pai* and *su-yeh*" to cause some mild sweating. If one was harmed by [inappropriate] eating and drinking, one applies a decoction prepared from *shan-ch'a, mai-ya,* and other [substances] to aid the digestion of the food. If one was affected by the influences of summerheat, one applies the "Six and one powder"[1] or the "Decoction with *kuang-huo*" to cool the heat. If one was harmed by wind-heat, one applies a "Decoction with *teng-hsin* and *chu-yeh*" to cool the fire. If one suffers from abdominal diarrhea, one applies a "Decoction with *ch'en-ch'a* and *fo-shou*" to harmonize the intestines and stomach. There are many such possibilities, and small mistakes will not result in any serious damage.

It may be, however, that while certain drugs appear to be only ordinary substances, they are, finally, [substances] that present [the possibility of] serious errors which one should consider. For example, in case of a pathocondition of abdominal pain and vomiting, this may be [due to] cold, or it may be [due to] heat, or it may also be [due to] summerheat or aggressive turbid influences. Now, if one sees this pathocondition and has [the patient] drink a "Decoction with *sheng-chiang*," [this drug] will — in case [the illness to be treated] is indeed a cold affection — not disperse the cold. Rather, a drug like *sheng-chiang* with its hot nature will enter into a fight with the cold influences. This is not a proper treatment, but there is still a rationale [involved] that might lead to success. If, however, [*sheng-chiang* were taken to treat] any of the other three pathoconditions [just mentioned], that would be quite dangerous.

I have seen people who had been hit by summerheat and who drank a bowl of strong *chiang* decoction. They died as fast as it took them to turn their cup. If one takes a *tzu-su* decoction, any cold will be dispersed immediately, and if [the illness was caused by] summerheat or ordinary heat, [the intake of *tzu-su*] would not cause any damage either. The reason is that *tzu-su* has a dispersing nature; it always disperses, regardless of which pathocondition is present. Hence, even [the application of] drugs whose effects are but very superficial [such as *tzu-su*], should be based, nevertheless, on a profound rationale. That is, one should be careful with these [drugs] too.

Whenever someone has a minor illness, and is able to pick some drugs that are very light and superficial in their [therapeutic] nature, and drink them according to the pathoconditions present, this person will take drugs but will not experience the [possibly] negative consequences of taking drugs. [In a way] he does not take [real] drugs yet has an effect as if he had taken drugs. Those working on nourishing their lives should consider this thoroughly.

Note

1.   The "Six and one" powder consists of six taels of *hua-shih* and one tael of *kan-ts'ao*.

腹内癰論

古之醫者無分内外又學有根柢故能無病不識後世

内外科既分則顯然為内症者内科治之顯然為外症

者外科治之其有病在腹中内外未顯然者則各執一

説各擬一方歷試諸藥皆無效驗輕者變重重者即殞

矣此等症不特外科當知之即内科亦不可不辨明眞

確知非已責即勿施治毋至臨危束手而後委他人也

腹内之癰有數症有肺癰有肝癰有胃脘癰有小腸癰

有大腸癰有膀胱癰惟肺癰咳吐腥痰人猶易辨餘者

或以為痞結或以為瘀血或以為寒痰或以為食積醫

藥雜投及至成膿治已無及外有不及成膿而死者病

者醫者始終不知何以致死此比比然也今先辨明癰

瘀血寒痰食積之狀凡痞結瘀血必有所因且由漸而

成寒痰則痛止無定又必另現痰症食積則必有受傷

之日且三五日後大便通即散惟外症則痛有常所而

遷延益甚金匱云諸脉浮數應當發熱而反淅淅惡寒

若有痛處當發其癰以手按上熱者有膿不熱者無

膿此數句乃内癰之眞諦也又云腸癰之為病身甲錯腹

皮急按之濡如腫狀腹無積聚身無熱是也若肝癰則

脇内隱隱痛日久亦吐膿血小腸癰與大腸癰相似而

位略高膀胱癰則痛在小腹之下近毛際著皮即痛小

便亦艱而痛胃脘癰則痛有虛實二種其實者易消若成

膿必大吐膿血而愈惟虛症則多不治先胃中痛眼火

而心下漸高其堅如石或有寒熱飲食不進按之尤痛

形體枯瘦此乃思慮傷脾之症不待癰成即死故凡腹

中有一定痛處惡寒倦卧不能食者皆當審察防成内

癰甚毋固循求治於不明之人以至久而膿潰自傷其

生也

23. On Intra-Abdominal Abscesses

In ancient times the physicians were not divided into [specialists of] internal and external [medicine], and, in addition, their learning was well founded. Hence, there was not a single illness with which they were not familiar. In later times, one distinguished the disciplines of internal and external [medicine. Ever since,] every pathocondition that is obviously located inside is treated through the discipline of internal [medicine], while every pathocondition that is obviously located on the outside is treated through the discipline of external [medicine].

For intra-abdominal illnesses that are neither clearly internal nor external, both [the disciplines of internal and external medicine] hold their own advice, and offer their own prescriptions. They test all their drugs, one after the other, but none of them is effective. Hence, minor [cases] develop into serious [problems], and serious [cases] end in death.

The knowledge of such pathoconditions should not be limited to the discipline of external [medicine]. Internal [medicine] should also be able to assess them exactly. If [a specialist of either discipline] realizes that [an illness] lies outside his expertise, he will not initiate a treatment, lest he be helplessly faced with a dangerous situation where he must call upon others for assistance.

Intra-abdominal abscesses are associated with many pathoconditions. There are lung abscesses, liver abscesses, stomach duct abscesses, abscesses in the small intestines, abscesses in the large intestines, and bladder abscesses. Only the abscesses of the lung, with [patients] coughing and vomiting foul phlegm, can be easily recognized by everyone. The others are identified either as congestions, or as stagnant blood, or as cold phlegm, or as food accumulations. When physicians indiscriminately toss their drugs [into their patients, these abcesses] will reach [a stage] where pus is generated. A cure is not achieved, and death may occur even before the generation of pus. Neither patients nor physicians have the slightest idea why [the illness] resulted in death. It is always the same.

Here, now, congestions of stagnant blood, or cold phlegm, or food accumulations should be distinguished first. In case of congestions and stagnant blood, there must be a cause. Also, these [conditions] develop gradually. In the case of cold phlegm, the onset of pain and its remission, are irregular. Also, there must be additional phlegm pathoconditions present. With food accumulations, there must be a specific day when the harm was received. Also, [these accumulations] dissolve after three to five days as soon as one's stools pass [again]. Only in the case of external pathoconditions is pain located somewhere permanently, and becomes worse and worse.

The *Chin-kuei* [*Yao-lüeh*] states, "Whenever the [movement in the] vessels is at the surface and frequent, [the patient] should develop heat. If, however, he shivers and has an aversion to cold, an abscess will develop at the location where one feels pain . . . . If one can feel heat in a swelling, it contains pus; where there is no heat, there is no pus."[1] These few sentences represent an accurate discourse on the nature of internal abscesses. [The same book] states further, "The illness of intestinal abscesses is accompanied by a scaly body; the abdominal skin is taut and feels, under pressure, soft like a swelling. No lumps [can be felt] in the abdomen, and the body shows no heat."[2] This is true.

In the case of liver abscesses, there is a very subtle pain in the flanks. After some time, [the patient] will vomit pus and blood. Abscesses in the small intestine resemble abscesses affecting the large intestine, except that they are located a little higher. Bladder abscesses are accompanied by pain below the lower abdomen, near the [pubic] hair line. They hurt as soon as one touches the skin and urination is difficult and causes pain.

Stomach duct abscesses may be of two types: depletion and repletion. Those accompanied by repletion are easy to dissolve. If they generate pus, the patient must vomit large amounts of pus and blood, and is healed. Only those [stomach duct abscesses] that are accompanied by a pathocondition of depletion can rarely be cured. In these cases, first the stomach hurts and is bloated. After some time, [the bloating and the pain] move gradually higher, upward to below the heart, and [the abdomen] is as hard as a stone. In some cases [the patient] experiences fits of cold and heat, and cannot eat or drink. The pain increases under pressure. The body is dry and emaciated. This is the same pathocondition that results when thinking and pondering damage one's spleen. [The patient] dies even before an abscess has developed.

Hence, whenever one has pain in one's abdomen at a fixed place, and if one has an aversion to cold, is tired and wants to lie down, and cannot eat, one should conduct a careful examination [as a precondition for an appropriate therapy] to prevent the formation of internal abscesses. And one should definitely not ask any person for treatment who does not know all this. Otherwise, [the treatment] would last until pus leaks out and one has jeopardized one's own life.

Notes

1.   See *Chin-kuei Yao-lüeh,* ch. 18, "Ch'uang-yung ch'ang-yung chin-yin ping mai cheng ping chih."

2.   Ibid.

圍藥論

外科之法最重外治而外治之中尤重圍藥凡毒之所

最忌者散大而頂不高蓋人之一身豈能無七情六慾

之伏火風寒暑濕之留邪飲食痰涎之積毒身無所病

皆散處退藏氣血一聚而成癰腫則諸邪四面皆會惟

圍藥能截之使不併合則周身之火毒不至矣其已聚

之毒不能透出皮膚勢必四布為害惟圍藥能束之使

不散漫則氣聚而外洩矣如此則形小頂高易膿易潰

矣故外治中之圍藥較之他藥為特重不但初起為然

即成膿收口始終賴之一日不可缺若世醫之圍藥不

過三黃散之類每試不效所以皆云圍藥無用如有既

破之後而仍用圍藥者則聾然笑之故極輕之毒往往

至於散越而不可收拾者皆不用圍藥之故也至於圍

藥之方亦甚廣博大段以消痰拔毒束肌收火為主而

寒熱攻提和平猛厲則當隨症去取世人不深求至理

而反輕議圍藥之非安望其術之能工也

24. On Drugs that Encircle

Among the [therapeutic] patterns of the specialty of [medicine concerned with] external [illnesses], external treatments are most important, and most [important] among [the various possibilities of] external treatment is the application of encircling drugs. The poisons that are to be feared are those dispersed over large areas without rising as a bump [at a specific location].

Now, in every human body the dormant fires of the seven emotions and six desires exist, or evil [influences] of wind, cold, summerheat or dampness remain hidden somewhere, or poisons have become stored through food and beverages, in phlegm or spittle. As long as the body has no illness, all these [fires, evil influences, and poisons] lie dispersed and hidden in many places. As soon, though, as [protective] influences and blood lump together and generate abscesses and swellings, the evil [influences] assemble from all sides. [In these situations,] only encircling drugs are able to intercept them and prevent their union. As a result, the fire or poison [that may come] from all regions of the body will not arrive here.

If the poisons have already gathered together and cannot leave [the body] through the skin, they will spread in all directions and cause harm everywhere. Only encircling drugs are able to tie them together and prevent them from spreading. They cause the influences to gather together and leak to the outside. This way, the [resulting abscesses] are small in size but [they accumulate and] rise as a bump. They easily develop pus, and [this pus] easily leaks out. The encircling drugs are particularly important in comparison with other drugs in external treatments. This is true not only with regard to [swellings] just emerging, but also where pus has already been generated, and where a wound is to be closed — one can rely on [encircling drugs] from beginning to end. One would not want to be without them for a single day.

The physicians of recent times apply only [prescriptions] such as "Three *huang* powder"[1] as encircling remedies, and each time they test [the abilities of these substances] they achieve no results. Hence they all say that encircling drugs are of no use. If someone applies encircling drugs after [an abscess] has already broken open, he will be laughed at by everyone. It appears quite often therefore, that even very light poisons may spread excessively [throughout the body], and cannot be brought under control because no one applies encircling drugs.

Prescriptions based on encircling drugs cover a broad [range of problems]. In general, though, their main task is to dissolve phlegm, to pluck poison, to tie together the flesh, and to contain fire. When it comes to [cases of] cold or heat, to [situations where one must] attack or support, or to [cases that are] mild or violent, one must take away or add [drugs to these prescriptions] as may be required by the pathocondition at hand. The people of recent times do not inquire into these principles thoroughly; on the contrary, they carelessly criticize the disadvantages of encircling drugs. How could they hope for a successful application of their art?

Note

1.   The "Three *huang* powder" contains, among other substances, the three "huang" drugs *hsiung-huang, huang-ch'in,* and *ta-huang.* Small amounts of this formula are to be blown in the patient's ear to cause any pus to discharge.

VI.
[Medical]
Literature
and
Disciplines

難經論

難經非經也以經文之難解者設為問難以明之故曰
難經言以經文為難而釋之也是書之旨蓋欲推本經
盲發揮至道剖晰疑義垂示後學真讀內經之津梁也
但其中亦有未盡善者其問答之詞有即引經文以釋
之者經文本自明顯引之或反遺其要以至經語反晦
或則無所發明或則與兩經相背或則以此誤彼此其
所短也其中有自出機杼發揮妙道未嘗見於內經而
實能顯內經之奧義補內經之所未發此蓋別有師承
足與內經並垂千古不知創自越人乎抑上古亦有此
書而越人引以為証乎自隋唐以來其書盛行尊崇之
者固多而無能駁正之者蓋業醫之輩讀難經而識其
大義已為醫道中傑出之流安能更深考內經求其異
同得失乎古今流傳之載籍凡有紕誤後人無敢議者

此比然也獨難經乎哉餘詳余所著難經經釋中

1. On the *Nan-ching*

The *Nan-ching* is not a classic. Its aim is to explain the difficult issues in the text of the Classic. Hence it poses questions concerning these difficult issues and then clarifies them. Therefore, it is called the *Nan-ching*. That is to say, it considers the text of the Classic as difficult, and explains it. The purpose of this book, therefore, is to investigate the original meaning of the Classic, to elucidate its ultimate principles, to dissolve doubtful aspects, and to provide guidance for students of later times.

It is, indeed, of great help for anyone who reads the *Nei-ching*. However, some parts of it lack final perfection. In the dialogues sometimes text passages from the Classic are quoted for explanation where the text of the Classic was quite clear originally. [In the *Nan-ching*,] however, either the decisive points are omitted, and the wording of the Classic is even obscured [by the commentary], or nothing is explained at all, or [the *Nan-ching*] contradicts the two [books of the *Nei-*]*ching*, or [the *Nan-ching*] misinterprets [the *Nei-ching*]. These are its shortcomings.

[The *Nan-ching*] contains several passages, and elucidates [a number of] subtle principles that did not appear in the *Nei-ching* but that are, in fact, suitable for clarifying some obscure meanings of the *Nei-ching* and for supplementing what had not been sufficiently developed in the *Nei-ching*. Hence, [the *Nan-ching*] can be considered as taking up an additional scholarly tradition that is well worth handing down together with the *Nei-ching* to eternity.

I am not sure whether [the *Nan-ching*] was compiled by Yüeh-jen. Maybe Yüeh-jen was introduced [as the author] simply to demonstrate that this book existed in antiquity. From Sui, T'ang times on, [the *Nan-ching*] received great attention; very many people highly appreciated it, and there was no one to approach it critically. As a consequence, medical practitioners read the *Nan-ching*, and after they had become familiar with its general meaning, they considered themselves outstanding [experts] of medicine already. How could they have [felt a need to] penetrate even deeper [into medicine] by investigating the *Nei-ching*, by searching for differences and agreement [between the *Nan-ching* and the *Nei-ching*], and by seeking to discover what was a gain and what was a loss [in the compilation of the *Nan-ching*]?

All writings handed down through the ages have deficiencies and errors; it is always the same, though no one dares to criticize [these errors]. Why should the *Nan-ching* be an exception? Further details can be found in my "Explanation of the *Nan-ching* on the Basis of the Classic."

Notes

1.   The *Nan-ching* was written at some time during the Eastern Han era, most probably in the first century A.D. Its unknown author systematized diagnostic, etiological, and therapeutic concepts of the medicine of systematic correspondence; most important is a consistent integration into diagnosis and needle therapy of the assumption of the circulation of blood and ch'i. Beginning with the Sung era, authors no longer appreciated the fact that the *Nan-ching* had been written to overcome the heterogeneous and unsystematic contents of the *Huang-ti Nei-ching* scripture. They attempted to reconcile the differences between the two books by pointing out that both meant, in fact, the same. With the onset of the so-called Han-studies movement of Chinese conservatives in the Ch'ing era, the *Nan-ching* was understood not as an independent and innovative work but as a commentary on the *Nei-ching*. Writers like Hsü Ta-ch'un accepted the contents of the *Nan-ching* as correct where they agreed with the *Nei-ching*, and as false where they disagreed. See P.U. Unschuld, *Nan-ching: The Classic of Difficult Issues*, Berkeley, Los Angeles, London: University of California Press, 1986.

傷寒論

仲景傷寒論編次者不下數十家因致聚訟紛紜此皆
不知仲景作書之旨故也觀傷寒叙所述乃為庸醫誤
治而設所以正治之法一經不過三四條餘皆救誤之
法故其文亦變動不居讀傷寒論者知此書皆設想懸
擬之書則無往不得其義矣今人必改叔和之次序或
以此條在前或以此條在後或以此症因彼症而生或
以此經因彼經而變互相詰屬孰知病變萬端傳經無
定古人因病以施方無編方以待病其原本次序既已
散亡庶幾叔和所定為可信何則叔和序例云今搜採
仲景舊論錄其症候診脈聲色對病真方有神驗者擬
防世急則此書乃叔和安有此書且諸人所編果
原本不如此抑思苟無叔和安有此書且諸人所編果
能合仲景原文否耶夫六經現症有異有同後人見陽

經一症襍於陰經之中以為宜改入陽經之內不知陰
經亦有此症也人各是其私反致古人圓機活法泯沒
不可問矣凡讀書能得書中之精義要訣歷歷分明則
任其顛倒錯亂而我心自能融會貫通否則徒以古書
紛更互異愈改愈晦矣

2. On the *Shang-han* [*Lun*]

No fewer than tens of writers have published editions and [different] arrangements of [Chang] Chung-ching's *Shang-han Lun*,[1] and all they have achieved is ambiguous interpretations and confusion. The reason is that no one understood the message intended by [Chang] Chung-ching when he wrote his book.

If one takes a close look at the contents of the preface to the *Shang-han* [*Lun,* one realizes that] no more than three or four paragraphs of that classic were written to replace erroneous treatments conducted by common physicians with outlines of what [Chang Chung-ching] considered to be proper therapeutic patterns. All the remaining [paragraphs of this book present] patterns for rescuing [someone who has been harmed by an] erroneous [therapy]. Hence the text of [the *Shang-han Lun*] is quite heterogeneous, and does not stick [to one particular topic].

All those readers of the *Shang-han Lun* who realize that this book contains a purely hypothetical discourse will not fail to grasp its meaning. Nowadays, everyone feels obliged to change the order [of the paragraphs in the *Shang-han Lun* as it was handed down] by [Wang] Shu-ho. In some [editions], a specific paragraph is at the beginning of [the book], while it is placed at the end in other editions. In some editions a specific pathocondition emerges from a certain other pathocondition; in other [editions] a specific conduit undergoes changes following [changes in] a certain other conduit. [The authors of all these different editions] abuse each other, and no one seems to know that illnesses may appear in countless variations, and that there is no fixed order in their transmission through the conduits.

In ancient times, people designed their prescriptions in response to an illness; they did not prepare a prescription and then wait for an [appropriate] illness. The order [of the paragraphs] of the original text [of the *Shang-han Lun*] has long been lost, but the way it was reconstructed by [Wang] Shu-ho is quite trustworthy.[2]

How is this? In his preface [Wang] Shu-ho states:

Now I have collected [Chang] Chung-ching's old discourse, and I have recorded his [statements on the] signs of pathoconditions, on the examination of the [movement in the] vessels, as well as on the [diagnostic significance of] voice and complexion, [and I have gathered] those of [his] authentic prescriptions [that are designed to] confront an illness directly [and] that show miraculous effects. They should relieve our time from urgent needs.

[As can be seen from these words], this book was compiled by [Wang] Shu-ho, but through the ages people have cast their doubts upon it, arguing that the original text was different. If it had not been for [Wang] Shu-ho, though, how could this book exist at all? Also, how could any of the editions prepared by all the people [in later times] come close to the original text of [Chang] Chung-ching?

Some of the pathoconditions produced by [illness in any of] the six conduits differ from each other, while some resemble each other. When later people saw a specific pathocondition associated with the yang conduits listed [by Wang Shu-ho among illnesses] in the yin conduits, they transferred [the description of this pathocondition to the section on illnesses in] the yang conduits because they did not know that this particular pathocondition could also be related to [illnesses in] the yin conduits.

Everyone considers only his private opinion to be correct, and this has resulted [in the fact that] the truly inspired and adaptable patterns applied by the ancients are dead and utterly forgotten. Whenever I study a text and am able to grasp its essential meaning and basic message, with every detail being clear and evident, my heart will be in a position to bring [all these details] together and reach a thorough understanding, regardless of how disorderly and confused they may be. Otherwise, the discrepancies and contradictions in an ancient text will cause one merely to ever more rearrange it and thereby to ever more obfuscate it.

Notes

1.   The *Shang-han Lun,* "On Harm Caused by Cold," was written by Chang Chi, style-name Chung-ching, (142-220). It comprises ten chapters and was taken from a sixteen chapter work by Chang Chi entitled *Shang-han Tsa-ping Lun,* "On Harm Caused by Cold and Various Other Illnesses," in the course of a revision conducted in 1065.

2.   Wang Hsi (210-285), whose style-name was Shu-ho, revised Chang Chi's *Shang-han Tsa-ping Lun.* Wang Hsi is also known for his compilation of the first known work exclusively focusing on pulse diagnosis, the *Mai-ching.* (See Chapter 4 of this section).

金匱論

金匱要略乃仲景治雜病之書也其中缺略處頗多而
上古聖人以湯液治病之法惟賴此書之存乃方書之
祖也其論病皆本於內經而神明變化之其用藥悉本
於神農本草而融會貫通之其方則皆上古聖人歷代
相傳之經方仲景間有隨症加減之法其脈法亦皆內
經及歷代相傳之真訣其治病無不精切周到無一毫
游移參錯之處實能洞見本源審察毫末故所投必效
如桴鼓之相應真乃醫方之經也惜其所載諸病未能
全備未知有殘缺與否然諸大症之網領亦已粗備後
之學者以此為經而參考推廣之已思過半矣自此以
後之書皆非古聖相傳之真訣僅自成一家不可與金
匱並列也

3. On the *Chin-kuei* [*Yao-lüeh*]

The *Chin-kuei Yao-lüeh*[1] is a book compiled by [Chang] Chung-ching, on the treatment of various illnesses. Many passages in this [book] are incomplete; but the fact that the patterns of the Sages of high antiquity describing how to treat illnesses by means of decoctions survive [to the present] is due entirely to this book.

Its discourses on illnesses are all based on the *Nei-ching*, and yet, at the same time, represent a most lucid transformation [of the *Nei-ching* doctrines]. Its applications of drugs are entirely based on the *Shen-nung Pents'ao*,[2] and represent a perfect accumulation and understanding [of the contents of the latter]. Its prescriptions are all classical prescriptions handed down through the ages from the Sages of high antiquity.

Occasionally [Chang] Chung-ching [offers] patterns for adding [drugs] to, or taking [drugs] away from [a prescription] in accordance with the pathoconditions [present in a particular situation]. Similarly, his methods [of examining the movement in the] vessels are all grounded in true instructions either from the *Nei-ching* or handed down through the ages.

Every single one of [Chang Chung-ching's] illness therapies is skillful and adequate; not even one passage is marked by insecurity or confusion. [This book] is certainly well suited both to make one comprehend the origins and to investigate the minutest detail [of any illness]. Hence, any use [of drugs based on] this [book] must be followed by success, just as the beating of a drum is followed by a sound. It is indeed the classic of medical prescriptions.

Unfortunately, the list of illnesses it deals with is incomplete, and I do not know whether [the *Chin-kuei Yao-lüeh* as it exists today] is just a fragment or not. However, the system of all the more important pathoconditions outlined [in this book] is close to complete. Those students in later times who considered it a classic, examined it closely, and extended its [ideas to cases they wished to treat], had already done a major part of their thinking. None of the books [published] after the [*Chin-kuei Yao-lüeh*] represented the true instructions handed down from the ancient Sages any longer. [Their authors] created schools of their own; they cannot be listed together with the *Chin-kuei* [*Yao-lüeh*].

Notes

1.   *Chin-kuei Yao-lüeh*, "A Summary of the Important [Contents] of the Golden Chest," is the short title of *Chin-kuei Yao-lüeh Fang-lun*, "On the Most Important Prescriptions of the Golden Chest," compiled by Chang Chi (142-220). Chang Chi's *Shang-han Tsa-ping Lun* was renamed *Chin-kuei Yü-han Yao-lüeh Fang*, "The Most Important Prescriptions of the Golden Chest and Jade Container," after its revision by Wang Shu-ho (210-285). In a later revision, in 1065, all prescriptions concerning "harm caused by cold" were taken out of the text, and the remainder was then renamed *Chin-kuei Yao-lüeh Fang-lun*.

2.   The *Shen-nung Pen-ts'ao Ching*, "Shen-nung's Classic on Materia Medica," is the oldest known herbal of China. It was compiled probably during the first or second century A.D. See P. U. Unschuld, *Medicine in China: A History of Pharmaceutics*, Berkeley, Los Angeles, London, University of California Press, 1986: 17-43.

脈經論

王叔和著脈經分門別類條分縷晰其原亦本內經而
漢以後之說一無所遺其中旨趣亦不能盡一使人有
所執持然其滙集羣言使後世有所考見亦不可少之
作也愚按脈之為道不過驗其血氣之盛衰寒熱及邪
氣之流在何經何臟與所現之症參觀互考以究其生
尅順逆之理而後吉凶可憑所以內經難經及仲景之
論脈其立論反若甚疎而應驗如神若執脈經之說以
為某病當見某脈某脈當得某病雖內經亦間有之不
如是之拘泥繁瑣也試而不驗於是或各脈之不準或
各病之非真或方藥之不對症而不知皆非也蓋病
有與脈相合者有與脈不相合者兼有與脈相反者同
一脈也見於此症為宜見於彼症為不宜同一症也見
某脈為宜見某脈為不宜一病可見數十脈一脈可現

數百症變動不拘若泥定一說則從脈而症不合從症
而脈又不合反令人徬徨無所適從所以古今論脈之
家彼此互異是非各別人持一論得失相半總由不知
變通之精義所以愈密而愈疎也讀脈經者知古來談
脈之詳密如此因以考其異同辨其得失審其真偽窮
其變通則自有心得若欲泥脈以治病必至全無把握
學者必當先參於內經難經及仲景之說而貫通之則
胷中先有定見後人之論皆足以廣我之見聞而識力
愈真此讀脈經之法也

4. On the *Mai-ching*

In his *Mai-ching,*[1] Wang Shu-ho arranged different [topics] in separate sections, and the individual paragraphs [of his book] are marked by clarity and detail. He based [the contents of his book] on the *Nei-ching,* and he also took into account all doctrines developed during and after the Han. Hence, the essential thoughts [Wang Shu-ho gathered in his *Mai-ching*] could not be homogeneous, [and could not] give the people something at hand they could grasp firmly.

Still, his bringing together all types of teachings, thereby allowing later generations to examine them in comparison, is an achievement that one would not want to miss. In my own view, the doctrine of the [movement in the] vessels only includes examining whether a [patient's] blood or influences are present abundantly or insufficiently, and through which conduit or through which viscus cold, heat, or [any other] evil influences flow. This [information] has to be compared to the [patient's] pathoconditions to find out which principle [is involved in that patient's illness — the principle of mutual] generation or destruction [among the five phases, or that of influences] moving in accordance with or contrary to [their normal direction].

Once this [has been clarified], reliable [predictions] are possible on the auspicious or inauspicious [character of the ailment]. Because the *Nei-ching,* the *Nan-ching,* and also the discourses on the [movement in the] vessels written by [Chang] Chung-ching [offer these guidelines], their doctrines show miraculous results even though they appear — in contrast [to those of the *Mai-ching*] — rather unsystematic.

If one adopts the teaching of the *Mai-ching,* one will believe that in case of a specific illness a specific [movement in the] vessels should appear, and that a specific [movement in the] vessels should be associated with a specific illness. Although such [relationships] also occur in the *Nei-ching,* [the *Nei-ching*] does not cling to these [correspondences] as tenaciously [as does the *Mai-ching*].

If one tries [the teachings of the latter in therapy] and earns no success, one will blame this either on an abnormality of the [movement in the] vessels, or on a misidentification of the illness, or on the lacking correspondence of the drugs in one's prescriptions with the [patient's] pathoconditions — without realizing that all these [attempts at explaining the failure of one's treatment] are beside the point. The fact is that there are illnesses that are in agreement with the [patient's movement in the] vessels, and there are others that do not agree with the [patient's movement in the] vessels. There are even [such illnesses] that are contradicted by the [movement in the patient's] vessels. One and the same movement in the vessels may appear together with one specific pathocondition that seems fitting, but it may also appear together with another pathocondition, and seem out of place. Or, one and the same pathocondition may be accompanied by one specific [movement in the] vessels that is fitting, but it may also be accompanied by another [movement in the] vessels that seems out of place. One and the same illness may be accompanied by tens of [different movements in the] vessels, and one and the same [movement in the] vessels may be associated with hundreds of pathoconditions.

[These relationships] change and are not fixed. If one clings to merely one doctrine, though, one may take a patient's [movement in the] vessels as one's guideline and find that his pathoconditions do not agree. Or, one may start from [a patient's] pathoconditions and realize that the [movement in his] vessels does not agree. In contrast [to what one would expect, the clear-cut doctrine of the *Mai-ching*] lets those people [who apply it in therapy] become perturbed, and leaves them without proper advice to follow.

Those experts who discussed the [movement in the] vessels through the ages have all contradicted one another, and they all differed in what they considered right and wrong. They all cling to their specific doctrine, and their advantages and errors balance each other. All this results from their ignorance of the essential meanings of changing relationships [among movements in the vessels, pathoconditions, and illnesses], and, the more detailed [their discourses become], the further away [they move from perfection]. Those readers of the *Mai-ching* who are fully aware of this all too detailed nature of all the discourses since antiquity on [the movement in] the vessels, and who, therefore, examine agreement and contradictions [between these different discourses], as well as distinguish what is useful from what is wrong, who differentiate between true and false, and who penetrate all the changing relationships [alluded to above], will reach a profound understanding. If one clings, though, to the [movement in the] vessels in order to [gain the information needed to] treat an illness, one will never reach a state of security.

Students [reading the *Mai-ching*] must consult the *Nei-ching*, the *Nan-ching*, and the doctrines of [Chang] Chung-ching. And, as a result, they will acquire a firm perspective in their bosom. Everything stated by people who came after [the three authoritative sources just mentioned] is worthwhile only to broaden our perspective, and help our knowledge to become ever more accurate. That is the way one should read the *Mai-ching*.

Note

1.   The *Mai-ching*, "Classic of the [Movement in the] Vessels," was written by Wang Shu-ho (210-285). It is based on materials from Chang Chi's work, the *Nan-ching*, the *Nei-ching*, and, possibly, earlier sources.

千金方外臺論

仲景之學至唐而一變仲景之治病其論臟腑經絡病
情傳變悉本內經而其所用之方皆古聖相傳之經方
並非私心自造閒有加減必有所本其分兩輕重皆有
法度其藥悉本於神農本草無一味游移假借之處非
此方不能治此病非此藥不能成此方精微深妙不可
思議藥味不過五六品而功用無不周此乃天地之化
機聖人之妙用與天地同不朽者也千金方則不然其
所論病未嘗不依內經而不無雜以後世臆度之說其
所用方亦皆採擇古方不無兼取後世偏雜之法其所
用藥未必全本於神農兼取雜方單方及通治之品故
有一病而立數方亦有一方而治數病其藥品有多至
數十味者其中對症者固多不對症者亦不少故治病
亦有效有不效大抵所重專在於藥而古聖製方之法

不傳矣此醫道之一大變也然其用意之奇用藥之巧
亦自成一家有不可磨滅之處至唐王燾所集外臺一
書則纂集自漢以來諸方滙萃成書而歷代之方於焉
大備但其人本非專家之學故無所審擇以為指歸乃
醫方之類書也然唐以前之方賴此書以存其功亦不
可泯但讀之者苟曾中無成竹則眾說紛紜羣方淆雜
反茫然失其所據故讀千金外臺者必精通於內經仲
景本草等書曾中先有成見而後取其長而舍其短則
可資我博採之益否則反亂人意而無所適從嗟乎千
金外臺且然況後世偏駁雜亂之書能不惑人之心志
哉等而下之更有無稽杜譔之邪書尤不足道矣

5. On the *Ch'ien Chin Fang* and the *Wai T'ai Pi-Yao*

The understanding of [Chang] Chung-ching's [doctrine] underwent a significant modification during the T'ang dynasty. [Chang] Chung-ching's treatment of illnesses, his discourses on the viscera and bowels, on the conduits and network [vessels], and on the changes in the nature of an illness — all this was based on the *Nei-ching*. The prescriptions he applied were all classical prescriptions handed down by the Sages of antiquity, and were never construed from his own imagination.

Whenever he added [drugs] to or took [drugs] away from [these prescriptions], he certainly had a good foundation [to act upon], and the weights and proportions [of the ingredients of his prescriptions] were all calculated on the basis of specific patterns. His drugs were grounded in the *Shen-nung Pen-ts'ao;* not a single substance was chosen without justification or good reason. Hence, a certain illness could be cured only with a certain prescription, and a certain prescription could be filled only with certain drugs.

The subtleties and mysteries [of his doctrine] cannot be discussed exhaustively! Although he never applied [in one therapy] more than five or six substances, the effects [of his prescriptions] were always all-encompassing. The secrets of the creation harbored in heaven and earth, the marvels of the Sages [are integrated in his work which] will be as everlasting as heaven and earth [themselves].

The *Ch'ien Chin Fang*[1] is different. Its discourses on illnesses are still grounded in the *Nei-ching*, but some of them are also mixed with the speculative teachings of later generations. For the prescriptions applied [in the *Ch'ien Chin Fang*, its author made] use of ancient prescriptions too, but he always took advantage of the one-sided and confused patterns of later times also. The drugs he employed were not all based on Shen-nung. [The author] made use both of prescriptions based on various drugs, and of formulae based on one single [drug], and he also employed cure-all substances. Hence there are instances [in his work] where several prescriptions are listed for the treatment of one single illness, and [there are other instances where] one single prescription was recommended for the treatment of several illnesses. He applied many drugs — up to some tens [of drugs — in his prescriptions], and included in [his prescriptions] are certainly many that were focused directly on the pathoconditions [to be treated]. But, there were also not a few that were not. Hence, the treatment of illnesses [with these prescriptions] is sometimes effective, and it is sometimes not.

Generally speaking, the emphasis [of the *Ch'ien Chin Fang*] is mainly on drugs; it no longer transmitted the patterns of prescription design introduced by the Sages of antiquity. This was a major modification of the principles of medicine. And still, the marvels of the use of drugs [in the *Ch'ien Chin Fang*], and its ingenious ideas, have led to the formation of a school of its own, some aspect of which will last eternally.

In his compilation of the *Wai-t'ai* [*Pi-yao*][2] the T'ang [author] Wang T'ao gathered all prescriptions since the Han, and collected them in one book. As a result, [this work represents] a complete compilation of all prescriptions through the ages. But the man [who wrote this book] had no expert training himself. Hence, he did not carry out any studies and made no selections to provide [his readers] with any guidance. His work is just a reference book with contents ordered by subjects. Still, his merits will last forever, since it is only for this book that prescriptions up to the times of the T'ang are today still extant at all. A reader, however, who has not yet made up his mind may completely lose whatever he has relied upon so far by the mix of doctrines and by the heterogeneity of prescriptions [in the *Wai-t'ai Pi-yao*].

Hence, anyone reading the *Ch'ien Chin* [*Fang*] or the *Wai-t'ai* [*Pi-yao*] should be most familiar with such books as the *Nei-ching*, [the works of Chang] Chung-ching, as well as the [*Shen-nung*] *Pen-ts'ao*. If someone has a firm opinion first, and only then makes use of the advantages, and rejects the shortcomings [of the *Ch'ien-Chin Fang* and of the *Wai-t'ai Pi-yao*], he will benefit from selecting [his prescriptions] from a large number. Otherwise [these books are] only suited to confuse the thoughts of the people, and no standards to be followed exist.

Alas! This being the case with the *Ch'ien-Chin* [*Fang*] and the *Wai-t'ai* [*Pi-yao*], all the biased and unsystematic books of subsequent times were definitely merely able to delude the minds of the people. And below these are some evil writings that are unfounded and trumped up to a degree that cannot be told in words.

Notes

1.   *Ch'ien Chin Fang*, "Prescriptions Worth Thousands in Gold," is a designation of two prescription works written by Sun Ssu-mo (581-682), the *Pei-chi Ch'ien Chin Yao-fang*, "Important Prescriptions for Urgent Use Worth Thousands in Gold," and the *Ch'ien Chin I-fang*, "Additional Prescriptions Worth Thousands in Gold."

2.   The *Wai-t'ai Pi-yao*, "Important [Prescriptions] from the Outer Terrace," was written by Wang T'ao in 725. It is based on the prescription works of sixty T'ang and pre-T'ang authors.

活人書論

宋人之書能發明傷寒論使人有所執持而易曉大有

功於仲景者活人書為第一蓋傷寒論不過隨舉六經

所現之症以施治有一症而六經皆現者并有一症而

治法迥別者則讀者茫無把握矣此書以經絡病因傳

變疑似條分縷晰而後附以諸方治法使人一覽了然

豈非後學之津梁乎其書獨出機杼又能全本經文

無一字混入已意豈非好學深思述而不作足以繼往

開來者乎後世之述傷寒論者唐宋以來已有將經文

刪改移易不明不貫至近代前條辨尚論編等書又復

顛倒錯亂各逞意見互相辨駁總由分症不清欲其強

合所以日就支離若能參究此書則任病情之錯綜反

覆而治法仍歸一定何必聚訟紛紜致古人之書愈講

而愈晦也

6. On the *Huo-Jen Shu*

Among all the books compiled by Sung authors that were successful in elucidating the [contents of the] *Shang-han Lun*, that gave the people firm guidelines at hand, that were easily comprehensible, and that represented great achievements with regard to [the propagation of the work of Chang] Chung-ching — [among all these books] the *Huo-jen Shu*[1] takes the first place.

The *Shang-han Lun* lists treatments only in the course of its presentation of those pathoconditions that appear in association with one of the six conduits. However, any reader [of the *Shang-han Lun*] will be left utterly without any guidance if he is confronted with an identical pathocondition that may appear in association with all six conduits, or if [he meets] one and the same pathocondition that must be treated quite differently [depending on the specific illness it may represent]. This [*Huo-jen Shu*] book lists, in detailed and clearly distinguished sections, [all that is necessary concerning] the conduits and the network [vessels], the causes of the illnesses, the transmission and changes [of illnesses in the organism], as well as concerning doubtful [situations]; and, then, offers all types of prescriptions and therapeutic patterns, so that everyone is well informed on first glance. How could it not serve as a bridge or ford for students of subsequent times?

[Also,] this book was written in an extraordinary style, and it is based entirely on the text of the Classic. Not a single word has entered [this book] without good reason, or was based on [the author's] personal opinion. Is not this [an example of] fondness for study and of deep thought, of transmission rather than making,[2] able to carry on past traditions and open the way for those who follow![3]

Among those who have transmitted the *Shang-han Lun* in later times, ever since the T'ang and the Sung, there were already those who cut down and changed the text of the Classic. They neither understood nor penetrated [the contents of the original book]. And such books as the [*Shang-han Lun*] *T'iao-pien*[4] or the *Shang Lun Pien*,[5] published only shortly prior to our own time — they really turned everything upside down, creating only errors and confusion. Each of them pursuing its own way, they were all engaged in mutual contradictions and arguments. All this results from the fact that the [authors of these books] were unable to distinguish clearly between [individual] pathoconditions, and that they preferred to force them together. As a result, [the contents of their books] turned increasingly sectarian day by day.

If [these authors] had been able to consult and study this book [i.e., the *Huo Jen Shu*], then, despite all the heterogeneity and variations among the illnesses, the therapeutic patterns would have been definite. None of all the contradictory explanations would have been necessary, which lead to the fact that the more the books of the ancients are discussed, the more obscure [their contents] become.

Notes

1. This is an abbreviation of *Lei-cheng Huo-jen Shu* 類証活人書, "The Book with Symptoms Arranged in Groups to Keep Man Alive," title of a text compiled by Chu Kung 朱肱 in 1108.

2. To be "a transmitter but not a maker" was said of Confucius [Lun Yü, 7:1].

3. A phrase coined by Hsü Ai 徐愛 (1487-1517), a disciple and brother-in-law of Wang Shou-jen 王守仁 (1472-1529), in his book *Ch'uan Hsi Lu* 傳習錄.

4. This book was published in 1592 by Fang You-chih 方有执, who was convinced that the *Shang-han Lun* of Chang Chi had lost its original characters through subsequent revisions and commentaries by Wang Shu-ho and Ch'eng Wu-i 成無已 (11th century).

5. The *Shang Lun Pien* was published in 1648 by Yü Ch'ang 喻昌 on the basis of the *Shang-han Lun T'iao-pien*, introducing a highly systematized etiology.

太素脈論

診脈以之治病其血氣之盛衰及風寒暑濕之中人可
驗而知也乃相傳有太素脈之說以候人之壽夭窮通
智愚善惡纖悉皆備夫脈乃氣血之見端其長而堅厚
者為壽之徵其短小而薄弱者為夭之徵清而有神為
智之徵濁而無神為愚之徵理或宜然若善惡已不可
知窮通則與脈何與然或得壽之脈而其人或不謹於
風寒勞倦患病而死得夭之脈而其人受護調攝得以
永年又有血氣甚清而神志昏濁者形質甚濁而神志
清明者即壽夭智愚亦不能盡驗況其他子又書中更
神其說以為能知某年得某官某年得財若干父母何
人子孫何若則更荒唐矣天下或有習此術而言多驗
者此必別有他術以推測而倖中借此以神其說耳若
盡於脈見之斷斷無是理也

7. On the *T'ai-Su Mai* [*Fa*]

If one examines the [movement in the] vessels in order to treat an illness, one may check and know whether someone's blood or influences are present in abundance or have faded away, and whether he was hit by wind, cold, summer-heat, or dampness. However, there have also been transmitted the *T'ai-su* doctrines of the [movement in the] vessels whereby, supposedly, one may examine whether a person will live long or die young, and whether he will have success in life, or failure; and whether he is knowledgeable or ignorant, good or bad — all this [it is claimed] is contained in great detail [in the *T'ai-su Mai Fa*[1]].

Now, the movement in the vessels is the clue to the condition of blood and influences, and it may be legitimate and reasonable [to state the following]. [Movements that come] in long strides, firm, and thick, are signs of long life. [Movements that come] in short intervals, are minor, thin and weak, they are signs of early death. A clear [movement in the vessels] and the presence of a [clear] spirit are signs of wisdom, while a turbid [movement in the vessels] and the absence of a [clear] spirit are signs of stupidity. However, it is impossible to know [from the movement in the vessels] whether someone is good or bad. And what do success and failure have to to with one's [movement in the] vessels?

It may well be that one feels a [movement in the] vessels indicating long life, but the person [displaying such movement in the vessels] may not care about wind-cold or fatigue, [and thus] contract an illness and die. Or one may feel a [movement in the] vessels indicating early death, but the person [displaying such a movement in the vessels] may take great care of his life and live forever! Or, blood and influences may be very clear, but [the same person's] mind may be confused and turbid; or someone's physical appearance is turbid, and his mind is clear and brilliant. In such cases it is equally impossible to find out whether [a person] will enjoy long life or die early, or whether he is intelligent or stupid. How much more does this apply to all the other [data one is supposed to get through examining the movement in the vessels by means of the *T'ai-su* method]!

Still, in this book, the [*T'ai-su*] doctrine is credited with even more miraculous [achievements]. Supposedly, it is possible to know [in advance] in which year someone will get which official position, or in which year someone will acquire a fortune, and of what size, what kind of people his father and mother are, and how his children and grandchildren will be. This, however, is even greater nonsense [than the claims previously listed]! Those in the empire who practice this technique with their statements proving to be true must rely on some additional technique from which they draw their conclusions and then, luckily, hit the mark. They draw on the [*T'ai-su* method] to make their statements sound miraculous. There is absolutely no reason to assume that all this [information] could become manifest in the [movement in the] vessels.

Note

1.   This book is no longer extant. Allegedly, the text was found in a stone-chamber in the final year of the T'ang dynasty. However, the *Ssu K'u Ch'üan-shu Tsung-mu* 四庫全書總目 notes that the doctrine transmitted by this book emerged only during the Northern Sung. Hence, this text, which is of unknown authorship, must have been compiled at that time, or later.

婦科論

婦人之疾與男子無異惟經期胎産之病不同且多癥瘕之疾其所以多癥瘕之故亦以經帶胎産之血易於凝滯故較之男子為多故古人名婦科謂之帶下醫以其病總屬於帶下也凡治婦人必先明衝任之脈衝脈起於氣街（在毛際兩旁）並少陰之經挾臍上行至胷中而散任脈起於中極之下（臍旁四寸下）以上毛際循腹裏上關元又云衝任脈皆起於胞中上循背裏為經脈之海此皆血之所從生而胎之所由繫明於衝任之故則本原洞悉而後其所生之病千條萬緒可以知其所從起更參合古人所用之方而神明變化之則每症必有傳受不概治以男子泛用之藥自能所治輒效矣至如世俗相傳之邪說如胎前宜涼産後宜溫等論夫胎前宜涼理或有之若産後宜溫則脫血之後陰氣大傷孤陽獨熾又瘀血未淨結為蘊熱乃反用姜桂等藥我見時醫以此殺人無數觀仲景先生於産後之疾以石羔白薇竹茹等藥治之無不神效或云産後瘀血得寒則凝得熱則行此大謬也凡瘀血凝結因熱而凝者得寒降而解因寒而凝者得熱降而解如桃仁承氣湯非寒散而何未聞此湯能凝血也蓋産後瘀血熱結為多瘀成塊更益以熱則煉成乾血永無解散之日其重者陰涸而即死輕者成堅痞癥瘕勞等疾惟實見其真屬寒氣所結之瘀則宜用溫散故凡治病之法不本於古聖而反宗後人之邪說皆足以害人諸科皆然不獨婦科也

8. On Gynecology

There is no difference between illnesses affecting females and those affecting males, except for illnesses related to the monthly period, to pregnancy, and delivery. Also, [women] more often suffer from obstruction. The reason they suffer from obstructions more often is also related to the blood associated with the monthly period, pregnancy and delivery. This blood lumps together easily, so [females suffer from obstructions] more often than males. Hence, the ancients called gynecology the "medicine below the belt,[1]" because all the illnesses [falling within the range of this discipline] are located below the belt.

For the treatment of females, one must first know everything about the throughway and controller vessels. The throughway vessel emerges from the thoroughfare of influences[2] — on both sides of the [pubic] hairline. It moves upward on both sides of the navel together with the minor-yin conduit, until it enters the chest and disperses. The controller vessel emerges from below the central peak — four inches below[3] the navel — moves up to the [pubic] hairline, and continues inside the abdomen up to the *kuan-yüan*.[4]

According to another source, both the throughway and controller vessels emerge from the uterus, and move upwards inside the backbone. They constitute the sea [feeding] all conduits and vessels; all blood is generated in and emerges from them, and the foetus is tied to them.

If one knows everything about the throughway and controller [vessels], one will have a thorough understanding of the source and foundation [of human existence], and no matter how many variations of illness brought forth by this [source] may appear, one will be able to know from where they emerged. And if one studies in comparison with [these illnesses] the prescriptions employed by the ancients, and knows perfectly how to modify and alter them [for each individual], then there will be a [proper] tradition for treating each pathocondition, and one does not thoughtlessly apply drugs suited for the treatment of males, so that any therapy will show immediate results.

There are some unorthodox doctrines [in gynecology], that are based on popular tradition, as, for instance, such theories that [a woman] before delivery should take cooling [drugs], and after she has given birth, she should take warming [drugs]. Now, there is some reason for [a woman] to take cooling [drugs] before delivery. But when it is said that she should take warming [drugs] after she has given birth [to a child, one should consider the following]. After such a loss of blood [as is experienced during delivery], the yin influences have received great damage, and the solitary yang flares up alone. Also, stagnant blood that has not yet been cleared away may congeal and create accumulations of heat. I have seen physicians, [who only employ the fashions of their own] time, killing countless persons by applying, [in such a situation], drugs such as *chiang* and *kuei* — contrary [to what is really required].

If one takes a look at Mr. [Chang] Chung-ching and how he treated illnesses arising after delivery, he applied drugs such as *shih-kao*,[5] *pai-wei*, and *chu-ju*,[6] and he always achieved miraculous successes.

Sometimes it is said: "After delivery, the stagnant blood will congeal if cold is added [to the body], and it will move again if heat is added." That is a great error! Any stagnant blood that has lumped together because of heat will move down and dissolve if cold is added. And [any stagnant blood that] has lumped together because of cold will move down and disperse as soon as heat is added. Take for example, the "Decoction with *t'ao-jen* supporting the influences." What else could it be than [a remedy] to dissolve through cold? I have never heard that this decoction may cause blood clotting. The fact is that stagnant blood often lumps together after delivery because of heat [rather than because of cold]. When blood stagnates due to heat, this generates lumps. If even more heat is added, the blood must dry up, and it will never again dissolve or disperse. In serious cases, the [patient's] yin [influences] will dry up, with death as a consequence. In minor cases, such illnesses as obstruction and extreme fatigue will result. Only such cases of stagnant [blood] that are truly accumulations of cold influences may be treated with warm and dispersing [drugs]. All therapeutic methods that are not based on the [teachings of the] ancient Sages but follow the unorthodox teachings of later men are only suited to harm the people. This applies to all [medical] disciplines alike, not only to gynecology.

Notes

1.   The earliest known usage of the term *tai-hsia i* for "gynecologist," "gynecology" is in the Pien Ch'io 扁鵲 biography of the *Shih-chi* 史記 of 90 B.C., ch. 105.

2.   The "thoroughfare of influences," *ch'i-ch'ung*, is the name of an insertion point.

3.   The text has *p'ang* "near." "Central peak," *chung-chi*, is the second lowest insertion point on the controller vessel.

4.   An insertion point for needles three inches below the navel.

5.   The character 羔 kao is an error for 膏.

6.   The character 莊 is an error for 茹.

334

痘科論

今天下之醫法失傳者莫如痘疹痘之源藏於臟腑骨脈而發於天時所謂本於臟腑骨脈者凡人受生之初陰陽二氣交感成形其始因火而動則必有渣滓未融之處伏於臟腑骨脈之中此痘之本源也然外無感召則伏而不出及天地寒暑陰陽之氣滲庚日積與人身之臟腑氣血相應則其毒隨之而越此發於天時者也而天時有五運六氣之殊標本勝復之異氣體既稟受不同感發又隨時各別則治法必能通乎造化之理而補救之此至精至微之術也奈何以寒涼伐之毒藥刼之哉夫痘之源不外乎火固也然內經云火鬱則發之其過天時炎熱火甚易發發者清解固宜若冬春之際為寒束則不起發發而精血不充則無漿漿而精血不繼即不斃則溫散提托補養之法缺一不可豈得概用

寒涼至其用蚯蚓桑蟲全蝎等毒藥為禍尤烈夫以毒攻毒者謂毒氣內陷一時不能托出則借其力以透發之此皆危篤之症千百中不得一者乃視為常用之藥則無毒者反益其毒矣病家因其能知死期故死而不怨孰知眼彼之藥無有不死非其識見之高乃其用藥之靈也故症之生死全賴氣血當清火解毒者則清火解毒當培養氣血者則溫托滋補百不失一矣嗚呼謬說流傳起於明季至今尤甚惟以寒藥數品按日定方不效則繼以毒藥如此而已夫以至變至微之病而立至定至粗之法於是羣以為痘科最易不知殺人亦最多也

9. On the Speciality of Pox [Medicine]

Nowhere is the loss of the tradition of medical patterns — marking our present time — as obvious as in the field of smallpox. The sources of the pox lie hidden in the body's viscera and bowels, bones and vessels. Their outbreak depends on the seasons. When it is said that [the pox] originates from the viscera and bowels, bones and vessels [this means the following]: At the beginning of man's receiving his life, the two influences of yin and yang meet each other and generate one's physical form. The initial movement is stimulated by fire, and there must be regions [in the body] where unfused sediments [accumulate]. These [sediments] lie hidden inside the viscera and bowels, bones and vessels. They constitute the origins and sources of the pox. As long as there is no stimulus from outside, the [pox] remains hidden forever and will never come out. But as soon as the celestial and terrestrial influences of cold and summer-heat, that is, of yin and yang, have lost their harmony and gather [in unbalanced proportions] in man day after day, and react with his body's viscera and bowels, influences and blood, then, as a result, the poison [stored in his body] leaves [its shelter]. Any such outbreak is, therefore, related to seasonal [factors].

Now, the course of the seasons is marked by variations [depending on the] five [calendrical] movements and six [changing] influences, and by differences in the effects of the six influences on man, as well as their respective periods of strength and recovery[1]. Hence there are differences in [an individual's] endowment with influences and physical constitution, and there are seasonal variations in the passive appropriation [of external influences] and the outbreak [of an illness]. A therapeutic method must, therefore, penetrate the principles of creation and it must supplement and support [creation]. This is the most refined and the most subtle art [in medicine].

How could it be appropriate, then, to attack [the pox] with cold or cool [substances], or to invade their [hiding places] with toxic drugs? Well, fire is the one and only source [of pox]. This is certain! The *Nei-ching* states, "When fire is depressed, effuse it!" It is most obvious that a fire [in the body] will be effused very easily at times of burning heat. Hence it is quite appropriate to dissolve [such a fire] by means of cooling [therapies]. If, however, in winter or during spring the influences are cold or restrained, [the fire underlying the pox] will not emerge. If it emerges at a time when essence and blood are deficient, the [pox] will not contain any thick fluid. If there is thick fluid [in the pox because essence and blood were present in ample quantities], and if essence and blood then do not continue [to be present in ample quantities], then there will be no skin marks. Hence one must consider all [therapeutic] methods such as warming, dispersing, supplementing and nourishing, but how could it be justified to employ cold or cool [drugs] indiscriminately?

The application of toxic drugs such as earthworms, silkworms, or whole scorpions, causes even greater disaster. Those who attack a poison with a poison say that one makes use of the strength of [a poison] to effuse toxic influences that have sunk deeply [into the body] and could not be expelled [from the body] by other means. Such dangerous pathoconditions, [however,] will not appear even once in hundreds or thousands of cases, so that if one regards [toxic substances] as the normal drugs [with which to treat pox], one adds — contrary [to one's intentions] — poison where there is no poison in the first place. And because the families of the patients [realize] that the [physicians] know in advance when [the patients] will have to die, these deaths are not followed by any complaints. They simply do not know that everyone who takes the drugs of these [physicians] is bound to die, and that this is not to be regarded as evidence of the high level of knowledge and experience of these [physicians], but as reflecting the magnificence of their application of drugs!

Whether a pathocondition is fatal or not depends entirely on the [condition of the patient's] influences and blood. Whenever [this condition] requires that a fire is to be cooled and a poison is to be dissolved, one [must select the appropriate drugs to] cool the fire and dissolve the poison. Once there is a situation where one must strengthen and nourish [the patient's] influences and blood, then one should employ warming, supporting, nourishing and supplementing [drugs], and one will not lose one [patient] in a hundred.

Alas! All these false doctrines that are currently transmitted emerged only at the close of the Ming and today they are most [influential]. All they do is to take a few cold drugs and specify a prescription in accordance with the [patient's condition]. If it shows no effects, the [therapy] is continued with toxic drugs, and that is it. That is to say, for illnesses that are most flexible and most subtle, they establish the most inflexible and the crudest [therapeutic] patterns. This way, everyone believes that the speciality of pox [medicine] is easier than any other [speciality], and no one knows that it kills more people than any other [speciality].

Note

1.   The text has *piao pen sheng fu*. In this context *piao* refers to the six environmental influences: wind, heat, dampness, dryness, cold and fire. *Pen* refers to the three yin and three yang influences reflecting the impact of the six environmental influences. The concepts of *sheng*, "dominance," and *fu*, "recovery," refer to the interdependence of opposites. In this paragraph Hsü Ta-ch'un alludes to ideas outlined in *Su-wen* treatise 74, most likely added to the *Su-wen* during the T'ang era or later.

337

附種痘說

種痘之法此仙傳也有九善焉凡物欲其聚惟痘不

欲其聚痘未出而強之出則毒不聚一也凡物欲其

多痘欲其少強之出必少二也凡物欲其大痘欲其

小強之出必小三也不感時痘之戾氣四也擇天地

溫和之日五也擇小兒無他病之時六也其痘苗皆

取種出無毒之善種七也凡痘必漿成十分而後毒

不陷種痘之漿五分以上即無害八也凡痘必十二

朝成靨并有延至一月者種痘則九朝已回九也其

有種而死者深用悔恨不知種而死者則自出斷無

不死之理不必悔也至於種出危險之痘或生痘毒

此則醫家不能用藥之故種痘之人更能畧知治痘

之法則尤為十全矣

10. Addendum: The Doctrine of Pox Planting

The pattern of planting the pox[1] has been transmitted by immortals. There are nine [criteria proving that someone who applies this technique is an] expert.

One wishes all types of things to accumulate; only the pox are something one does not wish to accumulate. Before the pox have broken out, one forces them to break out. As a result, [their] poison does not accumulate. This is the first [achievement proving a practitioner to be an] expert.

One wishes all things to be many; only the pox one wishes to be few. When they are forced to leave [the body], they must be few. That is the second [achievement proving a practitioner of this technique to be an] expert.

All things one wishes to be big; only the pox one wishes to be small. When they are forced to break out, they must be small. That is the third [achievement of an] expert [of this technique].

After the pox have been planted into a person, [this person] will never be affected by the violent influences of a pox epidemic. That is the fourth [achievement of an] expert [of this technique].

One selects, [for carrying out the procedure of planting the pox], a day when [the influences of] heaven and earth are warm and balanced. That is the fifth [achievement of an] expert.

One selects small children at the time when they have no other illness. That is the sixth [achievement of an] expert.

For pox seeds [to be planted] one takes only good ones that have broken out as a result of a planting, and do not contain any poison. That is the seventh [achievement of an] expert.

All pox must develop thick fluid so that no poison will sink into [the body] afterward. If at least fifty percent of all planted pox develop thick fluid no damage [to the patient] is to be expected. That is the eighth [achievement of an] expert.

All pox must develop skin marks on the twelfth morning; in some cases this takes as long as a month. The pox planted [into the body] already recede on the ninth morning. That is the ninth [achievement of an] expert.

If a child dies after a planting [of pox], and [its relatives] display regret as a result, [this means that] they do not know that when someone dies after a planting [of pox] the reason is that [the illness] has broken out independently, and that [in such a case] there is absolutely no way to escape death. Hence one must not display regret. If, after a planting, dangerous pox breaks out, or if [the patient] develops pox poison,[2] this means that the physician did not know how to apply drugs. Those who plant pox should also know a little about the methods for treating the pox. Then they would be one hundred percent effective.

Note

1.　"Planting the pox" refers to the process of variolation, an effort to prevent the outbreak of smallpox by artificially inoculating children with scabs obtained from smallpox patients. Even though legend has it that this technique was already practiced in China around the year 1000, the earliest indisputable evidence dates from the sixteenth century. See Fan Hsing-chun 范行準 : *Chung-kuo Yü-fang I-hsüeh Ssu-hsiang Shih*, Peking, 1955, 110ff. 中國預防醫學思想史.

2.　"Pox poison" refers to an illness where following an affliction with pox secondary pathoconditions emerge, such as blindness.

幼科論

幼科古人謂之啞科以其不能言而不知病之所在也此特其一端耳幼科之病如變蒸胎驚之類與成人異者不可勝舉非若婦人之與男子異者止經產數端耳古人所以另立專科其說精詳備自初生以至成童其病名不齊以百計其治法立方種種各別又婦人之與男子病相同者治亦相同若小兒之與成人即病相同者治亦迥異如傷食之症反有用巴豆硼砂其餘諸症多用金石峻厲之藥特分兩極少耳此古人真傳也後世不敢用而以草木和平之藥治之往往遷延而死此醫者失傳之故至於調攝之法病家能知之者千不得一蓋小兒純陽之體最宜清涼令人非太煖即太飽而其尤害者則在於有病之後而數與之乳乳之為物得熱則堅紉如棉絮況兒有病則食乳甚稀乳亦不食則愈充滿一與之吮則迅疾湧出較平日之下咽更多前乳未消新乳復充填積胃口化為頑痰痰火相結諸脈皆閉而死矣譬如常人平日食飯幾何當病危之時其食與平時不減安有不死者哉況兒虛如此全賴乳養若復禁乳則餓死矣不但不肯信反將醫家詬罵其餘之不當食而食與當食而反不與之食種種失宜不可枚舉醫者豈能坐守之使事事合節耶況明理之醫能知調養之法者亦百不得一故小兒之所以難治者非盡不能言之故也

11. On Pediatrics

In ancient times the people called pediatrics the "mute speciality" because [the patients] cannot speak, and there is no way to know the location of an illness. This is the one outstanding characteristic [of pediatrics]. In pediatrics there are innumerable illnesses — such as transformation and steaming, or foetus fright — that have no parallel in adults. This is different from the few [illnesses] distinguishing females and males, and that are limited to [issues related to] menstruation and delivery. The reason why the ancients established pediatrics as a separate speciality can be explained quite clearly.

The illnesses [that may affect a child] between coming to life and boyhood are counted in the hundreds, and there are many, many different therapeutic patterns and prescriptions. Also, if females and males suffer from identical illnesses, the treatment should be identical too. But if small children and adults suffer from an identical illness, their respective treatments should be different. For instance, in case of pathoconditions of harm received from food, one applies — contrary [to what one would give adults] — pa-tou and p'eng-sha, and in case of all other pathoconditions one employs aggressive drugs from the realms of minerals and stones — albeit in extremely small doses. This is a genuine tradition from the time of the ancients. In later times, though, the people no longer dared to use [these ancient patterns]; they treated [the children] with mild and balanced drugs from the realms of herbs and trees. Only too often [an illness] is protracted [this way] and ends in death.

The only reason is that physicians have lost the tradition. And the patients, not even one in a thousand of them knows the patterns for balancing and nourishing [the organism of the little ones]. The fact is, small children have a body of pure yang and it is most appropriate to provide them with cooling [substances]. Today's people, though, if they do not [dress their children] too warmly, they overfeed them. What makes things particularly bad is the fact that after an illness [the children] are given large amounts of milk.

Milk is an item that turns into a pliable but tough [substance] — like cotton — when heated. Also, when a child is sick it consumes very little milk, and if it does not consume milk over an extended period of time, [the breast of its mother] will fill up increasingly. Once [the child] sucks again, [the milk will] quickly gush forth, and [the child] will swallow even more than on a normal day. The milk [it took] before is not yet digested, and new milk is filled in on top of it — [the milk] accumulates at the entrance to the stomach, and is transformed into obstinate phlegm. When this phlegm comes into contact with the fire [in the child], all vessels will be closed and death occurs. For example, adults consume, on a normal day, a certain amount of rice. If at times of critical illness they do not decrease their intake of food in comparison with a normal day, how could they avoid death? But if one were to ask the patients not to [have a sick child] consume any milk, they would angrily respond: "Milk is like water; how could it be harmful to consume it? Also, a child as depleted as this, and totally dependent on the nourishment gained from the milk would starve if one were to prohibit any further consumption of milk!" Hence [the parents] are not only unwilling to believe a physician [who tells them not to give milk to a sick child], they even abuse him.

All the other cases where they [have the children] eat what they should not eat, and where they do not give them to eat what they should eat — all these examples where they miss what is appropriate — cannot be listed here. How could a physician always sit by their sides and guard them, so that everything has its order? Also among physicians themselves, there is not one in a hundred who knows the principles and is familiar, at the same time, with the patterns for balancing and nourishing [an organism]. Hence, the fact that small children cannot talk is not by far the only reason for the difficulties [these physicians encounter] in treating them!

瘍科論

瘍科之法全在外治其手法必有傳授凡辨形察色以
知吉凶及先後施治皆有成法必讀書臨症二者皆到
然後無誤其升降圍點去腐生肌呼膿止血膏塗洗熨
等方皆必純正和平屢試屢驗者乃能應手而愈至於
內服之方護心托毒化膿長肉亦有真傳非尋常經方
所能奏效也惟前方則必視其人之強弱陰陽而為加
減此則必通於內科之理全在學問根柢然又與內科
不同蓋前方之道相同而其藥則有某毒主某症
主某方非此不效亦另有傳授焉故外科總以傳授為
主徒恃學問之宏博無益也有傳授則較之內科為尤
易惟外科而兼內科之症或其人本有宿疾或患外症
之時復感他氣或因外症重極內傷臟腑則不得不兼
內科之法治之此必平日講於內科之道而通其理然

後能兩全而無失若不能治其內症則並外症亦不可
救此則全在學問深博矣若為外科者不能兼則當另
請名理內科為之定方而為外科者參議於其間使其
藥與外症無害而後斟酌施治則庶幾兩有所益若其
所現內症本因外症而生如痛極而昏暈膿欲成而生
寒熱毒內陷而脹滿此則內症皆由外症而生只治其
外症而內症已愈此又不必商之內科也但其道甚微
其方甚衆亦非淺學者所能知也故外科之道淺言之
則惟記前方數首合膏圍藥幾料已可以自名一家若深
言之則經絡臟腑氣血骨脈之理及奇病怪疾千態萬
狀無不盡識其方亦無病不全其珍奇貴重難得之藥
亦無所不備雖遇極奇極險之症亦了然無疑此則較
之內科為更難故外科之等級高下懸殊而人之能識
其高下者亦不易也

12. On the Speciality of Ulcer [Therapy]

All patterns of the speciality of ulcer [therapy] are based on treatments directed at the [patient's] exterior; and its manual methods must be learned from a teacher. Generally, fixed patterns exist for examining [a patient's] physical appearance and for observing his complexion in order to recognize whether [the prognosis of his illness] is good or bad, and in order to initiate a treatment at some earlier or later [stage in the development of his ailment]. If only two [conditions] are fulfilled, that is, if one studies the literature and follows [a patient's] pathoconditions, [no treatment] will be wrong.

[In the speciality of external therapies, though,] all prescriptions must be straightforward and balanced [in their ingredients], no matter whether they are supposed to rise or descend [in the body], whether they are meant to encircle [an illness], or whether they are applied to etch [the skin]; whether they are supposed to eliminate what is rotten, or to create new flesh; to evoke pus, or to stop bleeding; and whether they are to be applied as ointments, through washing, or by means of poultices. Numerous trials provide one with numerous experiences, and in the end one will achieve cures as soon as one moves one's hand. Reliable traditions also exist for those prescriptions that must be taken internally, [for example,] to protect one's heart[1], or to lift away poison[2] for the purpose of transforming pus or for growing [new] flesh, [in cases, that is,] where the ordinary prescriptions from the classics cannot achieve any good results. But for concocting such prescriptions, it is necessary to take into regard whether the person [to be treated] is strong or weak, what the balance of his yin and yang [influences] is like, and to add [drugs] or to take [substances] away from [a standard formula accordingly].

This, then, must be done in correspondence to the principles of the speciality of internal [therapies], and should be based entirely on [literary] scholarship. But there are also some differences with regard to the speciality of internal [therapies].

The basic doctrine of preparing prescriptions through boiling [their ingredients] is identical [in the specialities of external treatment and of internal treatment], but there are different teachings [in the former] saying that a specific poison is mastered by a specific drug, and that a specific pathocondition is mastered by a specific prescription, and that no effects can be obtained if these [specific relationships among poisons and their antidotes, pathoconditions and specific prescriptions] are not [taken into consideration].

This [knowledge] is handed on by teachers separately [from the tradition of literary scholarship]. That is to say, the speciality of external [therapies] is mostly based on [specific knowledge] transmitted by a teacher.

To rely solely on [literary] scholarship — as broad as it may be — is of no use [in this field]. If one has [such special knowledge] transmitted by a teacher, [the speciality of external therapies] appears rather easy in comparison with the speciality of internal [therapies]. However, it may be that [pathoconditions related to] the speciality of external [therapies] appear together with pathoconditions related to the speciality of internal therapies. Be it that the respective person had some dormant illness already, or be it that while he suffered from some external pathocondition he was affected by some additional [evil] influences [internally], or be it that an external pathocondition developed into such a serious condition that it harmed the [body's] viscera and bowels internally — all such cases must be treated by a simultaneous application of patterns of the speciality of internal [therapies with patterns of external therapy]. Hence it is essential that [everyone intending to apply external therapies] make it a habit to study the doctrines of the speciality of internal [therapies] and to penetrate its principles so that afterwards he will be perfect in both fields, without committing any mistakes.

If one is unable to cure internal pathoconditions, he will be equally unable to save [those who suffer from] external pathoconditions. [Success or failure in this regard] is based entirely on the depth and broadness of one's [literary] scholarship. If a specialist in external [therapies] is unable to [treat internal pathoconditions] equally well, he will have to call in someone with a reputation in the speciality of internal [therapies] to design a [suitable] prescription. But before it is applied in treatment, the specialist in external [therapies] will have to check all the ingredients of such [a prescription] to make sure that none of the drugs could have any negative effect on an external pathocondition. This way, both [the specialist in external and the specialist in internal therapies] may achieve positive results.

If an internal pathocondition emerges out of an external pathocondition — if, for instance, extreme pain causes someone to faint, or if emerging pus causes fits of cold and heat, or if poison sinks into [the body] and causes swellings — in all such instances, the internal pathoconditions arose out of external pathoconditions, and one has merely to cure the external pathoconditions and the internal pathoconditions will heal by themselves. Here, then, there is no need to draw on the speciality of internal [therapies] as well.

Still, the basic doctrines [of the speciality of external therapies] are quite subtle, and its prescriptions are quite numerous, and someone with but a shallow training can not be considered knowledgable. Superficially speaking, the doctrine of the speciality of external [therapies] is such that one only has to memorize how to concoct a few prescriptions, and one merely has to bring a few substances together to create an ointment or some encircling remedy, and he then can call himself a specialist. In more subtle terms, [the doctrine of the speciality of external therapies] includes the principles of the conduits and network [vessels], of the [body's] viscera and bowels, of the influences and of the blood, of the bones and of the vessels. No matter how strange the illnesses or how unusual the ailment, and no matter in which of thousands or tens of thousands of variations they may appear, one must always know the [appropriate] prescription so that no illness remains uncured. And no matter whether the drugs are rare, or strange, valuable or difficult to obtain, they all must be on hand. And even if one is confronted with some extremely uncommon or extremely critical pathocondition, one must understand it and have no doubts. Seen from this perspective [the speciality of external therapies] is much more difficult than the speciality of internal [therapies]. Hence there are significant differences in the standards of [those practicing] the speciality of external [therapies], and it is not easy for any [common] person to know who [may be ranked] high or low.

Notes

1.   "To protect the heart" is a phrase referring to a specific internal therapy designed to prevent the poisonous influences of certain ulcers from spreading internally and "attacking the heart." See, for example, *Wai-k'o T'u-shou* 外科圖説 (1834) by Kao Wen-chin 高文晉, ch. 1, "Hu Hsin San" 護心散 This prescription was first recorded in the *I-hsüeh Ju-men* 一學入門, ch. 7, of Li Ch'an 李梴 of 1575, about 180 years prior to Hsü Ta-ch'un's writing the present text.

2.   "To lift away poison" refers to a therapeutic pattern whereby drugs are consumed to strengthen the proper influences and the blood of a patient in order to expel the poison of an ulcer to the outside, thus preventing it from "sinking into the depth" of the organism. This technique is also known as *nei-t'o*, "internal support," and dates to ch. 7 of the *I-hsüeh Ju-men* of 1575.

347

祝由科論

祝由之法內經賊風篇岐伯曰先巫知百病之勝先知
其病所從生者可祝而已也又移精變氣論岐伯云古
恬憺之世邪不能深入故可移精祝由而已今人虛邪
賊風內著五臟骨髓外傷孔竅肌膚所以小病必甚大
病必死故祝由不能已也由此觀之則祝由之法亦不
過因其病情之所由而宣意導氣以釋疑而解惑此亦
必病之輕者或有感應之理若果病機深重亦不能有
效也古法今已不傳近所傳符咒之術間有小效而病
之大者全不見功蓋岐伯之時已然況後世哉存而不
論可也

13. On the Speciality of Exorcising the Cause [of an Illness]

In the *Nei-ching*, in the treatise "Destroyer Wind," Ch'i Po says on the pattern of exorcising the cause [of illness]:[1]

> The shamans of former times knew how to overcome all types of illnesses. First they had to know why an illness had emerged; then they were able to exorcise [the cause], and [the illness] was healed.[2]

Also, in the treatise "On Moving the Essence and Transforming the Influences," Ch'i Po states:

> In the tranquil times of antiquity, the evil was unable to penetrate deeply [into a body]. Hence one could move [a patient's] essence and exorcise the cause [of his illness, and the illness] was cured. Today's people [are harmed by] the depletion evil and by the destroyer wind, which attach themselves to the five viscera and to the bones and the marrow internally, and damage the orifices, the flesh, and the skin externally. Hence minor illnesses inevitably become serious, and major illnesses result in death. To exorcise the cause [of an illness] is therefore of no use.[3]

Judged on the basis of these [statements], the pattern of exorcising the cause [of an illness] is nothing but [an attempt to recognize] the origins of an illness and then to redirect [a patient's] sentiments and guide his influences so as to solve all doubts and to eliminate all uncertainties. It is quite reasonable that minor illnesses react to this [approach]. However, no results are to be expected once an illness has developed into a serious problem.

The ancient patterns [of exorcising the cause of an illness] are no longer transmitted today. Occasionally the techniques of exorcising by means of amulets, as transmitted in more recent times, show some minor effects, but no positive results whatsoever appear when major illnesses are concerned. This was obviously already the case at the time of Ch'i Po, and it applies all the more to later periods. [The method] may be left to persist, but it is not necessary to discuss it.

Notes

1.   A "speciality of exorcising the cause [of an illness]" was an official part of the traditional Chinese medicine of the imperial court and in the academies until the establishment of the Ch'ing dynasty. Listed as the thirteenth speciality, it included demonology and magic. Hsü Ta-ch'un's psychological rationalization of this branch of health care, and his avoidance of any reference to its magico-demonological contents, reflect his conservative Confucian world view. Unofficially, though, *chu yu k'o* has continued to exist well into the twentieth century, and has served to provide treatments directed at the patient's psyche, or mind — an approach neglected by orthodox naturalistic traditional Chinese medicine. See also P. U. Unschuld, *Medicine in China: A History of Ideas,* pp. 215-223.

2.   *Ling-shu,* treatise 58: "Tsei-feng."

3.   *Su-wen,* treatise 13: "I Ching Pien Ch'i lun."

獸醫論

禽獸之病由於七情者少由於風寒飲食者多故治法

較之人為猶易夫禽獸之臟腑經絡雖與人殊其受天

地之血氣不甚相遠故其用藥亦與人大略相同但其

氣粗血濁其所飲食非人之飲食則藥亦當別有主治

不得盡以治人者治之矣如牛馬之食則當用消草之

藥犬豕之食則當用消糠豆之藥是也又有專屬之品

如猫宜烏藥馬宜黃藥之類而其病亦一獸有一獸獨

患之病此則另有專方主治餘則與人大段相同但必

劑大而力厚之方取効為易其中又有天運時氣之不

同變化多端亦必隨症加減此理亦廣博深奧與治人

之術不相上下今則醫人之醫尚絕傳況獸醫乎

14. On Veterinary Medicine

The illnesses of animals are rarely caused by one of the seven emotions; they are mostly caused by wind or cold, or [inappropriate] intake of liquids and food. Hence in comparison with [the illnesses of] man, the patterns [of veterinary medicine appear to be] quite easy. Although the viscera, and the bowels, the conduits and the network [vessels] of animals differ from those of man, the way they receive blood and influences from heaven and earth is not too far [from that of man]. Hence the use of drugs [against the illnesses of animals] is, generally speaking, identical with [the use of drugs against the illnesses of] man.

But the influences [of animals] are unrefined, and their blood is turbid, and what they eat and drink differs from what humans eat and drink. Hence there are different drugs applied in the treatment [of animal illnesses], and not always can those [drugs be employed] for treatments that are used to treat [the illnesses of] man. If, for instance, [an illness has emerged in a] cow or horse due to their food, one must apply drugs that [aid in the] digestion of grass. Or if a dog or a pig [have fallen ill] due to their food, one must apply drugs that [aid in the] digestion of chaff and beans.

Also, there are some special relationships between certain substances [and certain animals]; thus, cats should be treated with *wu-yao,* and horses should be treated with *huang-yao,* to name [but two] examples.[1] Then there are illnesses that affect but one specific type of animal; and there are special prescriptions mastering those illnesses that affect only one type of animal.

In all other respects, [veterinary medicine] is generally identical with human [medicine]. The prescriptions, though, must consist of larger doses, and their strength must be greater. [If these conditions are met,] it is easy to achieve positive results. [The illnesses of animals] may appear in many variations according to different celestial phases and seasonal influences [governing a special time of the year]. Here too [just as in humans] one has to add [drugs] to, or take [substances] away from, [standard prescriptions] in accordance with the pathoconditions [of each individual case]. Hence the principles [of veterinary medicine and human medicine] are equally comprehensive and subtle, and it is impossible to rank one or the other higher.

The physicians of today have been cut off from the [ancient] tradition of [human] medicine; how much more does this apply to veterinary medicine!

Note

1.   The *Pen-ts'ao Kang Mu* 本草綱目 of 1596 by Li Shih-chen 李時珍 states in its monograph on *mao* 貓, "cats," in ch. 51: "When cats have an illness, *wu-yao* is forced into them with water." *Huang-yao*, also called *huang-yao-tzu* 黃藥子, was recorded as a drug useful for the illness of horses at least since the *Pen-t'sao T'u Ching* 本草圖經 of 1061. It is not clear whether the fact that both drug names refer to colors (*wu-yao*, "black drug"; *huang-yao*, "yellow drug") is coincidental or serves to express theoretical relationships between the animals mentioned and the five colors.

VII. History

四大家論

醫道之晦久矣明人有四大家之說指張仲景劉河間
李東垣朱丹溪四人謂為千古醫宗此真無妄談也
夫仲景先生乃千古集大成之聖人猶儒宗之孔子河
間東垣乃一偏之學丹溪不過斟酌諸家之言而調停
去取以開學者便易之門此乃世俗之所謂名醫也三
子之於仲景未能望見萬一乃躋而與之並稱豈非絕
倒如扁鵲倉公王叔和孫思邈輩則實有師承各操絕
技然亦僅成一家之言如儒家漢唐諸子之流亦斷斷
不可孔子並列況三人哉至三人之高下劉則專崇內
經而實不能得其精義朱則平易淺近未覩本原至於
東垣執尚理脾胃之說純用升提香燥意見偏而方法
亂貽誤後人與仲景正相反後世頗宗其說皆由世人
之於醫理全未夢見所以為所惑也更可駭者以仲景

有傷寒論一書則以為專明傷寒金匱要略則以為不
可依以治病其說荒唐更甚吾非故欲輕三子也蓋此
說行則天下惟知竊三子之緒餘而不深求仲景之學
則仲景延續先聖之法從此日衰而天下萬世天札載
途其害不小故當丞正之也

1. On the "Four Great Masters"

For a long time already the path of medicine has been obscured by darkness. Among the people of the Ming dynasty one spoke of "four great masters," referring to Chang Chung-ching, Liu Ho-chien, Li Tung-yüan, and Chu Tan-hsi. They were said to have established "everlasting schools of medicine." This is truly nonsense based on ignorance.

Mr. [Chang] Chung-ching is, in fact, a sage who gathered [data] and arrived at conclusions that will last forever. [His position in medicine] equals that of Confucius in Confucianism. [Liu] Ho-chien and [Li] Tung-yüan left only one-sided teachings, and [Chu] Tan-hsi did nothing but consider the words of all the others. He modified here and there, discarded [some statements] and selected [some others], and opened a convenient and simple gate for beginning students. These, then, are those whom all the world calls "famous physicians."

Actually, these three authors, if compared with [Chang] Chung-ching, were unable to recognize one [principle] out of ten thousand [that he saw], and it is absolutely inappropriate to promote [the former] and name them together with the latter! Take, for example, people like Pien Ch'io, Ts'ang-kung, Wang Shu-ho, or Sun Ssu-mo. They truly adopted a doctrine from a teacher, and each of them commanded superior scholarship, and yet they all established teachings merely reflecting one idiosyncratic school. They resemble the many authors in the Confucian school who followed each other from the Han through the T'ang dynasties; definitely none of them could be named together with Confucius himself. How much more does this apply to the three men [mentioned above]!

Now, what are the achievements of these three men? Liu [Ho-chien] revered nothing but the *Nei-ching;* the fact is, he was unable to grasp its essential meaning. Chu [Tan-hsi's ideas are] flat and shallow; he never saw the sources. And [Li] Tung-yüan stuck all his life to his doctrine on how to regulate spleen and stomach. He advocated [nothing] but the use of [drugs with an] aromatic and dry [nature], only [unfolding a] rising effect [in one's body]. His views were unbalanced, and his patterns for designing a prescription were chaotic. He misled posterity! This was in direct contrast to [Chang] Chung-ching, and when later generations so enthusiastically venerated his doctrines, this was only because the people of these [later] generations had not the slightest idea of the [true] principles of medicine, and hence they were led astray!

Even more appalling is the fact that because [Chang] Chung-ching wrote the book "On Harm Caused by Cold," (i.e. the *Shang-han Lun*) [all people] believe that [the] only thing he knew was harm caused by cold, and

357

they think they cannot rely on [his other book,] the *Chin-kuei Yao-lüeh,* for treating illnesses. Such kind of talk is even more inappropriate!

It would be wrong [to assume] that I am stubbornly intending to despise these three authors. The fact is, though, that their doctrines have become popular, and the entire country knows only how to take hold of the remnants produced by these three authors while no one searches in depth for the teachings of [Chang] Chung-ching. As a result, the patterns of the earlier Sages, transmitted by [Chang] Chung-ching, have lost strength day by day, and those who die young in the empire will fill the streets for all ages to come. Hence, the harm [generated] by these [three scholars] is severe, and an immediate correction [of this situation] is necessary.

醫家論

醫之高下不齊此不可勉強者也然果能盡智竭謀小
心謹慎猶不至於殺人更加以詐偽萬端其害不可窮
矣或立奇方以取異或用僻藥以惑眾或用參茸補熱
之藥以媚富貴之人或假托仙佛之方以欺愚魯之輩
或立高談怪論驚世盜名或造假經偽說瞞人駭俗或
明知此病易曉偽說彼病以示奇如冬月傷寒強加香
薷於傷寒方內而愈以為此暑病也不知香薷乃強加
人之法也如本係熱症強加乾姜於涼藥之內而愈以
為此真寒也不知彼之乾姜乃泡過百次而無味者也
於外科則多用現成之藥尤不可辨其立心尤險先使
其瘡極大令人驚惶而後治之并有能發不能收以至
斃者又有偶得一方如五灰膏三品一條鎗之類不顧
人之極痛一概用之哀號欲死全無惻憫之心此等之

人不過欲欺人圖利即使能知一二亦為私欲所汩沒
安能奏功故醫者能正其心術雖學不足猶不至於害
人況果能虛心篤學則學日進學日進則每治必愈而
聲名日起自然求之者眾而利亦隨之若專於求利則
名利必兩失醫者何苦舍此而蹈彼也

2. On Physicians

Nothing can be done about the fact that inequalities exist between physicians of higher and lower qualities, but as long as [those of lower quality] devise [their therapies] as carefully as possible, and act with utmost care and caution, they will not necessarily kill their patients. If, however, all types of irregular and deceptive practices are added [to lower quality], tremendous damage must result.

Some [physicians] create strange prescriptions just to be different. Some employ unusual drugs to delude the masses. Some use drugs like [jen-]shen and [lu-]erh, supplementing one with heat, to please the rich and noble. Some pretend to apply prescriptions from immortals or Bodhisattvas in order to cheat the uneducated. Some make lofty speeches and offer queer doctrines to impress the world and steal themselves a name. Some fabricate false classics and illegitimate teachings, this way deceiving the people and startling the ordinary man.

Or, they will know very well that a certain illness they are presented with offers no difficulties, hence they falsely claim it to be another illness in order to demonstrate unusual [skills]. For instance, if someone has been harmed by cold during the winter months, they add, without any need, [the drug] hsiang-ju to a prescription against harm caused by cold. When the illness is cured the [patients] believe it was caused by summerheat because they do not know that hsiang-ju [in such a case] serves only to deceive the people[1]. Or, [with] a pathocondition [that] is basically related to heat, without any need, they add kan-chiang to [a prescription based on] cooling drugs, and [the illness] is healed. [The patients] believe it was truly a case of cold, and they do not know that this kan-chiang had been boiled in water more than a hundred times already, and that it no longer contained any flavor [that might have exerted any effect].

In the speciality of external [therapies, these physicians] often employ drugs prepared beforehand so that it is even more difficult to distinguish [the ingredients of a prescription]. Their intentions here are especially dangerous. First, they cause the ulcers [of their patients] to develop as large as possible, so that these people are frightened to hell, and only then do they treat them. Also, they know [drugs] that open [abscesses] but do not cause [the resulting lesions] to close, with the effect that [some patients even] die! Or they may, by chance, get hold of such prescriptions as the "Five Ashes Paste"[2] or the "Three Substances One Spear,"[3] and employ them without distinction, even if the patients suffer from utmost pain. [The patients] may wail bitterly and they may be about to die, [but these physicians] have absolutely no compassion. Such people have nothing in mind but to cheat the people and to acquire riches. And even if they know one or two things, they are misled to such a degree by their personal greed that they can hardly achieve any positive effects!

Physicians whose training is insufficient may still avoid harming people as long as they are able to follow proper principles. And if they are able to remain modest, and if they attach great importance to studying, their knowledge will progress every day, and each of their therapies will result in a cure. Hence their fame and reputation will increase and many people will seek [their help] as a consequence — with riches following them. If one searches for nothing but riches, one will miss both fame and riches. Why do the physicians increase their own problems by neglecting the one and going for the other?

Notes

1.   *Hsiang-ju* was recorded as being effective against summerheat for the first time by Chu Tan-hsi 朱丹溪 in his *Pen-ts'ao Yen-i Pu-i* 本草衍義補遺 of the early 14th century. Li Shih-chen criticized the indiscriminate and widespread application of *hsiang-ju* against summerheat by the professional physicians.

2.   The "Five Ashes Paste" was prepared from *tsao chai hui* [ashes of jujube/date wood], *sang chai hui* [ashes of mulberry wood], *ching-chieh hui* [ashes of Herba Schizonepetae], *ch'iao-ai kan tzu hui* [ashes of buckwheat stalks], and *t'ung-tzu ku hui'* [ashes of elm seed shells]. To these basic ingredients, other substances were added in the process of the preparation of this formuala, including *pan-mao* [mylabris beetle], *ch'uan-shan chia* [pangolin scales], *yao-shih hui* [ashes from a kiln], and *ju-hsiang* [Gummi Olibanum]. The resulting paste was to be applied to swellings and tumors. The first known recording of this prescription appears in the *Shen-shih Tsun-sheng Shu* of 1767, ten years after the publication of Hsü Ta-ch'un's *I-hsüeh Yüan Liu Lun*. If Hsü Ta-ch'un referred to the same formula as listed in the *Shen-shih Tsun-sheng Shu*, this formula may already have been known in an unrecorded folk tradition for some time.

3.   The "Three Substances One Spear" formula was recorded first in the *Wai-k'o Cheng-tsung* of 1617. It was prepared from *ming-fan* [common alum, alumite], *p'i-shih* [arsenic], and *hsiung-huang* [realgar] in addition to *ju-hsiang* [Gummi Olibanum]. From these ingredients a spear-like stylus was prepared for insertion into the lesions to be treated.

醫學淵源論

醫書之最古者內經則醫之祖乃岐黃也然本草起於

神農則又在黃帝之前矣可知醫之起起於藥也至黃

帝則講夫經絡臟腑之原內傷外感之異與夫君臣佐

使大小奇偶之制神明夫用藥之理醫學從此大備然

其書講人身臟腑之形七情六淫之感與針灸雜法為

多而製方尚少至伊尹有湯液治病之法然亦得之傳

聞無成書可考至扁鵲倉公而湯藥之用漸廣張仲景

先生出而雜病傷寒專以方藥為治遂為千古用方之

祖而其方亦俱原本神農黃帝之精義皆從古相傳之

方仲景不過集其成耳自是之後醫者以方藥為重其

於天地陰陽經絡臟腑之道及針灸雜術徃徃不甚考

求而治病之法從此一變唐宋以後相尋彌甚至元之

劉河間張潔古等出未嘗不重內經之學凡論病必先

叙經文而後採取諸家之說繼乃附以治法似為得旨

然其人皆非通儒不能深通經義而於仲景制方之義

又不能深考其源故其說非影響即支雜各任其偏而

不歸於中道其尤偏駁者李東垣為甚惟以溫燥脾胃

為主其方亦毫無法度因當時無眞實之學盜竊虛名

故其教至今不絕至明之薛立齋尤浮泛荒謬猶聖賢

之學變而為腐爛時文何嘗不曰我明經學古者也然

以施之治天下果能如唐虞三代者乎既不知神農黃

帝之精義則藥性及臟腑經絡之源不明也又不知仲

景制方之法度則病變及施治之法不審也惟曰某病

則用某方如不效改用某方更有一方服至二三十劑

令病者遷延自愈者胸中毫無把握惟以簡易為主自

此以降流弊日甚而枉死載途矣安得有參本草窮內

經熟金匱傷寒者出而挽救其弊以全民命乎其害總

由於習醫者皆貧苦不學之人專以此求衣食故祇記
數方遂以之治天下之病不復更求他法故其禍遂至
於此也

3. On the Origin and History of Medicine

The oldest medical book is the *Nei-ching*, and Ch'i Po is, therefore, the father of medicine. But the *Pen-ts'ao* dates back to Shen-nung, and [Shen-nung] lived prior to Huang-ti. Hence it is obvious that medicine arose from [the application of] drugs. By the time of Huang-ti, one discussed the origins of the conduits and network [vessels], of the viscera and bowels, as well as the differences between harm caused from the inside and influences affecting [the body] from the outside. The principles underlying the application of drugs were well known by then, and the structure of prescriptions was based on the composition of ruler, minister, aide, and messenger [substances], as well as large or small, uneven or even [numbers of ingredients].

From that time on medicine was more or less complete. In the literature the shape of the human body and of its viscera and bowels, as well as the effects of the seven emotions and six excesses [on human health],[1] and the various methods of needling and cauterization were dealt with relatively often, while the design of prescriptions was still only rarely mentioned. By the time of I Yin,[2] the method of treating illnesses by means of liquid decoctions had come into existence, but it was transmitted only orally and no books [of that period] are available for reference.

By the time of Pien Ch'io[3] and Ts'ang-kung,[4] the application of boiled drugs had gradually spread more widely, and when Mr. Chang Chung-ching appeared, and [wrote his book] *Tsa-ping Shang-han* [*Lun*], he relied on nothing but prescriptions and drugs for treating [illnesses]. He became forever the father of the use of prescriptions. The prescriptions [he described in his books] were all grounded in the ideas of Shen-nung and Huang-ti; [Chang] Chung-ching had done no more than to collect — from all the prescriptions handed down from antiquity — those that had proven to be effective.

Ever since, physicians have regarded prescriptions and drugs as more important [than anything else], and mostly they have not taken great pains any longer to study the ways of heaven and earth, of yin and yang, of the conduits and network [vessels] and of the viscera and bowels, as well as the various techniques of needling and cauterization. Hence the patterns of treating illnesses underwent significant changes at the same time, and this was particularly so after the T'ang and Sung. By the time of the Yüan, when Liu Ho-chien,[5] Chang Chieh-ku[6] and others appeared, the study of the *Nei-ching* was emphasized by everyone. Each time these [authors] discussed an illness [in their books], they first quoted from the text of the Classic; then they took into account what all the experts [of later centuries] had said; and, finally, they added the therapeutic pattern which seemed to be the very best. But these people were not accomplished scholars; they were unable to penetrate deeply the meaning of the classics and they failed to investigate thoroughly the conceptual origins underlying the design of prescriptions by [Chang] Chung-ching. Hence their doctrines showed no effects [in actual therapy]; they were irrelevant.

Each of these [author-physicians] was preoccupied with his own biases only, and none of them found his way back to the central stream [of ancient medicine]. The most one-sided and confused [doctrine] of them all was offered by Li Tung-yüan.[7] He concentrated on [therapies intended to] warm and dry the spleen and stomach, and his prescriptions did not adhere to any ancient pattern whatsoever. However, since no genuine scholarship existed at his time anyway, he could steal for himself some empty fame, and, as a result, his teachings have found adherents until our own time. Later, Hsüeh Li-chai[8] of the Ming was even more superficial and marked by errors [in his writings]. It was as if the scholarship of the Sages and exemplary men had been transformed into rotten and putrid texts lasting no longer than the period [in which they were written].

Still, all [these authors] claimed: "I understand the classics, and I have studied [the heritage from] antiquity." When they applied [their shallow knowledge] to treat the empire, how could their results ever be on a par with the achievements of Yao and Shun,[9] and the three ancient dynasties? They were unfamiliar with the subtle meanings [in the work] of Shen-nung and Huang-ti; and hence the sources of [all knowledge on] the nature of drugs and [the actions of drugs on the body's] viscera and bowels, conduits and network [vessels] remained unknown to them. They were unfamiliar with the patterns guiding [Chang] Chung-ching in the design of his prescriptions, and hence they did not study the changes in the courses of illnesses and the patterns underlying his therapy. They said only: In case of a certain illness use a certain prescription, and if it shows no effects use a certain other prescription. Also, they had the patient consume twenty to thirty doses of one and the same prescription, protracting an illness until it healed by itself. Since they were absolutely insecure as to what actions they had to take, they always chose an unproblematic way.

Ever since, evil practices have spread, and [the spirits of] those who died as a result of [the physicians'] crimes fill the streets. When will someone finally appear who consults the *Pen-ts'ao*, who thoroughly investigates the [contents of the] *Nei-ching*, and who is familiar with the [prescriptions outlined in the] *Chin-kuei* [*Yao-lüeh*] as well as in the *Shang-han* [*Lun* to such an extent] that he could correct all these evil practices and help the people enjoy their allotted lifetime to the full! The entire problem results from the fact that medicine [today] is practiced by people who are poor and have no training and who have nothing in mind but to make a living. Hence they memorize merely a few prescriptions and with these they go out to cure the illnesses of the empire. They make no effort to search for further [therapeutic] patterns, and, as a result, they have caused all the misfortune that we see today.

Notes

1.   See paragraph I.5, p. 69, for the "seven emotions" and "six excesses."

2.   A legendary personality; supposedly the author of a treatise entitled *I Yin T'ang-yeh Ching* ("I Yin's Classic On Decoctions").

3.   A name referring to one or possibly several historic itinerant physicians of about the sixth century B.C. Pien Ch'io is credited by legend with the introduction of acupuncture in China although his biography in ch.105 of the *Shih-chi* refers to him as having needled only one insertion point on the head.

4.   An official of the second century B.C. famous for his medical skills. A biography and list of treatments he performed is in ch.105 of the *Shih-chi*.

5.   Liu Ho-chien (1110-1200), with the personal name Liu Wan-su, is the founder of the *han-liang p'ai*, the "school of cooling." For him and the following two Sung-Chin-Yüan scholars see *Medicine in China: A History of Ideas*, pp.172 ff.

6.   Chang Chieh-ku (fl.1180), with the personal name Chang Yüan-su, contributed significantly to the theorization of drug use. He was the teacher of Li Kao (see below).

7.   Li Kao (1180-1251), with the personal name Li Tung-yüan, continued the efforts of Chang Yüan-su to establish a theoretical basis for the application of drugs. He is also known as the founder of the *pu t'u p'ai*, the "school of supplementing the soil," [i.e., of supplementing the influences of spleen and stomach].

8.   Hsüeh Li-chai (fl.1550), with the personal name Hsüeh Chi, was a Ming follower of Chu Chen-heng (1281-1358) and Li Kao; he attempted to synthesize the views of these two scholars. See *Medicine in China: A History of Ideas*, pp. 198-200.

9.   Two pre-historic rulers of China's legendary Golden Age.

考試醫學論

醫為人命所關故周禮醫師之屬掌於冢宰歲終必稽
其事而制其食至宋神宗時設內外醫學置教授及諸
生皆分科考察陞補元亦彷而行之其考試之文皆有
程式未知當時得人何如然其慎重醫道之意未嘗異
也故當時立方治病猶有法度後世醫者大概皆讀書
不就商賈無資不得巳而為衣食之計或偶涉獵肆中
勦襲醫書或托名近地時醫門下始則欲以欺人久之
亦自以為醫術不過如此其誤相仍其害無盡岐黃之
精義幾絕矣若欲斟酌古今考試之法必訪求世之實
有師承學問淵博品行端方之醫如宋之教授令其嚴
考諸醫取則許掛牌行道既行之後亦復每月嚴課或
有學問荒疎治法謬誤者小則撤牌讀書大則飭使改
業教授以上亦如周禮醫師之有等其有學問出眾治

効神妙者侯補教授其考試之法分為六科曰針灸曰
大方曰婦科曰幼科曰痘科曰眼科曰外科其能諸科
皆通者曰全科通一二科者曰兼科通一科者曰專科
其試題之體有三一曰論題出靈樞素問發明經絡臟
腑五運六氣寒熱虛實補瀉逆從之理二曰解題出神
農本草傷寒論金匱要略考訂藥性病變製方之法三
曰案自述平日治病之驗否及其所以用此方治此病
之意如此考察自然言必本於聖經治必遵乎古法學
有淵源而師承不絕矣豈可聽涉獵杜譔全無根柢之
人以人命為兒戲子

4. On Examinations in Medicine

Medicine is decisive for human life. Hence [we read in] the *Chou Li* that the teachers of medicine were supervised by the prime minister. By the end of the year, their activities were evaluated and this had a bearing on the amount of provisions they were granted. By the time of Sung [emperor] Shen-tsung,[1] study courses for internal and external medicine were set up, and both professors and students were promoted, and given positions, according to [the results of] examinations in each of the specialities. This [system] was taken over and continued by the Yüan. The texts of the examinations were standardized, and I do not know the quality of the persons selected as worthy [of promotion] this way. Still, [these attempts at judging professors and students by examinations] reflected the same idea [as was expressed in the *Chou Li*], namely an appreciation of the practice of medicine as something that is of importance and needs great care. Hence the formulation of prescriptions and the treatment of illnesses in those times still followed the patterns [of antiquity].

Ever since, though, most of the physicians have been unsuccessful students [for an official career], and they lack the capital to become traders. Hence they have no other way but to [take up medicine for] earning their livelihood. Some of them browse through the [book-]shops in search of [ancient] medical texts they aim to plagiarize; others pretend to belong to the school of a physician who just happens to be fashionable. In the beginning they merely wish to cheat people; after a while, though, they come to believe that there is no more to medicine anyway. Hence they just continue their mistakes, and the damage they cause finds no end.

The transmission of the subtle ideas [from the works] of Shen-nung and Huang-ti almost terminated. If one were to consider [what might have been suitable] patterns underlying the examinations conducted through the ages, one should search for those physicians of today who truly received [their knowledge] from a [capable] teacher, whose scholarship is both profound and broad, and whose conduct is upright and respectable. Take, for example, the professors of the Sung era. They had to examine critically all physicians and select those who could be granted permission to hang up a signboard and to practice their profession. Once the [physicians had passed those examinations], they were still critically evaluated each month. If someone's knowledge proved to be confused, and if his therapeutic patterns were marked by errors, he was asked, if his defects were minor, to take off his signboard and study the literature; or, if [his mistakes were] serious, he was ordered to move into another occupation.

The professors themselves were ranked in different categories just as the medical teachers of the *Chou Li*. Those [physicians] who demonstrated superior scholarship, and whose therapies showed miraculous effects, became candidates for promotion to professorship. The examinations were divided into the following six specialities. [First,] needling and cauterization. [Second,] comprehensive prescriptions. [Third,] gynecology. [Fourth,] pediatrics and pox [therapy. Fifth,] ophthalmology, [and sixth,] external [therapy]. Those who passed all specialities were named "[qualified in] all specialities." Those who passed one and a second speciality were called "[qualified in a] combination of specialities." Those who passed only one speciality were called ["qualified in a] single speciality."

The examinations were grouped into three sections. The first was called "discourse." Here [the candidates] had to elucidate, on the basis of the *Ling-shu* and the *Su-wen*, the principles of the conduits and network [vessels], of the viscera and bowels, of the five [calendrical] movements and six [changing] influences [during the year], of cold and heat, of depletion and repletion, of supplementing and draining, as well as of acting contrary to, or following [some given rule]. The second was called "explanation." Here [the candidates] had to [demonstrate] on the basis of the *Shen-nung Pen-ts'ao*, the *Shang-han Lun*, and the *Chin-kuei Yao-lüeh*, [that they were able to] investigate and correlate the patterns underlying the nature of drugs, the changes in the course of an illness, and the structure of a prescription. The third [section] was called "case." Here [the candidates] had to tell of their successes or failures in treating illnesses in their daily routine, and why they had employed a particular prescription to treat a particular illness.

There is no doubt that those who are examined this way will base all their words on the classics compiled by the Sages, and that they will treat [illnesses] in accordance with the patterns developed in antiquity. Their knowledge is deeply grounded [in history], and the transmission from teacher to students is never interrupted. How could one tolerate that there are people who — lacking any authoritative basis — browse through fictitious [doctrines], and who treat human life as merely a toy?

Note

1.   Lived A.D. 1076 - 1100.

醫非人人可學論

今之學醫者皆無聊之甚習此業以為衣食之計耳孰知醫之為道乃古聖人所以洩天地之祕奪造化之權以救人之死其理精妙入神非聰明敏哲之人不可學也黃帝神農越人仲景之書文詞古奧搜羅廣遠非淵博通達之人不可學也凡病之情傳變在於頃刻真偽一時難辨一或執滯生死立判非虛懷靈變之人不可學也病名以千計病症以萬計臟腑經絡內服外治方藥之書數年不能竟其說非勤讀善記之人不可學也又內經以後支分派別人自為師不無偏駁更有怪僻之論鄙俚之說紛陳錯立淆惑百端一或誤信終身不返非精鑒確識之人不可學也故為此道者必具過人之資通人之識又能屏去俗事專心數年更得師之傳授方能與古聖人之心潛通默契若今之學醫者與前

數端事事相反以通儒畢世不能工之事乃以全無文理之人欲頃刻而能之宜道之所以日喪而枉死者徧天下也

5. On the Fact that Not Everyone is Suited to Study Medicine

Today, all those who study medicine are rather poor, and they adopt this occupation in order to earn a livelihood. How could they know that the profession of medicine was something by which the Sages revealed the secrets of heaven and earth, and by which they appropriated the powers of the creation in order to save humanity from death? The principles [of medicine] are most sophisticated, and only persons who are highly intelligent should study them. The style and contents of the writings of Huang-ti, Shen-nung, [Ch'in] Yüeh-jen,[1] and [Chang] Chung-ching are old and mysterious, and cover a wide range of investigations, and only such persons whose understanding [of ancient literature] is both profound and broad should study them. The transmission of illnesses [through the body], and the changes the nature [of illnesses] may undergo,[2] occur within the shortest periods of time; genuine and false [conditions] are difficult to distinguish offhand; and a single hesitation may decide [a patient's] survival or death. Only such persons who are open-minded and whose minds are flexible should study [all this].

The names of illnesses go into the thousands; the pathoconditions associated with illnesses go into the ten thousands. And many years are not enough to study the contents of all the books on the viscera and bowels, conduits and network [vessels], on the intake [of remedies] and on external therapy, as well as on prescriptions and drugs. And only such persons who are willing to read with diligence, and who have a good memory, should study [all this].

Also, after the *Nei-ching* [was written], different schools [of thought] emerged; everyone became his own teacher, and there was no one who was not one-sided one way or the other. Heterodox discourses appeared, and vulgar doctrines [were published]. Confusing statements were made and mistakes established. These confusions were a hundredfold. If anyone happened to adopt an erroneous belief, he never realized this for his entire life. Therefore, only such people who are critical and go for genuine knowledge should study [medicine]. Hence anyone taking up the profession [of medicine] must surpass others in his natural gifts, and he must leave others behind in his knowledge. He should be able to leave all common affairs aside, and concentrate his mind [on his study] for many years. And if he is, in addition, taught by an [expert] teacher, he will be able to reach a secret penetration and tacit understanding of the intentions of the ancient Sages.

Those, however, who study medicine today correspond to none of the many points listed above. If something that even an erudite scholar cannot achieve in his lifetime is approached by people who lack any accomplishments, and who wish to become experts instantaneously, then no wonder the profession [of medicine] weakens day by day, and those who were killed through the crimes [of physicians] fill the entire world.

Notes

1. A second name of Pien Ch'io, the alleged author of the *Nan-ching*.

2. The order of the characters here should be *fang ping ch'ing chih ch'uan pien*.

名醫不可為論

為醫固難而為名醫尤難何則名醫者聲價甚高敦請
不易即使有力可延又恐往而不遇即或可遇其居必
非近地不能旦夕可至故病家凡屬輕小之疾不即延
治必病勢危篤近醫束手舉家以為危然後求之夫病
勢而人人以為危則真危矣又其病必遷延日久屢易
醫家廣試藥石一誤再誤病情數變已成壞症為名醫
者豈真有起死回生之術哉病家不明此理以為如此
大名必有回天之力若亦如他醫之束手亦何以異於人
哉於是望之甚切責之甚重若真能操人生死之權者
則當之者難為情矣若此病斷然必死則明示以不治
之故定之死期飄然而去猶可免責倘此症萬死之中
猶有生機一線若用輕劑以塞責致病人萬無生理則
於心不安若用重劑以背城一戰萬一有變則謗議蜂

起前人誤治之責盡歸一人雖當定方之時未嘗不明
白言之然人情總以成敗為是非既舍我之藥而死其
咎不容諉矣又或大病差後元氣虛而餘邪尚伏善後
之圖尤宜深講病家不知失於調理愈後復發仍有歸
咎於醫之未善者此類甚多故名醫之治病較之常醫
倍難也知其難則醫者固宜慎而病家及旁觀
之人亦宜曲諒也然世又有獲虛名之時醫到處誤人
而病家反云此人治之而不愈是亦命也有殺人之實
無殺人之名此必其人別有巧術以致之不在常情之
內矣

6. On the Impossibility of Being a Famous Physician

To be a physician is certainly difficult, but to be a famous physician is even more difficult. Why is that? A famous physician is one with a great reputation. It is not easy to call him by just sending him a cordial invitation; one must have sufficient resources to have him come. Still, it is to be feared that one visits him and is not received; but then, it may also be that he receives one. His residence must be far away; it is impossible to leave in the morning and reach him at night. Hence patients suffering from minor ailments will never ask him for treatment. Only when the strength of the illness is definitely quite dangerous, and when the physicians nearby are completely helpless, and when everyone thinks a dangerous situation has emerged, then will one request his help, because if everyone thinks an illness is dangerous it is truly dangerous. Also, the illness in question must have lasted for some time already, and [the patient must] have changed his physician a number of times, and he must have tried a wide range of herbal and mineral drugs. One mistaken [treatment] has followed another, and the nature of the illness has changed several times until, finally, destructive pathoconditions emerge.

But how could any famous physician be in possession of a technique truly able to raise the dead and bring them back to life? The patients who do not understand the principles [of medicine] assume if someone has such a great name, he must be powerful enough to cause heaven to to turn backwards, and if [a famous physician] is as helpless [vis-a-vis such hopeless conditions] as the other physicians, what distinguishes him from [ordinary] people? Hence [the patients] place great hope in him, and burden him with extreme responsibility.

If there was indeed [a physician] who had grasped the powers to decide about human life and death, he would be embarrassed to accept the task laid before him. If the illness in question must end in death, he will make it very clear why he does not treat it. He will determine the time of [the patient's] death, and then immediately leave him. This way he avoids being blamed for [the patient's passing away].

If a particular pathocondition includes a minimal chance of survival — even against ten thousand odds — and a physician employs but a mild preparation as a perfunctory performance of his duties but with the effect that there is no possibility for the patient to survive, this will [only] leave him with a troubled mind. But if he employs a powerful preparation to fight with the back against the wall in a situation where there is one chance in ten thousand that the course of events may be changed, then [in case of failure,] slanderous criticisms will emerge like swarms of bees, and the entire responsibility for [the results of] mistaken treatments applied by others before will now be concentrated on him alone. He may state the reasons for his approach as clearly as possible at the time he formulates his prescription, [but] human nature always judges right or wrong on the basis of success or failure. Hence if [the patient] dies with my drugs in his mouth, I will not be allowed to escape the blame.

Also, it often happens that after a severe illness was cured, the [patient's] original influences are depleted and some remnant evil [influences] still lie hidden [in the body. In such a situation,] thorough attention should be given to a [suitable] regimen for recovery. The patients do not know this, and they fail to adjust [their way of living to their condition]. The [illness] was cured but breaks out anew, and again the blame is laid on the physician for not being sufficiently qualified. Such situations occur quite often. Hence, in comparison, it is twice as difficult for a famous physician to treat illnesses than for an ordinary physician.

Being aware of these difficulties, a physician cannot be careful enough. The patients and the bystanders, however, should be more understanding. Still, there are those physicians who are able to acquire some unjustified fame. Wherever they go, they [harm] the people through erroneous treatments. But the patients say, "If this man treated [my illness] and it was not cured, it must be fate." Hence [these physicians] do indeed murder people, but they are not called murderers. Persons who achieve this must be skilled in techniques other than [medicine]. [Their activities] remain outside the normal circumstances.

邪說陷溺論

古聖相傳之說揆之於情有至理驗之於疾有奇效然
天下之人反甚疑焉而獨於無稽之談義所難通害又
立見者人人奉以為典訓守之不敢失者何也其所由
來矢矣時醫之言曰古方不可以治今病嗟乎天地之
風寒暑濕燥火猶是也生人七情六慾猶是也而何以
古人用之則生今人用之則死不知古人之以某方治
其病者先審其病之確然然後以其方治之若今人之
所謂某病非古人之所謂某病也如風火雜感症類傷
寒實非傷寒也乃亦以大劑桂枝湯汗之重者吐血狂
躁輕者身熱悶亂於是罪及仲景以為桂枝湯不可用
不自咎其辨病之不的而咎古方之誤人豈不謬乎所
謂無稽之邪說如深秋不可用白虎白虎乃傷寒陽明
之藥傷寒皆在冬至以後尚且用之何以深秋已不可

用又謂痢疾血症皆無止法夫痢血之病屬實邪有瘀
者誠不可止至於滑脫空竭非止不為功但不可
塞其火邪耳又謂餓不死之傷寒夫傷
寒論中以能食不能食驗中寒中風之別其中以食不
食辨症之法不一而足況邪方退非扶其胃氣則病變
必多宿食欲行非新穀入胃則腸中之氣必不下達但
不可過用耳執餓不死之說而傷寒之禁其食而餓死
者多矣此皆無稽之談而吃不殺者乃指人之患痢非噤口而
能食者則其胃氣尚強其病不死故云然非謂痢疾之
人無物不可食執吃不殺之說而痢疾之過食而死者
多矣此皆無稽之談不可枚舉又有近理之說而謬解
之者亦足為害故凡讀書議論必審其所以然之故而
更精思歷試方不為邪說所誤故聖人深惡夫道聽塗
說之人也

7. On Being Trapped in Heterodox Doctrines

If one examines the doctrines transmitted among the Sages for their contents, they prove to be most logical, and if they are tested on illnesses, they are most effective. The people of today, however, contrary [to what one should expect], are very suspicious of [these ancient doctrines]. Only such statements that are totally unfounded, and whose meaning is difficult to comprehend, while the damage they cause becomes obvious immediately — [only such statements] are readily accepted by everyone, as if these were canonical guidelines that must be observed and must not be ignored. Why?

The origins of this [situation] already date back a long time. The physicians who merely follow the fashions of their own days say: "Ancient prescriptions are unsuited to treat today's illnesses."[1] Alas! The wind and the cold, the heat and the dampness, the dryness and the fire of heaven and earth are the same today [as in antiquity]! And the seven emotions and six desires in the life of man — they, too, are the same today [as in antiquity]. How, then, is it possible that [patients] survived when the ancients applied their [prescriptions], and that [patients] die when these [prescriptions] are applied by the people of today?

Obviously, it is unknown that the ancients, when they employed a specific prescription to treat a specific illness, first of all investigated the exact nature of that illness and only then applied that prescription to treat it. It may well be that when the people of today speak of a certain illness, and when it is not the same illness the ancients [had in mind] when they spoke of it — for instance, if [a patient] was affected by wind and fire, the resulting pathocondition resembles a harm caused by cold, but is not really a harm caused by cold — and when [the people of today] treat [this condition] with large doses of the "Decoction with *kuei-chih* " to have [the patient] sweat [just as Chang Chung-ching did to treat harm by cold], then in severe cases [the patient] will split blood and turn crazy, and in milder cases he develops fever and shows signs of depression and confusion. Given these [outcomes of treatments with *kuei-chih* decoction], Chang Chung-ching is blamed, and it is believed that *kuei-chih* decoctions cannot be used [in the present case]. The blame is not sought with oneself for not having exactly interpreted the illness; the blame is put on the ancient prescription for [harming] people through mistaken [treatments]. This is so wrong!

[Earlier, I] had spoken of heterodox doctrines that are totally unfounded. An example [is the statement that] late in autumn one should not apply *pai-hu*. *Pai-hu* is a drug against harm caused by cold, [and it is effective in the] yang-brilliance [region]. Harm caused by cold always occurs after winter solstice, and then this drug may be applied. Why should one already stop using [this drug] in late autumn?

Also, it is said that no patterns exist to stop a pathocondition of diarrhea associated with [an anal loss of] blood. Well, those illnesses of diarrhea associated with [an anal loss of] blood belong to [the condition of] repletion evil associated with stagnant [blood]; they certainly cannot be stopped immediately, but if they are not stopped before the anus prolapses, and [the patient] is totally exhausted, this is not [a sign] that one was unable to stop [the diarrhea], but represents a failure to block a fire evil.

Other [examples of unjustified doctrines appear in] such statements as, "Harm caused by cold will not be fatal if [the patient] is kept hungry"; or "Diarrhea will not be fatal as long as [the patient] eats." In the *Shanghan Lun*, [a patient's] ability or inability to eat served to clarify whether he was struck by cold or by wind. And a number of patterns existed, on the basis of whether [a patient] consumed food or not, to distinguish, within these [two illnesses themselves], among various pathoconditions. Also, in a situation when the evil [influences] are just about to retreat, if one fails to support the influences put forth by the stomach, the illness will change into many [secondary illnesses]. If one wishes to move stagnant food [out of the body], without having new grains enter the stomach, the influences in the intestines will be unable to descend. Of course, one cannot apply [this method] excessively. If, however, one merely sticks to the doctrine of "[The patient] will not die as long as he is hungry," and prohibits the intake of food to all those who were harmed by cold, many [patients] will starve to death.

When it is said that diarrhea will not kill as long as [the patient continues to] eat, that refers to the fact that if someone suffers from diarrhea but is still able to open his mouth and ingest food, then the influences put forth by his stomach are still strong, and his illness is not fatal. It does not mean that patients suffering from diarrhea can eat just about everything! If one sticks to the doctrine of "[Diarrhea] will not be fatal [as long as] the patient eats," then there will be many who die because they ate too much during their diarrhea.

I cannot list here all such unfounded statements one by one. Also, there are some doctrines that come close to the principles [of antiquity]. But because they are interpreted erroneously, they too just serve to cause harm. Hence, whenever one reads books and encounters discourses critical [of antiquity], one must first investigate the reasons for such [criticisms], and then carefully examine [the statements themselves]. This way, one will not be misled by heterodox doctrines. Hence the Sages of antiquity deeply detested all those people who told on the road what they had heard by the way!

Note

1.   A statement ascribed to Chang Yüan-su (fl. 1180), the initiator of the Sung-Chin-Yüan theorization of drug use.

涉獵醫書誤人論

人之死誤於醫家者十之三誤於病家者十之三誤於之死誤於醫家者十之三誤於病家者十之三誤於旁人涉獵醫書者亦十之三蓋醫之為道乃通天徹地之學必全體明而後可以治一病若全體不明而偶得一知半解輒以試人輕淺之病或能得效至於重大疑難之症亦以一偏之見妄議用藥一或有誤生死立判矣間或偶然倖中自以為如此大病猶能見功益復自信以後不拘何病輒妄加議論至殺人之後猶以為病自不治非我之過於是終身害人而不悔矣然病家往往多信之者則有故焉蓋病皆不知醫之人而醫者寫方即去見有稍知醫理者議論鑿鑿又關切異常情面甚重自然聽信誰知彼乃偶然繙閱及道聽塗說之談彼亦未嘗審度從我之說病者如何究竟而病家已從之矣又有文人墨客及富貴之人文理本優偶爾檢點

醫書自以為已有心得旁人因其平日稍有學問品望倍加信從而世之醫人因自己全無根柢辨難反出其下於是深加佩服彼以為某乃名醫尚不如我遂肆然為人治病愈則為功死則無罪更有執一偏之見恃其文理之長更著書立說貽害後世此等之人不可勝數嗟乎古之為醫者皆有師承而又無病不講無方不通文理之長更著書立說貽害後世此等之人不可勝數一有邪說異論則引經據典以折之又能實有把持所治必中故餘人不得而參其末議今之醫者皆全無本領一書不讀故涉獵醫書之人反出而臨乎其上致病家亦鄙薄醫者而反信夫涉獵之人以致害人如此此獵之人久而自信益真始誤他人繼誤骨肉終則自誤其全在醫中之無人故人人得而操其長短也然涉其身我見甚多不可不深省也

8. On Browsing Through the Medical Literature and [Harming] People with Mistaken [Treatments]

Three out of ten patients die as a result of mistakes committed by physicians; three out of ten patients die as a result of mistakes committed by themselves; and another three out of ten patients die as a result of mistakes committed by outsiders who happen to have browsed through medical literature. The profession of medicine requires an understanding of heaven and earth. One must be familiar with the entire field, and only then will one be able to treat a single illness. If one is not familiar with the entire field, and has merely a very limited knowledge, and uses [this limited knowledge in treating] people, one may well be successful as long as only light and superficial illnesses are concerned. But when it comes to serious pathoconditions that are hard to identify and difficult [to cure], and one resorts to one's one-sided views, and employs drugs following some meaningless opinion, the moment one commits a mistake [the patient's] survival or death have been decided.

It may well be that in [such serious cases] one achieves success by sheer luck, but one will be convinced that it is one's own ability that allows for successes even in case of illnesses of such severity, and one's self-confidence increases. Subsequently, one offers one's unfounded remarks on any illness. And after one has killed a patient, one assumes the illness could not be cured; it was not my fault. Hence one harms people all one's life without ever regretting it. However, there is a reason why the patients believe such [practitioners] again and again.

The fact is that the patients are people who do not know anything about medicine, and the physicians just write a prescription and then leave [the patients] again [without spending any time explaining their therapy]. When [the patients] meet someone who knows a little about medical principles, and offers clearcut discourse and discussion, they will believe what they hear, especially if he displays extraordinary concern and if emotions and face are involved. Who knows that this talk is based on superficial reading and stands for nothing but gossip!

Before those [people offering such clearcut discourse and discussion] have considered what will happen to the patients following their advice, the patients will have already followed them. Also, there are rich and high-ranking literary men and people whose understanding of [classical] literature is basically excellent. It so happens that they thumb through some medical books and believe [themselves] to have acquired a thorough knowledge already. Because these people are usually respected for a certain degree of scholarship, outsiders will be especially willing to believe [their words] and follow [their advice].

The physicians of our day, though, lack any solid foundations themselves and, hence, in discussions [with these browsers], contrary [to what one should expect], they come out even below them. The former, then, pay [the latter] even greater respect, and the [latter] think: He is a famous physician, but he is not as good as I am. As a result, they recklessly treat other people's illnesses, and if [these illnesses] heal, they consider this their own achievement. If [the patient] dies they have done no wrong. They cling only more strongly to their one-sided views and rely on their good understanding of literature. They go on and write books and establish doctrines of their own, and thusly bequeath harm even to later generations. There are so many such people — one cannot count them.

Alas! All those who practiced medicine in ancient times had received [their knowledge] from a teacher, and there was no illness they did not investigate, and there was no prescription they did not understand. As soon as they encountered some heterodox doctrine or abnormal discourse, they would rely on the classics and quote [ancient] codes to destroy them. They were truly able to get a grasp on [medicine], and when they treated [an illness], they always achieved success. Hence, others had no way they could interfere. Today's physicians possess no skills. They do not read a single book. Hence those who merely browse through medical literature appear — contrary [to what one should expect] — on top of them. As a result, the patients, also, despise the physicians and believe in those browsers instead, with the effect that the people are harmed to such an extent [that we witness today].

All this is to be blamed on the fact that no [suitable] persons enter medicine, and that, as a consequence, everyone is able to pass judgment. Those browsers, though, believe themselves to be increasingly right after some time. In the beginning they [harm] other people through their mistaken [treatments]. Then they [harm] their relatives through their mistaken [treatments]. In the end they [harm] themselves through their mistaken [treatments]. I have seen very many such [cases]; one should think about this thoroughly!

病家論

天下之病。誤於醫家者固多。誤於病家者尤多。醫家而誤。易良醫可也。病家而誤。其弊不可勝窮。有不問醫之高下。即延以治病。其誤一也。有以耳為目。聞人譽某醫即信為真。不考其實。其誤二也。有平日相熟之人。務取其便。又慮別延他人。覺情面有虧。而其人又叨任不辭。希圖酬謝。古人所謂以性命當人情。其誤三也。有遠方邪人假稱名醫。高談闊論。欺騙愚人。遂不復詳察。信其欺妄。其誤四也。有因至親密友。或勢位之人。薦引一人。勉強延請。其誤五也。更有病家戚友。偶閱醫書。自以為醫書頗通。每見立方。必妄生議論。私改藥味。善則歸己。過則歸人。或各薦一醫。互相毀謗。遂成黨援。甚者各立門戶。如不從己。

反幸災樂禍以期必勝。不顧病者之死生。其誤七也。又或病勢方轉。未收全功。病者正疑見效太遲。忽而讒言蜂起。中道變更。又換他醫。遂至危篤。反咎前人。其誤八也。又有病變不常。朝當桂附。暮當芩連。又有純虛之體。其症反宜用硝黃。大實之人。其症反宜用參朮。病家不知以為怪僻。不從其說。反信庸醫。其誤九也。又有吝惜錢財。惟賤是取。況名醫皆自作主張。不肯從我。反不若某某等和易近人。柔順受商。酬謝可略。扁鵲云。輕身重財不治。其誤十也。此猶其大端耳。其中更有用參附則喜。用攻劑則懼。服參附而死則委之命。服攻伐而死則咎在醫。使醫者不敢對症用藥。更有製藥不如法。煎藥不合度。服藥非其時。更或飲食起居。寒暖勞逸。喜怒語言。不時不節。難以枚舉。

383

小病無害。若大病則有一不合。皆足以傷生。然則

爲病家者當何如。在謹擇名醫而信任之。如人君之

用宰相。擇賢相而專任之。其理一也。然則擇賢之

法若何。曰必擇其人品端方。心術純正。又復詢其

學有根柢。術有淵源。歷考所治。果能十全八九。

而後延請施治。然醫各有所長。或今所患非其所長

。則又有誤。必細聽其所論切中病情。和平正大。

又用藥必能命中。然後託之。所謂命中者。其立方

之時。先論定此方所以然之故。服藥之後。如何效

驗。或云必得幾劑而後有效。其言無一不驗。此所

謂命中也。如此試醫。思過半矣。若其人本無足取

。而其說又怪僻不經。或游移恍惚。用藥之後。與

其所言全不相應。則即當另覓名家。不得以性命輕

試。此則擇醫之法也。

9. On Patients

It is certain that many illnesses in the world are mistreated by physicians, but those mistreated by the patients themselves are even more. Mistakes committed by a [bad] physician can be [corrected], if one moves on to a good physician instead. The mistakes committed by the patients result from so many wrong ways of behavior that they cannot all be listed.

For instance, when they invite a physician without inquiring before whether [his abilities are to be classed] high or low, that is one of the mistakes [committed by patients].

When they take their ears for their eyes; that is, when they believe as true what they hear other people say about a certain physician, and do not check the facts themselves, that is another mistake.

Or it may be that one has been well acquainted with someone for some time already and takes advantage of him because it is most convenient. Also, one thinks if one called in someone else [one's acquaintance would interpret this as] a lack of respect. This acquaintance, though, happily accepts this duty because he hopes for a reward. The ancients called such [behavior]: To give one's life as a favor. It is a third mistake that may be committed by patients.

Or some evil person comes from far away and falsely calls himself a famous physician. He cheats ignorant people with high-flown talk, and the latter do not examine him carefully but believe in his swindle. That is a fourth mistake.

It may also be that some very close relative or intimate friend, or someone in a powerful position, has recommend someone [as a suitable healer], and it is difficult to reject their favor. If one, therefore, invites under pressure [the person recommended], this is a fifth mistake [patients may commit].

Or relatives or friends have casually studied some medical texts and believe themselves to be experts in medical literature. Every time they see that a prescription was set up, they offer their unfounded remarks and on their own account exchange its drugs. If the outcome [of such intervention] is good, they take it for their own credit; if they make a mistake, they will blame it on others.

Or, various physicians were recommended and now defame each other. Factions emerge, and if worse comes to worst each of them creates his own party. Those whom the patient does not follow rejoice — contrary [to what one should expect] — at the misfortune of the others, hoping that this will make them winners. They do not care whether the patient dies or survives. This is a seventh mistake.[2]

Or the condition of the illness has just taken a turn [for the better], but [the treatment] has not yet resulted in complete success. The patient begins to doubt [his therapy] just at that moment, [believing] that the results are too slow. All of a sudden [the physician] is met by all types of slander, and a new direction is taken in the middle of the way. Also, the physician is changed, and when it comes to a critical situation, as a result, the blame — contrary [to the actual facts] — is laid on the former. This is an eighth mistake.

Also, an illness may undergo an unusual change. Hence it is appropriate [that the patient consumes] *kuei*[-*chih*] or *fu*[-*tzu*] in the morning, and [*huang-*]*ch'in* or [*huang-*]*lien* at night.[1] Or, someone's body is truly marked by depletion but his pathoconditions require, contrary [to one's expectations], an intake of *hsiao-huang*. Someone whose body is strong and marked by repletion suffers from pathoconditions that require — contrary [to what he expected] — an application of [*jen-*]*shen* or [*pai-*]*chu*. The patient does not understand [the reasons for this treatment] and considers it strange. He does not follow the advice given to him but listens to some quack. That is a ninth mistake.

Or it may be that [a patient] is a miser and takes advantage only of what is cheap. Now, famous physicians are used to making their own proposals; they do not listen to me [the patient]. They are very unlike those people from nearby who are easy to get on with, and with whom one can discuss things and whose rewards can be calculated in advance. Pien Ch'io has said, "Those who disregard their body and who emphasize wealth must not be treated." This is a tenth mistake.

[The mistakes listed above] represent but a general outline. [Other mistakes that could also be] included are [the patients'] joy over the application of [*jen-*]*shen* and *fu*[-*tzu*],[3] and their fears when it comes to preparations designed to attack. When they die after they have consumed [*jen*] *shen* or *fu*[-*tzu*], it is blamed on fate; when they die following the intake [of drugs intended] to attack, then this is blamed on the physician. This, however, has the effect that the physicians no longer dare to apply drugs according to pathoconditions. Furthermore, it happens that [the patients] do not prepare the drugs in accordance with the patterns [ordered by the physician], that they fail to boil the drugs according to the rules, and that they do not take them at the times specified. The patients' drinking and eating, their rising and resting, their [exposure to] cold and warmth, their fatigue and their idleness, their joy and their anger, as well as their ways of talking; nothing happens in time, and nothing is properly regulated. It would be difficult to list [all these wrong ways of behavior] one by one. As long as minor illnesses are concerned, no harm may result. But in case of serious illnesses, each single deviation from [the rules] will be sufficient to injure [the patient's] life. How, then, should the patients proceed?

It is essential to carefully select a renowned physician and then trust him. This is just like the use of a prime minister by a sovereign. [The sovereign] selects an able and virtuous statesman and then entrusts him the office. The principle is the same. But what is the [correct] method guiding the selection of an able and virtuous [physician]? One must select a person with an upright character. His ideas and his skills must be pure and correct. Furthermore, one must examine whether his learning has a solid foundation, and whether his expertise is profound. One must check his therapies over a period of time. If he is able to cure eight or nine [cases] out of ten, then one may invite him to conduct a treatment [of oneself].

However, all physicians are especially skilled in some area or other. And it would be a mistake again to have someone treat an illness one suffers from that is not within the realm of his special expertise. One must carefully listen whether his statements are to the point of the nature of an illness; he must be even-tempered and upright. Also, his application of drugs must hit the mark. Only then can one entrust [a treatment] to him. When [I] just said "[must] hit the mark," [I meant] at the time he designs a prescription, he must first point out the reasons for designing this particular prescription, and [he must] predict what kind of effects it will have once [the patient] has consumed the drugs. Or he may say, [the patient] has to take several doses before [the prescription] will show its effects. Each of these statements must prove to be true. That is [what I meant when I] said "[must] hit the mark."

If one has tested a physician this way, the major part of the problem is already solved. If the person [chosen as a physician] was not worth choosing in the beginning, and if what he says is strange rather than based on the classics, or if he demonstrates insecurity in his approach, and is confused, and if the effects of his drugs do not correspond at all to what he said before, then one must look for some renowned specialist instead. One should not risk one's life carelessly. This, then, is the method for selecting a physician.[4]

Notes

1.   *Kuei-chih* and *fu-tzu* are drugs with hot thermo-influences; *huang-ch'in* and *huang-lien* are drugs with cold thermo-influences.

2   None of the editions consulted had a "sixth mistake" in this list of altogether ten mistakes.

3.   *Jen-shen* and *fu-tzu* are referred to by Hsü Ta-ch'un as prototypes of mildly supplementing drugs, i.e., the opposite of drugs directly attacking an illness.

4.   This paragraph was significantly shortened and altered in its contents in the 1778 *Ssu K'u Ch'üan-shu* version of the text. It is reproduced here in its original length from the Wu chou Publishing Co. edition, Taipei, 1969.

醫者誤人無罪論

人命所關亦大矣。凡害人之命者。無不立有報應。乃今之爲名醫者。既無學問。又無師授。兼以心術不正。欺世盜名。害人無算。宜有天罰以彰其罪。然往往壽考富厚。子孫繁昌。全無殃咎。我殆甚不解焉。以後日與病者相周旋。而後知人之誤藥而死。半由於天命。半由於病家。醫者不過依違順命以成其死。並非造謀之人。故殺人之罪。醫者不受也。何以言之。夫醫之良否。有一定之高下。而病家則于醫之良者。彼偏不信。醫之劣者。反信而不疑。言補益者以爲良醫。言攻散者以爲庸醫。言溫熱者以爲有益。言清涼者。以爲傷生。或旁人互生議論。或病人自改方藥。而醫者欲其術之行。勢必曲從病家之意。病家深喜其和順。偶然或愈。醫者自矜其功。如其或死。醫者不任其咎。病家亦自作主張。隱諱其非。不復咎及醫人。故醫者之曲從病家。乃邀功避罪之良法也。既死之後。聞者亦相傳。以爲某人之病。因誤服某人之藥而死。宜以爲戒矣。及至自己得病。亦復如此。更有平昔最佩服之良醫。忽然自生疾病。反信平日所最鄙薄之庸醫。而傷其生者。是必有鬼神使之。此乃所謂命也。蓋人生死有定數。若必待人之老而自死。則天下皆壽老之人。而命無權。故必生疾病。使之不以壽而死。然疾病之輕重不齊。或其人善自保護。則六淫七情之所感甚輕。命本當死。而病淺不能令其死。則命又無權。於是天生此等之醫。分布於天下。凡當死者。少得微疾。醫者必能令其輕者重。重者死。而命之權於是獨重。則醫之殺人。乃隱然奉天之令。

389

以行其罰。不但無罪。且有微功。故無報也。惟世
又有立心欺詐。買弄聰明。造捏假藥。以欺嚇人。
而取其財者。此乃有心之惡。與前所論之人不同。
其禍無不立至。我見亦多矣。願天下之人細思之。
眞鑿鑿可徵。非狂談也。

10. On the Fact that It Is Not a Crime When Physicians [Harm Patients Through] Mistaken Treatments

Human life is something most important. Everyone who harms a human life receives his retribution immediately. Today's renowned physicians, though, have no scholarship, and they are not instructed by teachers. In addition, their thoughts are not correct; they cheat the world and steal for themselves a name. They harm innumerable people, and one would expect that heavenly punishment gives evidence of their crimes. But often enough they live a long life and become wealthy. Even their sons and grandsons live under prosperous circumstances. There is absolutely no retribution or blame.

[At first,] I could barely understand this. Later, after I had dealt with patients every day, I realized that half the people who die from mistaken drugs do so because of their heavenly fate, the other half because of the [behavior of the] patients [themselves]. The physicians have but the choice to act in accordance with [the heavenly] fate, intending to [have the patients] die; they certainly do not plot [their patients' death] and hence they cannot be punished for homicide.

Why do I say so? Well, there are clear cut differences in the hierarchy of good and bad physicians. But the patients do not at all trust the good physicians, while they trust and do not treat with suspicion those physicians who are bad. They categorize those as good physicians who speak of supplementing [therapies], and — in contrast — they regard those as quacks who advocate attacking and dispersing [treatments]. They believe those to be of benefit to them who speak of warming and heating [medications], and they assume that those will harm their lives who propose [drugs meant] to cool. Sometimes they exchange opinions with outsiders; sometimes the patients alter prescriptions and exchange drugs [prescribed by a physician] themselves. The result is that physicians who wish to practice their art are forced to bend to the ideas of their patients.

The patients, in turn, love such civil and obliging [physicians]. If they happen to be cured, the physicians boast of their own merits. If they die, the physicians are not to be blamed. Since the patients [or their] families gave out directives of their own, they [wish to] conceal their errors, and do not accuse their physician. That is to say, when the physicians bend to the [wishes of their] patients, this is certainly a good way to seek the credit for any successes [that may occur], and to escape responsibility for any failure. But once [the patients] have died, those who hear of it tell each other that such-and-such patient died because he took the wrong drugs prescribed by such-and-such person [treating him], and that one should beware of [this physician]. But when they fall ill themselves, they behave in the same way.

Then there are good physicians who have already been respected as such for a long time. Suddenly they fall ill themselves and, contrary [to what one might assume], they trust in those quacks whom they have always regarded with utmost contempt before. And when they have done harm to their lives this way, they must have been stimulated [to do so] by demons or spirits. That is the so-called fate.

The fact is that fixed dates exist for human life and death. If everyone were to live until he grew old and die by himself, then all people would enjoy longevity and fate would have no power. Hence [fate] must generate illnesses to cause people to die without reaching old age. But whether an illness is mild or serious is not always the same. Some people know how to take care of themselves; hence they are only mildly affected by the six excesses and seven emotions. Their original fate was to die, but their illness is not deep enough and hence cannot cause them to die. Again, fate would have no power. Hence heaven created this kind of physician and spread them all over the earth. All those who are scheduled to die and get only a minor ailment will [come upon] a physician who is definitely able to make mild cases turn serious, and to have serious cases end in death. Here, then, the power of fate reaches its full strength. When, therefore, physicians kill a person, they have secretly received an order from heaven to carry out its punishment. Hence they themselves do not only commit no crime, they even earn secret credit! Hence there is no retribution!

Only those who set out to cheat others, who create a clever facade and fabricate false drugs in order to deceive the people and appropriate their belongings, they have an evil mind and differ from the persons discussed above. Their [activities] are always met by immediate disaster. I have also seen many such cases already. I wish all people would carefully think about this. Indisputable evidence exists [for what I have said]; it is not just some crazy talk.[1]

Note

1.   This paragraph was significantly shortened and altered in its contents in the 1778 *Ssu K'u Ch'üan-shu* version of the text. It is reproduced here in its original length from the Wu chou Publishing Co. edition, Taipei, 1969.

Index